COVID-19 in Europe and North America

COVID-19 in Europe and North America

Policy Responses and Multi-Level Governance

Edited by
Veronique Molinari and Pierre-Alexandre Beylier

DE GRUYTER
OLDENBOURG

With the support of ILCEA 4.

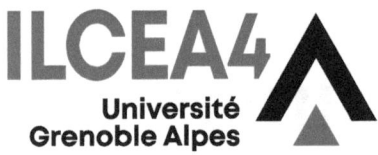

ISBN 978-3-11-074451-4
e-ISBN (PDF) 978-3-11-074508-5
e-ISBN (EPUB) 978-3-11-074516-0

Library of Congress Control Number: 2022930252

Bibliographic information published by the Deutsche Nationalbibliothek
The Deutsche Nationalbibliothek lists this publication in the Deutsche Nationalbibliografie;
detailed bibliographic data are available on the Internet at http://dnb.dnb.de.

© 2022 Walter de Gruyter GmbH, Berlin/Boston
Cover image: da-kuk/E+/Getty Images
Printing and binding: CPI books GmbH, Leck

www.degruyter.com

Table of Contents

Pierre-Alexandre Beylier and Véronique Molinari

COVID-19 in Europe and North America

Policy Responses and Multi-Level Governance

The Coronavirus disease 2019 (COVID-19)[1] pandemic, which appeared in the Republic of China in December 2019 before hitting the rest of the world in early 2020, started as a one-dimensional health crisis, evolving in the space of a few months from the status of "Public Health Emergency of International Concern" on January 30, 2020[2] to that of "pandemic," on March 11, 2020."[3] As the virus affected countries across the world in subsequent waves[4] (the term used to refer to the periods of increased transmission of the disease), the health crisis then rapidly turned into a socio-economic, humanitarian, and political crisis, testing governments and societies to an exceptional degree. As measures were taken to deal with the pandemic – from curfews to varying lockdown restrictions, or the mandatory wearing of face masks indoor and outdoor – debates as to the effectiveness of the various systems of territorial organization multiplied, raising in their wake issues of trust and good democratic governance.

---

1 Caused by the severe acute respiratory syndrome coronavirus 2 (SARS-CoV-2).

2 As declared by the Emergency Committee convened by the WHO Director-General on January 30, 2020, "Statement on the second meeting of the International Health Regulations (2005) Emergency Committee regarding the outbreak of novel coronavirus (2019-nCoV)," accessed September 19, 2021, https://www.who.int/news/item/30-01-2020-statement-on-the-sec ond-meeting-of-the-international-health-regulations-(2005)-emergency-committee-regarding-the-outbreak-of-novel-coronavirus-(2019-ncov).

3 "WHO Director-General's opening remarks at the media briefing on COVID-19—11 March 2020," World Health Organization," March 11, 2020, accessed September 19, 2021, https://www.who.int/director-general/speeches/detail/who-director-general-s-opening-remarks-at-the-media-briefing-on-covid-19--11-march-2020.

4 There is no strict definition for when a wave starts and ends according to the Office of National Statistics. The estimated dates are provided using the reproduction rate (R), the growth rate, and the positivity rate, "Coronavirus (COVID-19) Infection Survey technical article: waves and lags of COVID-19 in England, June 2021," June 29, 2021, accessed September 19, 2021, https://www.ons.gov.uk/peoplepopulationandcommunity/healthandsocialcare/conditionsanddiseases/articles/coronaviruscovid19infectionsurveytechnicalarticle/wave sandlagsofcovid19inenglandjune2021.

Pierre-Alexandre Beylier, Associate Professor, Univ. Grenoble Alpes, ILCEA4, 38000 Grenoble, France.
Véronique Molinari, Professor, Univ. Grenoble Alpes, ILCEA4, 38000 Grenoble, France.

https://doi.org/10.1515/9783110745085-001

Looking at neighboring countries and comparing their management of the epidemic with one's own has become a common feature. While in France, one of the most centralized states in Europe and one of the European countries that was most severely affected by the pandemic in the first half of 2020,[5] a majority of the population believed on the eve of the crisis that "the most effective level of action to improve things" in health matters was the national level,[6] many in the media came to praise decentralization, with Germany being regularly referred to as an example of efficiency in its fight against the coronavirus.[7]

Yet, decentralized governments have differed considerably in the way they have been tackling the crisis, partly because of varying institutional arrangements. As pointed by Yvonne Hegele and Johanna Schnabel, federations do not all follow the same political models. Differences may have to do, among others, with constitutional powers or the policy-making process itself.[8] Health-related matters can thus be in normal times the responsibility of the federal government or that of the states/*Länders* and be subject to more or less coordination between the different decision-making levels. The same variations are to be observed in regionalized systems (such as Spain or Italy), and even within a same devolution system (with, in the case of the United Kingdom, differences between the Scottish Parliament and the Welsh *Senedd*). Besides, the decentralized approach that was praised by the French media was itself rapidly questioned in the countries where it was implemented, with federalism being variously denounced in the press from the very beginning of the crisis as inefficient to handle

---

5 Patrick Hassenteufel, "Handling the COVID-19 crisis in France: Paradoxes of a centralized state-led health system," *European Policy Analysis* 6, no. 2 (December 2020): 170 – 79, accessed September 19, 2021, https://doi.org/10.1002/epa2.1104.
6 57 %, as compared to 11 % for the local level (19 et 20 février 2020), "Les Français et les risques de conflit" – Opinionway avril 2020: 31, accessed August 17, 2021, https://www.opinion-way.com/fr/sondage-d-opinion/sondages-publies/economie/opinionway-pour-le-printemps-de-l-econo mie-vague-4-avril-2020.html.
7 Even in centralized states such as France, after an initial centralized reponse, a territorial-based approach was put in place, with lockdowns being imposed on those parts of the country that were the most affected by the virus. The country also witnessed the transfer of powers to regional authorities, such as *préfets*, who were given some latitude to impose stricter measures. Overall, this led to the emergence of internal borders, with free mobility being limited between regions and, even more tellingly, sanitary border-related controls – health pass or PCR tests – being imposed when entering Corsica.
8 Yvonne Hegele and Johanna Schnabel, "Federalism and the management of the COVID-19 crisis: centralisation, decentralisation and (non-)coordination," *West European Politics:* 2, accessed August 17, 2021, DOI: 10.1080/01402382.2021.1873529.

a pandemic and likely to lead to responses of a "hodgepodge nature" (US),[9] "a patchwork of measures" (Germany)[10] or, as an "outdated remedy" (Switzerland).[11]

The experience of COVID-19 showed in fact that, even in federal or strongly decentralized states, a crisis on that scale required the central government to play a leading role and ensure the design of general policy frameworks, action plans, the overall coordination of public policies, the reallocation of resources from the national budget, not to forget international relations. Generally speaking, coordination, cooperation, and communication were crucial to the effective handling of the crisis and increased efforts were required in terms of multilevel governance, thus testing various aspects of each administration's ability to work alongside central government. However – and that will be another of our concerns here –, tensions over the handling of the pandemic and strategies of blame-shifting allowed by the sharing of responsibilities may have added to already strained relationships between national and regional or federal governments. In some cases – within Spain and the United Kingdom notably – it may even seem to have acted as a catalyst for nationalist and separatist tendencies.

This volume was born from the wish of the editors and the contributors to analyze how such a deep crisis as the one represented by the COVID-19 pandemic could be used as a test for political systems of governance based on a separation or devolution of powers, whether in a context of federalism, devolution or regionalism, and, possibly, promote significant changes in inherited institutional dynamics. Publications of all kinds multiplied during this period, but focused essentially on health system responses and, more generally speaking, on how the crisis was tackled. Our aim here is not so much to focus on the management of the crisis as on its consequences in countries with similar decentralized political systems. For, while it may still be a little early to pass any definitive judgment about these states' ability in finding appropriate policy responses and handling the political, social, and economic implications of the new virus, the first 18 months of the pandemic have, to a very large extent, laid

---

9 Noah Feldman, "U.S. Federalism Isn't Great at Handling Pandemics," March 19, 2020, accessed April 7, 2021, https://www.bloomberg.com/opinion/articles/2020-03-19/coronavirus-pandemic-shows-challenges-of-u-s-federalism.

10 *Flickenteppich*, see Chapter 3 (Birte).

11 Translated from French "un remède périmé," Serge Gumy (editor-in-chief of the newspaper *La Liberté*), "L'union nationale a quelques fissures," *La Liberté*, March 13, 2020, accessed April 7, 2021, https://www.laliberte.ch/dossiers/les-opinions-du-redacteur-en-chef-de-la-liberte/articles/l-union-nationale-a-quelques-fissures-557251.

bare the way sub-national interventions coordinate or clash with national policies and strategies.

Our period of investigation will thus extend from the beginning of the pandemic in late January 2020 – when the first cases were reported in the United States – to the Summer of 2021. The choice has been to focus on a limited number of countries whose political systems are historically related and which share borders, or even belong to a greater union of some kind – the European Union, or the United States/Mexico/Canada Agreement, which superseded the North American Free Trade Agreement renegotiated by Donald Trump between 2018 and 2019 –, thus easily allowing for comparisons.

Challenging the nation-state

In the last few decades, with the advent of globalization, the nation-state has experienced an erosion of its sovereignty.[12] Not only has its power been challenged by the emergence of new actors and new institutions – supranational institutions, international organizations, and even, to a certain extent, multinational corporations – but it has also lost its ability to regulate certain fields, such as the economy, international trade or, in Europe, internal migrations.[13] This gradual loss of ground has led some authors to hypothesize on the "end of the nation-state"[14] or, at the very least, "the crisis of our nation-state system."[15]

If the power of the nation-state has been challenged from outside, it has also been challenged from within. In the post-World War II period, a number of highly centralized countries in Western Europe (France and Spain among others) began to consider centralization as inefficient and started implementing some kind of "territorial reorganization." Coupling the reform of the state with economic modernization,[16] they decentralized some of their institutions and thus gave space – and power – to a new territorial entity: the region. Although this was a way for

---

12 Martin Carnoy, "The Demise of the Nation-State?," *Theoria: A Journal of Social and Political Theory*, no. 97 (2001): 69-81.

13 Vincent Cable, "The Diminished Nation-State: A Study in the Loss of Economic Power," *Daedalus* 124, no. 2 (1995): 23-53.

14 Jean-Marie Guéhenno et Victoria Elliot, *The End of the Nation-State* (Minneapolis; London: University of Minnesota Press, 2000).

15 Rana Dasgupta, "The demise of the nation state," *The Guardian*, avril 5, 2018, https://www.theguardian.com/news/2018/apr/05/demise-of-the-nation-state-rana-dasgupta.

16 Malcolm Anderson, *Frontiers: territory and state formation in the modern world* (Malden, MA: Polity Press, 1997), 114.

centralized states to reform themselves, this dynamic was also a means to respond to the challenges of a fast-changing world.[17] Decentralization thus created a new level of government[18] and a "new territoriality."[19]

This reconfiguration of the political space gathered momentum and climaxed in the 1990s with the emergence of a new school of thought – new regionalism. As globalization contributed to the emergence of a "borderless world," in which governments became less powerful actors and borders less relevant[20] if not "obsolete barriers,"[21] scholars promoted a new approach to the territory, which gave more prominence to regions. Ohmae for instance believed that nation-states were to be gradually replaced by regional states.[22] The region thus appeared as "the ideal scale of policy intervention."[23] This idea echoed Denis de Rougemont's call for a "Europe of the regions."[24]

The rise of regions and regionalism

The definition of the "region" as a territorial entity is not clear, however. Originally, the region referred to an intermediate scale between the national and the local.[25] More recently, the term "region" has come to be associated with a

---

17 In the context of globalization, centralization was considered as an obstacle to economic development (Anderson, 113).

18 Michael Keating, "The Invention of Regions: Political Restructuring and Territorial Government in Western Europe," *Environment and Planning C: Government and Policy* 15, no. 4 (décembre 1997): 383, https://doi.org/10.1068/c150383.

19 Denis Duez et Damien Simmoneau, "Repenser la notion de frontière aujourd'hui. Du droit à la sociologie," *Droit et Société* 98 (2018): 46.

20 Ken'ichi Ōmae, *The Borderless World: Power and Strategy in the Interlinked Economy; [Management Lessons in the New Logic of the Global Marketplace]*, rev. ed. (New York, NY: HarperBusiness, 1999).

21 Gabriel Popescu, *Bordering and ordering the twenty-first century: understanding borders, Human geography in the new millennium: issues and applications* (Lanham, MD: Rowman & Littlefield Publishers, Inc, 2012), 25.

22 Ōmae, *The Borderless World*.

23 Anssi Paasi, *Handbook on the geographies of regions and territories, Research handbooks in geography series* (Northampton, MA: Edward Elgar Pub., Inc, 2018), 5.

24 François Saint-Ouen, "De l'Europe des États à l'Europe des Régions?," *Relations internationales*, no. 73 (1993): 23.

25 Fredrik Söderbaum et Timothy M. Shaw, eds., *Theories of New Regionalism* (London: Palgrave Macmillan UK, 2003), 6, https://doi.org/10.1057/9781403938794; Michael Keating, "Les régions européennes en question," *Pôle Sud* 46, no. 1 (2017): 21, https://doi.org/10.3917/psud.046.0021.

larger scale, which has to do with integration projects. Indeed, in the context of globalization and international competition, "inter-state regional organizations and institutions" have multiplied in the last few decades (e.g. the European Union, ASEAN, NAFTA),[26] thus bringing together different countries at the supra-national level. The very geographic definition of a region is also blurred and shifting: we have historical regions whose sub-national borders correspond to what used to be borders between states (e.g. Scotland/England), while in other cases regional boundaries were redrawn (e.g. post-Franco Spain or, more recently, France).[27] Whether we are looking at a micro-region or a macro-region,[28] the scale of the territory and its borders are not the only elements that define a region. In addition to the ambivalence of its geographic definition, the region itself is a multidimensional concept that can be understood in terms of economic competition, "functional processes," identity or governance.[29]

For the purpose of this book, we will examine the region as a sub-national entity which plays a role as a political actor. In other words, the region appears as "a political space where it provides an arena for political debate, a frame for judging issues and proposals, and a space recognized by actors as the level where decisions may legitimately be taken".[30]

Although the noun "region" conveys in itself this idea of governance – it is derived both from the noun "*regio*", which in Latin means "direction" as well as from the verb "*regere*," which means "to rule, to command"[31] – not all regions have the same powers. Some are mere administrative or historical divisions, with little power – that is the case for the example of English regions –, while others, as in Italy or Spain, both decentralized countries, are powerful, even autonomous in areas such as healthcare or culture. Regionalism tends to be a choice made after periods of centralization, as in the case of France, Spain, or the United Kingdom, which chose to transfer power to sub-national parliaments[32] through the process of devolution in the late 1990s. Federalism, on the other hand, was chosen by the United States, Canada, and Germany on their inception as a system which defines and distributes power to different lev-

---

26 Söderbaum et Shaw, *op. cit.*
27 Anderson, *Frontiers*, 106.
28 Söderbaum et Shaw, *Theories of New Regionalism*, 6.
29 Söderbaum et Shaw, 6; Keating, "Les régions européennes en question," 21.
30 Keating Michael, "The Invention of Regions: Political Restructuring and Territorial Government in Western Europe," *Environment and Planning C: Government and Policy* 12 (1997): 384.
31 Söderbaum et Shaw, *Theories of New Regionalism*, 6.
32 From a UK perspective the Welsh *Senedd* and Scottish Parliament are however considered as "national" from the Welsh and Scottish perspectives.

els of government and is based on shared institutions and shared responsibilities. As Delpérée puts it, "shared power is the golden rule of federalism." It gives sub-national entities competences in some areas and introduces a sharing of the institutional apparatus between the federal government and the sub-national governments.[33] Although competences are defined by constitutions, federalism is not set in stone; it is an evolutionary process that adapts to the context or the ideology of the time.[34]

The Reconfiguration of political space

Besides, regionalization did not happen "naturally." It was put in place with a specific agenda. In some cases, it was seen as a technocratic instrument, a way of "resolving the 'overloading' of the centralized state, and improving democracy."[35] In the 1960s, the "intermediate scale of government,"[36] whatever its denomination, began to be considered as more efficient by central governments. From the state's standpoint, the region was considered as the "key level of action."[37] But from the standpoint of the people, the region, by its smaller scale, was believed to induce their involvement in politics, in that they felt they could affect decisions more decisively.[38] These considerations were what prompted France to adopt a decentralized policy in the 1960s. In other cases, the latter amounted to a political strategy: in countries such as Spain or the United Kingdom, transferring more responsibilities to the sub-national level was considered as a way to put an end to separatist movements. As expressed by George Robertson, the Shadow Secretary of State for Scotland, when the issue was discussed within the British Labour Party in 1995: Devolution was expected to "kill Nationalism stone dead" (it manifestly did not).

Whatever the underlying motivations, upward and downward transfers of state powers have contributed to the emergence of new territorial entities with

---

33 Francis Delpérée, *Le fédéralisme en Europe*, *Que sais-je? 1953* (Paris: Presses universitaires de France, 2000), 4.
34 Jonathan Rodden, "Comparative Federalism and Decentralization: On Meaning and Measurement," *Comparative Politics* 36, no. 4 (2004): 489, https://doi.org/10.2307/4150172.
35 Frans Schrijver, *Regionalism after Regionalisation: Spain, France and the United Kingdom* (Amsterdam: Vossiuspers, 2006), 15.
36 Thomas Perrin, *Culture et eurorégions: la coopération culturelle entre régions européennes*, *Science politique* (Bruxelles: Éd. de l'Univ. de Bruxelles, 2013), 10.
37 Keating, "The Invention of Regions," 384.
38 Anderson, *Frontiers*, 112.

more power to deal with some issues, the consequence being that the institutional landscape in Europe and in North America is quite fragmented with different political systems that distribute power differently between the central governments and their sub-national level. This fragmentation and the redistribution of power linked with regionalist and decentralization policies have led to a reconfiguration of the political space and a "reterritorialization of economic, political, and governmental activity."[39] As a result, new dynamics and new games of power have emerged and this fragmentation of the jurisdictional landscape is bound to fuel tensions between the different levels of governments, each competing to assert its power, especially in countries where competences are not constitutionally defined – as opposed to federal states.

With the COVID-19 pandemic shaking our convictions and questioning the sustainability of our global system, arguments have been held as to which scale is better suited to respond to this issue. Given this "diversity of new forms of territorial action,"[40] this volume explores the responses that emerged in different European and North American countries in the first 18 months of the crisis, thus questioning the issue of multi-level governance.[41] Which levels were involved in the response to the pandemic? How did the different levels of government interact? Did they coordinate their responses or did clashing interests and positions fuel tensions? In that respect, has the COVID-19 pandemic been considered as an opportunity for some regional powers to prove that they are more suited than the central government in the handling of such a crisis – or even a case for more power, especially in regions that are animated by nationalist forces? Finally, to what extent has the question of regional governance shed new light on internal borders and crystallized tensions that might have not always been visible between different levels of government?

---

39 Keating, "The Invention of Regions."
40 Keating, 383.
41 Bache, Ian. et Flinders, Matthews (eds), *Multi-level Governance*, Oxford University Press, 2004; Brunet-Jailly, Emmanuel, "NAFTA, economic integration, and the Canadian-American security regime in the post-September 11, 2001 era: Multi-Level Governance and Transparent Border?", *Journal of Borderlands Studies*, 19:1, 2004, 123–142; Daniell, Katherine et Kay, Adrien "Multi-Level Governance: an Introduction" in *Multi-level Governance: Conceptual challenges and case studies from Australia*, Canberra, ANU Press, 2017; Poupeau, François-Mathieu, *Analyser la gouvernance multi-niveaux. Presses universitaires de Grenoble.* Presses universitaires de Grenoble, 2017, 978-2-7061-2682-6.

Federal Systems in Europe and North America

Modern federalism is a system of government that distributes power vertically by creating two scales, which share institutions, competences, and territories.[42] This shared sovereignty is inscribed in and defined by the constitution.[43] The corollary to this institutional organization is the existence of different "decision-making centers"[44] since the institutional apparatus is duplicated between the federal state and the sub-federal entity, which is sometimes called a state, a province, a *Land*, or a canton. To this diversity of denominations corresponds a diversity of functioning or, in other words, different degrees of power-sharing. Federalism can be more or less centralized, thus giving more or less autonomy to the sub-federal entities. Federalism in its modern form was born in America and, for a long time, developed only in former European colonies – the United States, Canada, Mexico, Brazil, Australia. It was not until the twentieth century that it started permeating Europe, where strong, centralized nation-states were the norm.[45] But each federalist project came with a specific ideology and specific interests that some groups wanted to defend or promote.

The origins of the system are to be found in the American Revolution and in the constitutional debate that followed the first attempt at a political union, the Confederation (1781–1789). When the rebellious colonies discussed the modalities of coming together in a political union, a passionate debate arose about how to distribute power and at which level between proponents of and opponents to a centralized government. The latter feared the emergence of an "American monarchy" and wanted power to be more decentralized so the states could retain a high degree of autonomy.[46] A more balanced approach was needed, especially after the failures of the Confederation, which had given almost all powers to the states. Therefore, federalism was found as a compromise between the two camps and the 1789 Constitution defined two kinds of powers: the powers and functions that were "delegated" to the federal government and those that

---

42 Francis Delpérée, *Le fédéralisme en Europe, Que sais-je? 1953* (Paris: Presses universitaires de France, 2000), 3.

43 François Vergniolle de Chantal, *Fédéralisme et antifédéralisme, Que sais je? 3751* (Paris: Pr. Univ. de France, 2005), 4.

44 Delpérée, *Le fédéralisme en Europe* (2000), 3.

45 Vergniolle de Chantal, *Fédéralisme et antifédéralisme*, 5.

46 Vergniolle de Chantal, 11.

were "prohibited" to either the federal government or the states – in order, in the latter case, to "safeguard national unity" or to protect individual rights.[47]

The fact that the powers of the federal government are "delegated" is rather an upward transfer of power – as opposed to a downward transfer in the case of regionalization and devolution –, insofar as the sovereignty comes from the people and the states, who then grant power to the federal government. American federalism also encapsulates a certain distrust towards a powerful government – a distrust that dates back to the colonial period.[48] States retain authority over much of the economic and social lives of the citizens.[49]

However, American federalism has evolved since its inception. The Great Depression, which was triggered by the Wall Street Crash of 1929, led to a centralization of federal power, under the stewardship of Franklin D. Roosevelt, a trend that was reinforced into the 1960s in order to introduce social programs.[50] Subsequently, since the 1970s, with the rise of neo-conservatism, the concept of New Federalism has been put forward as a way to fight against "big government" and go back to the origins of the country as defined by the Constitution, which shows that federalism in the United States is still very much debated.[51] That debate is at the core of the analysis led by Nicole Huberfeld, Sarah Gordon, and David Jones in Chapter 1. For the authors, federalism and the fragmented nature of the US institutional landscape have "complicated the US response to the novel coronavirus." Under President Donald Trump, the federal government failed to formulate a centralized response, leaving a "leadership vacuum" that was filled by the states. Therefore, many of the decisions were taken on the state level, with responses varying from states that were in favor of strict measures to slow down the spread of the virus to others that favored economic concerns. At times – even within states – decisions diverged, leading to the emergence of "micro-federalism." However, many states were not well-equipped in terms of financial resources as well as infrastructures to respond to such a large-scale emergency. The authors emphasize the fact that the pandemic has exacerbated inequities between the states in terms of political ideology as well as in terms of social inequalities. In addition to the institutional fragmentation of the country, the pandemic has also revealed its socio-economic fragmentation.

---

47 Emmette S. Redford et al., *Politics and Government in the United States* (New York, NY: Harcourt, Brace & World Inc, 1965), 114-15.
48 Vergniolle de Chantal, *Fédéralisme et antifédéralisme*, 11.
49 Redford et al., *Politics and Government in the United States*, 115.
50 Vergniolle de Chantal, *Fédéralisme et antifédéralisme*, 23.
51 Vergniolle de Chantal, 25.

Since the American Revolution, Canada – at the time, British North America – has developed an ambivalent relationship with the United States, a blend of attraction and distrust. When it came to drafting a constitution in 1867,[52] the Founding Fathers rejected the idea of a Republic and instead modeled their political system on the British one, with a bicameral Parliament – the lower house being called the "House of Commons," as in the UK – and a Governor General, who is the representative of the British Monarch. At the same time, they opted for a federal system in order to divide power between the federal government and the provinces – and to grant Francophones a degree of "local autonomy," a way to make sure they would join the Confederation.[53] However, the kind of system that was put in place in Canada was different from the American federal system: first, the sovereignty of the country came from the government – and not from the provinces; then, the constitution defined a set of rules that gave the federal government more power; finally, the constitution defined "concurring" powers on which both the federal government and the provinces had jurisdiction.[54] All in all, Canadian federalism was originally highly centralized, a way to prevent a similar kind of Civil War that the United Stated had just experienced.[55]

However, Western expansion to the Pacific Ocean led to a territorial reconfiguration of the country, which forced Canada to rethink its federal system: given the size of the country and the diversity of its cultures – an East/West gap had emerged between the original Provinces and the new ones[56] in addition to the Francophone/Anglophone gap – Canada opted for a more decentralized system in 1906 called "intergovernmental federalism." The Provinces' Premiers started meeting with the Canadian Prime Minister in order to decide on the distribution of financial resources, an informal meeting that was given constitutional status in 1982 when the Canadian Constitution was repatriated.[57] As a result, the Canadian federal system is one of the most decentralized systems in the world and the provinces have a great deal of autonomy in terms of fiscal policy as well as in terms of the possibility of "opting out" of federal programs.[58]

---

52 Originally, Canada only had four provinces: Ontario, Quebec, New Brunswick, and Nova Scotia.
53 Jeffrey Keshen and Suzanne Morton, *Material Memory: Documents in Post-Confederation History* (Don Mills, Ont: Addison-Wesley, 1998), 1.
54 Vergniolle de Chantal, *Fédéralisme et antifédéralisme*, 41.
55 Keshen et Morton, *Material Memory*, 1.
56 In the years following Confederation in 1867, new provinces joined: British Columbia (1871), Prince Edward Island (1873), Yukon (1898) and Alberta and Saskatchewan (1905).
57 Vergniolle de Chantal, *Fédéralisme et antifédéralisme*, 42-43.
58 Vergniolle de Chantal, 44.

Given its particularly decentralized nature, Canadian federalism thus provides an excellent case study, and Charles Breton and Paisley Sim (Chapter 2) examine the "potential advantages" of this system in the context of a crisis like the COVID-19 pandemic. Provinces have a lot of autonomy in terms of healthcare, which allowed them to design different responses after an initial centralized response. The authors analyze how these responses varied, using a dataset that tracks 12 different public health measures. To illustrate these variations, they take the example of two specific measures – Manitoba's "essential goods" list and Quebec's curfew – to study the concept of "policy innovation and diffusion" – or the lack of it – between Provinces. The COVID-19 also led to the closing down of internal borders within Canada, with inter-provincial travel coming to a standstill. In that respect, the authors underscore two phenomena: the lack of vertical coordination on the part of the federal government on the one hand, and the "highly coordinated and institutionalized response" on the part of the Atlantic Provinces on the other hand. All in all, the response to the pandemic is shown to have been a rather smooth "mix of directives from provincial governments and the federal government," due to the "more cooperative and less acrimonious" nature of Canadian federalism as compared with American federalism.

While federalism was, therefore, already well-entrenched in North America in the early twentieth century, it was not until the end of the Second World War that it took its roots in Europe, where the model of a centralized nation-state had long prevailed.[59] Germany is probably an exception, having a strong tradition of federal government dating back to the founding of the Holy Roman Empire and adopted by the unified state in 1871 before being suppressed under the Nazi regime and restored after 1945. The German Constitution – also known as the Basic Law (*Grundgesetz*) – which came into effect in 1949[60] defines a two-tier system with the *Bund* – which represents the federal government – and the *Länder* – the German states, both levels of government being "almost equal partners."[61] The *Grundgesetz* also defines the powers granted to the *Bund* and those granted to the *Länder*. In that respect, the *Länder* are given jurisdictions over "local issues" such as local government, culture, education, public safety, and some areas of civil service and health care. There are also con-

---

59 Vergniolle de Chantal, 61-62.
60 It first applied to the Western Länder and, after the reunification, in 1990, to the Eastern Länder.
61 Arthur B. Gunlicks, "Theory and constitutional framework of German federalism," in *The Länder and German federalism* (Manchester University Press, 2003), 55, http://www.jstor.org.sid2nomade-2.grenet.fr/stable/j.ctt155j6k3.8.

current powers that are shared by both levels of government.[62] Besides, in addition to defining powers, the German constitution also deals with the implementation of federal legislation. Whereas the laws, which fall into federal jurisdiction, are passed by the German Parliament (*Bundestag*), each *Land* takes care of their implementation. This dual federalism, also known as administrative federalism, grants huge powers to the *Länder*; the constitution does not define a "strict separation of powers" but rather "a system of cooperation, interconnections and inter-relationships." As a result, there is a "functional division between federal legislative and *Land* administrative responsibilities."[63]

German federalism seems to be less rigid in its organization than American or Canadian federalism, and more democratic. There are indeed a lot of interplays between the federal government and the *Länder*, which requires dialogue and coordination. This specific dimension of the German political system has led scholars to call it "cooperative federalism."[64]

In this institutional context, Birte Wassenberg (Chapter 3) examines the German response, which was praised during the first wave for its effectiveness, and compares it to the French response. While at first, Germany opted for a decentralized approach, giving much latitude to the different *Länder*, France put into place a very centralized response, with a national lockdown and strict measures to limit travel. As a result, Germany was characterized at first by a "patchwork of measures" ranging from strict lockdowns to softer restrictions. But the institutional chaos that arose – along with a second wave, which hit Germany harder – led the country to follow a more centralized approach. Birte Wassenberg thus analyzes the actions taken by the different levels of government, while reflecting on how multi-level governance played into the pandemic in terms of coordination. In so-doing, she sheds light on some vertical and horizontal tensions that resulted from different opinions as to what the response should be between the different actors, providing one specific case study in order to show that multi-level governance was key in keeping the French/German border open by fostering cross-border cooperation between the *Länder* and the French Grand Est region.

Austrian federalism, finally, finds itself in a paradoxical situation in that the country "describe[s] [itself] as [a] federation while being so centrally dominated

---

62 Gunlicks, 56–58.
63 Gunlicks, 60-61.
64 Gunlicks, 61.

in design and practice as to be little short of [a] unitary state."[65] It is often described as "highly centralized" with the federation playing a prominent role, leaving only "restrictive fields of competences" to the *Länder*.[66] The Austrian federal system was founded in the aftermath of the First World War, when the Austrian-Hungarian empire was dismantled. Federalism was not initially favored as the two leading political parties – one having a stronghold in the large city of Vienna and the other being more powerful in the countryside – disagreed about what kind of system to put in place, a federal one or a unitary one. It took two years before a federal constitution was drafted in the Austrian Republic and came into effect, in November 1920.[67] In the immediate aftermath of WWII, when Austria was divided into four occupation zones and, like Germany, jointly occupied between the United States, France, the United Kingdom, and the Soviet Union, a similar debate arose. The country's Chancellor, Karl Renner, favored a unitary state but his government was only recognized by the Soviets. Under the pressure of the *Länder* that were occupied by "Western" powers/Allies, Renner promised to re-establish a federation, a condition for the recognition of his government by the Allies.[68] The inception of federalism in Austria therefore encapsulated tensions between diverging forces with, to a certain extent, the prevalence of the *Länder*.

Today Austria is highly centralized in theory, as defined by its constitution. Although, as in the United States, the "residual powers" – the powers that are not explicitly given to the federal government – are the responsibility of the *Land*, the federal government has competence over 100 areas as opposed to 15 for the *Länder*.[69] Besides, the *Land* governors are in charge of the execution of the federal laws, as is public administration, which has been defined as a

---

65 Hueglin and Fenna quoted in Ferdinand Karlhofer, "Austrian Federalism," in *Austrian Federalism in Comparative Perspective*, ed. Ferdinand Karlhofer and Günter Bischof, vol. 24 (University of New Orleans Press, 2015), 19, https://doi.org/10.2307/j.ctt1n2txpf.4.

66 Peter Bußjäger, "Austria's Cooperative Federalism," in *Austrian Federalism in Comparative Perspective*, ed. Günter Bischof and Ferdinand Karlhofer, vol. 24 (University of New Orleans Press, 2015), 12, https://doi.org/10.2307/j.ctt1n2txpf.6.

67 Karlhofer, "Austrian Federalism," 21.

68 Bußjäger, "Austria's Cooperative Federalism," 12.

69 As listed by Bußjäger, the *Land* competences include: some aspects of environmental protection, construction law, town and country planning, hunting, fishing, some aspects of agriculture, areas of youth and child welfare, nursery schools, sports, tourism, local government, local police, laws on land transfers, acquisition of real estate, and the preservation of landscape and natural heritage. It is important to note that in some areas, *Länder* only have jurisdiction over "some aspects."

"so-called indirect federal administration."[70] However, the system is also shaped by "instruments of informal cooperation" by the way of the Conference of *Land* Governors, which allows for much discussion between the central government and the *Länder*. This "practical operation" of Austrian federalism, to use Bußjäger's words, makes the system more cooperative than one would have thought at first sight.[71]

Caught in between centralized federalism and cooperative federalism, Austria started with a centralized – and apparently efficient – response to the COVID-19 pandemic before delegating responsibility to the *Länder*. Michelle Falkenbach (Chapter 4) seeks to understand the reasons for that choice, drawing attention to the chaos that resulted from this shift in scales of governance. Underlining how trust in political actors is a major component in times of crisis, and focusing on the different levels of governance as well as the involvement of opposition parties and the country's social partners within the decision-making process, the author analyzes how the general confusion associated to the management of the pandemic in Austria and the politics of "credit and blame" impacted public support and questioned the efficiency of "federalism by negotiation."[72]

Regionalism: the Cases of Spain and Italy

As compared to federalism, regionalism was not defined by the countries' constitutions. It is rather a process, the result of a transformation of the countries' "basic form of governance," with governments decentralizing their power and resources to sub-national governments or structures.[73] In Europe, the process started in the 1960s, when the countries that had a tradition of centralization – France, Spain, Italy – began to consider it as inefficient and oppressive.[74] In France, centralization had entailed a gap between Paris, a dynamic capital city, and the rest of the country. In Spain, centralization was associated with Franco's dictatorship, which had "suppressed regional authorities" because

---

70 Bußjäger, "Austria's Cooperative Federalism," 13.

71 Bußjäger, 11.

72 Bußjäger, 16.

73 Rodden, "Comparative Federalism and Decentralization: On Meaning and Measurement," 481.

74 Anderson, *Frontiers*, 114.

they represented a "danger for the unity of the country." In Italy, centralization was blamed for its inefficiency and its corruptive character.[75]

Defined as "the division of an area [...] into regions and the transfer of administrative and political responsibilities to those regions,"[76] regionalism is an administrative reorganization of the country, which sometimes also entails a political reorganization. It is also underlain by some forces: even though the objective of regionalism can be economic competitiveness, administrative effectiveness or political modernization – as stated above – regional boundaries are not chosen randomly. Most of the time, they correspond to old historical regions or nations with strong identities, such as Catalonia or the Basque Country.[77] As such, if strong identities and economic competitiveness collide, this can well lead to tensions, or even a desire for independence.

The two countries that have been retained for scrutiny in this volume – Spain and Italy – are both examples of highly decentralized states and the countries that were the most affected in Europe in the early months of the pandemic.

In the late 1970s, following a long period of authoritarian rule under General Franco combined with high centralization, Spain underwent a transition to democracy that was accompanied with "a process of deep decentralization and incipient federalization."[78] Today, the country is divided in 17 *Comunidades Autónomas* (Autonomous Communities – ACs), which all have substantial – even though varying – degrees of autonomy, including in financial terms, with, as a rule, all responsibilities not expressly attributed to the central state by the Constitution being devolved to them over 23 areas, including housing, transportation, education, public order, planning, urbanism and environmental protection, agriculture, culture, and, since 2002, healthcare. Shared competences between the center and the regions include education, social services, universities, municipal and provincial supervision.

While the country is constitutionally a unitary state, it is, in reality, in the eyes of many observers, a "quasi-federal" system,[79] in which various national-

---

75 Anderson, 112.

76 Schrijver, *Regionalism after Regionalisation*, 17.

77 Even when the divisions are merely administrative ones, such as the former Midi Pyrénées region or the newly merged Grand Est region in France, which had no "pre-existing political identity," a sense of identification can sometimes emerge in the long run (Anderson, *Frontiers*, 107-8).

78 Luis Moreno, "Decentralization in Spain," *Regional Studies* 36 (2002): 4, 399–408, DOI: 10.1080/00343400220131160.

79 Daniele Conversi, "Asymmetry in Quasi-federal and Unitary States," *Ethnopolitics* 6 (2007): 1, 121–24, DOI: 10.1080/17449050701233064; Laura Chaqués Bonafont and Anna M. Palau Roqué, "Comparing Law-Making Activities in a Quasi-Federal System of Government: The Case of

isms and regionalisms coexist. This state of affairs raises many questions as to both the management of the COVID-19 crisis and the impact the latter may have had on the relationships between the different levels of governance, in the early months of the pandemic. Juan M. Trillo Santamaría, Valerià Paül and Roberto Vila Lage (Chapter 5) provide elements of answer and show how the crisis in Spain was managed from a territorial perspective. Analyzing the six phases of the crisis management between March 2020 and June 2021, they confirm that internal Spanish borders between the 17 ACs were "resignified" and demonstrate the existence of constant tensions between the Spanish Government and the ACs Governments due to their divergent views on the distribution of territorial powers. Their analysis not only points to a virtual absence of effective mechanisms of coordination, collaboration, and cooperation between the different Spanish tiers of government, it also shows how various coexisting nationalisms and regionalisms have erected conflicting and overlapping borders at different scales.

Michel Martinez (Chapter 6) adds to this reflection on the management of the pandemic in Spain by establishing the different types of internal borders that were used in the different lockdowns and other measures of containment and explaining how the use or contestation of these "dividing lines" that testify to a territorial structure and a local and national network still under discussion may take on political significance for the different nationalist movements that are to be found in the country.

Less regionalized than Spain, more regionalized than France, Italy has a "peculiar quasi-federalist configuration" in which, next to the structures of the central State, is to be found a complex system of regional and local autonomies: five of its 20 Regions – characterized as "autonomous or special"[80] – thus have been conferred the exclusive power to legislate on a given list of subjects (such as foreign affairs and defense) while the remaining 15 Regions – defined as "ordinary"[81] – are conferred two types of legislative competences: "concurrent" (*i.e.* shared) competences, which are owned both by the state and the regions and include education, health care, civil protection, and culture, to be exercised within the principles set by the national laws; and "residual" competences in all the other areas. In chapter 7, Anna Malandrino and Giliberto Capano demonstrate how this peculiar configuration of the Italian system and the constitutional dis-

---

Spain," *Comparative Political Studies* 44, no. 8 (August 2011): 1089–19. https://doi.org/10.1177/0010414011405171.

80 Valle d'Aosta / Vallée d'Aoste, Trentino-Alto Adige / Südtirol, Friuli Venezia Giulia, Sardinia, and Sicily.

81 Piedmont, Lombardy, Veneto, Liguria, Emilia-Romagna, Tuscany, Umbria, Marche, Lazio, Abruzzo, Molise, Campania, Puglia, Basilicata, and Calabria.

tribution of the responsibility over health policies between the central and regional governments influenced the policymaking processes that took place between the first and the third waves of the COVID-19 pandemic and how intergovernmental relations evolved in that context. These processes, which were characterized by repeated shifts between phases that built up and scaled-down restrictions aimed at protecting public health, were, as their chapter will show, not free from conflict. Five dimensions of Intergovernmental relations will thus be under scrutiny: the level of conflict between different levels of government; the types of relationships involved (vertical vs horizontal); the capacity of these different levels to share common goals and practices; their level of agreement on policies and practices; and their ability to clearly define their respective roles.

Devolution

The United Kingdom provides us with one last and peculiar example of decentralization. The origin of Devolution, as the process is called, is to be found in the very nature of the country, a multinational state born from three successive – and more or less willing – unions between a larger and more powerful country, England, and its Celtic neighbors: Wales (1536), Scotland (1707), and Ireland (1801). The last two lost their Parliaments (Wales did not have one in the first place), and all were divided into constituencies that would enable them to send representatives to the English Parliament in London which became, *de facto*, the British Parliament. While some nationalist claims arose immediately and demands for "Home Rule" appeared as early as the nineteenth century, it was only in the late 1990s that a series of Acts of Parliament[82] created legislative and executive bodies in Scotland, Wales, and Northern Ireland, with powers to legislate over "devolved matters," while "reserved" matters, such as defense or foreign affairs, remained the responsibility of Westminster. Since then, devolution has never stopped transforming the governance of the UK as new settlements have subsequently been agreed on which have granted all three devolved institutions (the Scottish Parliament, the Northern Irish Assembly, and the Assembly of Wales – now Welsh Parliament / *Senedd*) greater scope for action.[83]

---

82 The Scotland Act 1998, the Government of Wales Act 1998, and the Northern Ireland Act 1998.
83 See for instance Scotland Act 2016 and Wales Act 2017.

While Devolution can be said to have given the UK some of the characteristics of a federal system, it is not, however, synonymous with federalism. The devolved territories could easily be compared to states (all the more so as they enjoy varying levels of tax-raising powers), and the governmental bodies based in London to federal organs, but that would amount to ignoring one essential aspect of the system: unlike federal or confederal systems of government, under which every constituent part of the state enjoys autonomy and sovereignty, the devolved powers of the "sub-national" authorities (Scotland, Wales, and Northern Ireland) ultimately reside in the central government, with Westminster remaining "sovereign." This also implies that the UK Parliament can still legislate in devolved areas – although, under the Sewel Convention, it does "not normally" do so without the explicit consent of the relevant devolved body.[84] Besides, as – in contrast to the arrangements typically found in federations – there is no written constitution in the UK and the devolved institutions are products of statute law issued by Westminster, the legislation that gave birth to the devolved parliaments or assemblies can be repealed or amended by Parliament in the same way as any statute. This means that devolution is, in theory, reversible.

When the COVID-19 pandemic broke out in the UK in February 2020, it was against a backdrop of already strained relationships between the UK government and the three devolved governments due to Brexit, which had not yet been settled. With, on the one hand, a nationalist government in Scotland (the Scottish National Party) and a Labour government in Wales[85] having to work hand in hand with the Conservative Johnson-led administration in London, and, on the other hand, the existence of divergent views over the management of the epidemic, one might expect the unity of the kingdom to have been further put to the test. As health was one of the powers devolved to Northern Ireland, Scotland, and Wales and many of the mechanisms used to try and contain the spread of the virus – restrictions on social gatherings, education, transport, and businesses – are also the responsibility of lawmakers in the devolved administrations, the differences in the way the four governments have managed the pandemic in their own territories contribute to illustrate the practical dimensions of devolution and the complexity of a multinational state.

---

84 David Torrance, "Introduction to devolution in the UK," BRIEFING PAPER Number CBP 8599, House of Commons Library, June 19 2019, accessed September 19, 2021, https://researchbriefings. files.parliament.uk/documents/CBP-8599/CBP-8599.pdf.
85 The specificity of the Northern Irish situation and the tensions linked with Brexit and the Northern Ireland Protocol make it difficult to include the Province in this study.

Fiona Simpkins (Chapter 8) thus shows how the Scottish Parliament's extensive devolved powers have allowed the SNP government both to provide a distinctive response to the coronavirus crisis and to communicate effectively with the Scottish public, giving them the opportunity to successfully build trust in its ability to manage a crisis and govern Scotland. The author's findings nevertheless prove wrong those who, early in the crisis, predicted that the cautious management of the pandemic and effective communication by First Minister Nicola Sturgeon, by increasing public trust in the Scottish Parliament, would also contribute to greater support for independence.

Daniel Wincott (Chapter 9) completes this analysis by providing an additional approach to the multi-level/devolved system that characterized the management of the pandemic in the UK. Taking a territorial politics perspective, and opting for an off-center interrogation of the UK state, his chapter builds on critiques of the conventional "unitary state" account of the UK state. His analysis shows how the UK government repeatedly failed to recognize the scope and limits of its own powers or the extent of the powers wielded by the devolved Welsh government – or local authorities and metro-mayors in England. Arguably focused on the needs and preoccupations of London and the South-East of England, even in the context of a pandemic emergency, the Johnson administration often also defaulted to an abrasive approach to other governments within the UK. Thus, the initial modest effectiveness of UK-Welsh government co-operation was always matched – it seems – by elements of fierce conflict.

As a conclusion, and since it embodies another level of government at the supranational level, the European Union (EU) provides us with an interesting example of interlocked scales and multi-level governance. It is therefore relevant to zoom out and study how COVID-19 was dealt with inside this macro-regional organization, which brings together no fewer than 27 members. Almost all the systems that will be examined in this volume concern countries which either share power with or have delegated power to sub-national entities. In other words, most case studies have to do with downward transfers of power. With the EU, we have the opposite process: states that have decided to come together, with an upward transfer of their sovereignty to supranational institutions, some areas falling under the "exclusive competences" of European institutions (e.g. trade, the customs union, monetary policy).[86] In terms of healthcare, however, the European Union does not have much power, as this competence remains

---

[86] EUR-Lex, "Glossary of Summary – Distribution of competences", accessed October 15, 2021, https://eur-lex.europa.eu/summary/glossary/competences.html.

in the hands of member states and the EU is only in charge of policies and actions in public health whose goals are to: "protect and improve the health of EU citizens; support the modernization and digitalization of health systems and infrastructure; improve the resilience of Europe's health systems [and] equip EU countries to better prevent and address future pandemics."[87] Examining at a macro-level the role played by the EU and by European institutions in a pandemic that affected all of its members and the coordination – or lack of it – is the topic of Sara Casella Colombeau's final chapter. The author approaches the pandemic by analyzing how internal borders within the Schengen area conveyed great importance during the first wave of the pandemic. This rebordering phenomenon – at cross-purposes with the concept of free mobility on which the EU was built – happened unilaterally on the part of most member states, without any consultation with European institutions or with their neighbors. Sara Casella Colombeau nuances the unprecedented character of this national reflex by contextualizing the situation and emphasizing other periods during which some member states had re-introduced controls beyond the limits stipulated by European laws. In the context of multi-level governance, she also examines, using post-Rokkannian literature, the tension that arose between the "EU political center" and France, a "national political center," and how EU institutions did their utmost in the following waves to remove border controls.

---

87 European Commission, "EU Health Policy," accessed October 15, 2021, https://ec.europa.eu/health/policies/overview_en.

Part 1: **Federal Systems in Europe and North America**

Nicole Huberfeld, Sarah H. Gordon, and David K. Jones

1 American Public Health Federalism and the Response to the COVID-19 Pandemic

Introduction

For the first year of the SARS-CoV-2 pandemic, the United States had the dubious distinction of being the global frontrunner in infection and mortality rates.[1] By January of 2021, COVID-19 became the number one cause of death in the U.S., with more Americans dying of COVID than World War II, the Vietnam War, and the Korean War combined. Many commentators blamed leadership failures for the lack of a coordinated response.[2] However, fundamental features of the American public health system complicated the launch of an effective and expe-

---

Note: We dedicate this chapter to David K. Jones, our dear friend and coauthor who suffered an untimely death on September 11, 2021. We co-authored the article but completed revisions after his passing, honoring the thoughtfulness and precision he brought to all of our multidisciplinary projects. David cared deeply about health equity and social justice, and this work carries the imprint of his recent research in a particularly disadvantaged place, the Mississippi Delta. David's research in the Delta on the health inequities experienced by Black and other historically oppressed populations provides an important backdrop for understanding the ways in which the novel coronavirus pandemic exacerbated challenges faced by poor people of color in the U.S. More broadly, David's scholarship considered how U.S. federalist structures shape health inequities and can impact the objectives of public health. This chapter serves as a testament to David's commitment to these studies.

1 Scottie Andrew, "The US has 4% of the world's population but 25% of its coronavirus cases," *CNN*, June 30, 2020, https://www.cnn.com/2020/06/30/health/us-coronavirus-toll-in-numbers-june-trnd/index.html.
2 The Editors, "Dying in a Leadership Vacuum," *New Eng. J. Med.*, October 7, 2020, https://www.nejm.org/doi/full/10.1056/NEJMe2029812?query=TOC; "The U.S. Is Missing Key Opportunities to End the COVID-19 Pandemic," *The Dose – Commonwealth Fund*, January 15, 2021, https://www.commonwealthfund.org/publications/podcast/2021/jan/us-is-missing-key-opportunities-end-covid-19-pandemic.

Nicole Huberfeld, Professor of Health Law, Ethics, and Human Rights at the School of Public Health and professor of law at the School of Law, Boston University.
Sarah H. Gordon, Assistant Professor in the Department of Health Law, Policy, and Management, at the School of Public Health, Boston University.
David K. Jones, Associate Professor in the Department of Health Law, Policy, and Management at Boston University's School of Public Health.

https://doi.org/10.1515/9783110745085-002

dient response to the pandemic, interacting with both short and long-term leadership failures to result in more than 33 million COVID-19 infections and over 589,000 excess deaths by May of 2021.[3] One key feature is federalism, the governance structure common to public health laws that divides responsibility for given policies between federal and state governments.

Federalism has commonly cited benefits such as tailoring of policies to local populations and experimenting through the smaller "laboratories of democracy" of states and localities. But the weaknesses of public health federalism came into sharp focus in the face of a global infectious disease outbreak. Federalism significantly increases the need for coordination between government officials and necessitates dependable leadership, increasing complexity and variability by relying on 51 governments rather than one and increasing risk by creating more room for error.

Leadership and federalism were intertwined in the U.S. response to the novel coronavirus pandemic. Federal laws rely on both federal and state participation in implementation of national goals in a public health emergency. The federal government can issue guidance and direct funding, but day-to-day public health measures are operationalized by over 2,000 state and local health departments. If each official does not play their role at every level, relief efforts can fail to materialize or generate inequitable responses across states and localities. In addition, emergency response builds on historical policy choices that created vulnerabilities in the public health system, such that preexisting health and economic conditions were intensified by a public health emergency. During the novel coronavirus pandemic, a disproportionately high number of infections and deaths occurred within the populations of Black, Hispanic, indigenous, and other people of color.[4] The communities hit hardest by novel coronavirus also faced exacerbation of existing income, housing, education, and other inequities, reflecting in part that health is a function of location.

This chapter briefly provides an overview of the American public health emergency framework and highlights key leadership challenges that occurred at federal and state levels throughout the first year of the pandemic. Then the chapter examines decentralized responsibility in American social programs

---

3 "COVID-19 Dashboard by the Center for Systems Science and Engineering (CSSE)," Johns Hopkins University, https://coronavirus.jhu.edu/map.html; Centers for Disease Control and Prevention, "United States COVID-19 Cases, Deaths, and Laboratory Testing (NAATs) by State, Territory, and Jurisdiction," accessed May 28, 2021, https://covid.cdc.gov/covid-data-tracker/#cases_total deaths.

4 "The COVID Racial Data Tracker," https://covidtracking.com/race (reporting "Nationwide, Black people are dying at 2.362 times the rate of white people").

and states' prior policy choices to understand how long-term choices affected short-term emergency response. Finally, the chapter explores long-term ramifications and solutions to the governance difficulties the pandemic has highlighted.

Public Health Emergency Authority

An emergency or other disaster prompts federal executive and legislative actions, especially when a multi-state or nationwide event is involved. A declaration of a public health emergency (PHE) triggers both presidential power unique to a crisis and coordinated action between the President, Congress, federal agencies, states, and localities. Each governmental player must participate with precision, engaging in certain actions in a specific order and at the right moment to address an emergency effectively.

Federal Actions

A patchwork of long-standing federal laws provides the President, Congress, and federal agencies with authority for federal emergency response, which are often enhanced by "relief bills" that Congress may enact to deliver short-term economic and other aid to people and states harmed by an emergency. Most federal legislative action involves indirect action through providing guidance and money to assist state and local efforts. Most direct actions occur at the state or local level, yet, federal response is necessary to emergency and disaster response.

In March 2020, Congress enacted two major relief bills, the *Coronavirus Aid, Relief and Economic Security Act (CARES Act)*[5] and the *Family First Coronavirus Response Act (Families First Act)*.[6] These laws offered loans to businesses, increased federal funding to states for Medicaid, and enhanced unemployment insurance benefits. Another, smaller relief bill passed in December 2020 offered a variety of economic boosts such as stimulus checks, rent relief, enhanced unemployment benefits, education funding, aid to small businesses, and vaccine funding.[7]

In an emergency, many people become eligible for Medicaid, a program that provides public health insurance to low-income people, including those who

---

5 Coronavirus Aid, Relief, and Economic Security Act, Pub. L. No. 116–136 (2020).
6 Families First Coronavirus Response Act, Pub. L. No. 116–127 (2020).
7 Consolidated Appropriations Act, 2021, Pub. L. No. 116–260 (2020).

lose their jobs. The program is governed by federal law but is funded by both the federal and state governments. The state portion of Medicaid costs is related to the state economy, ranging from about 46% in wealthier states like California and New York to about 15% in Mississippi.[8] At the same moment that state tax revenue declines and states often need to cut budgets, Medicaid enrollment spikes; so, Congress often increases its share of Medicaid funding during emergencies and disasters. The health and economic emergency brought on by the pandemic led Congress to include enhanced federal Medicaid funding to states in the *CARES Act* and the *Families First Act*, but these relief bills also required state "maintenance of effort" so enrollment could not be decreased or eligibility cut while states accept the extra money.

During a PHE, multiple federal agencies have distinct responsibilities, an approach that can work with strong leadership and good communication but risks a fragmented response even in the best of circumstances. The *Public Health Service Act of 1944* authorizes direct action by the Secretary of the Department of Health and Human Services (HHS) to prevent the entry and spread of communicable diseases from foreign countries and between states.[9] The Centers for Disease Control and Prevention (CDC), a sub-agency of HHS, is authorized to detain, examine, and release individuals crossing U.S. borders and traveling between states who may carry communicable diseases.[10] The Department of Homeland Security, the Federal Emergency Management Agency (FEMA), and the Transportation Security Administration also are responsible for federal response to emergencies and disasters.

Notably, the President and the HHS Secretary must both formally declare an emergency to produce the full range of federal aid. The President declares a National Emergency under the *National Emergencies Act* or issues major disaster declarations for states under the *Stafford Act* usually at a state governor's request.[11] When the President declares a National Emergency, federal assistance and coordinated relief can flow to affected areas, including public health infor-

---

8 Kaiser Family Foundation, "Federal Medical Assistance Percentage (FMAP) for Medicaid and Multiplier" (2021), https://www.kff.org/medicaid/state-indicator/federal-matching-rate-and-mul tiplier/?currentTimeframe=0&sortModel=%7B%22colId%22:%22FMAP%20Percentage%22,%22sort%22:%22desc%22%7D.
9 Public Health Service Act Section 361; 42 U.S.C. § 264.
10 42 C.F.R. Parts 70 & 71.
11 Robert T. Stafford Disaster Relief and Emergency Assistance Act, Public Law 100–707 (November 23, 1988) amending the Disaster Relief Act of 1974, Public Law 93–288 (codified in scattered sections of title 42 of the U.S. Code); National Emergencies Act, Pub. L. 94–412 (1976), codified at 50 U.S.C. §§ 1601–1651.

mation and data; assistance with distribution of food, medicine, and other supplies; and direct support to "save lives" as needed.[12] The President's National Emergency declaration prompts action from agencies like FEMA and HHS.[13] In addition, the HHS Secretary's public health emergency declaration facilitates regulatory relief that makes state response actions easier.[14] Both National Emergency and PHE declarations must be renewed regularly if an emergency continues. Disaster declarations can last longer.

Early in the pandemic response, the Trump administration moved to enact international travel restrictions and to provide funding and resources for "Operation Warp Speed" vaccine development efforts. However, on the whole, President Trump did not readily exercise the special power federal laws give to the President to address emergencies, creating a leadership vacuum that other officials had to fill. The President waited to declare a national emergency, despite knowing the novel coronavirus pierced U.S. borders – his first declaration was issued on March 13, 2020 and effective as of March 1 – so West Coast states contending with early outbreaks had little federal assistance at the time they began to address novel coronavirus. The President's messaging to the public regarding the severity of COVID-19 and the effectiveness of mitigation efforts was inconsistent and at times inaccurate. President Trump made fabulist claims such as sunlight and injected bleach could kill the virus and ignored mask-wearing and other state or local rules during public events,[15] modeling noncompliance with state and local containment efforts.[16] The White House also obstructed dissemination of scientific information.[17] The President was hospitalized with COVID-19

---

12 42 U.S.C. § 5121, 5192(a).

13 42 U.S.C. §§ 5122, 5191, 5192.

14 42 U.S.C. § 247d.

15 Timothy Bella, "'Shameful, dangerous and irresponsible': Nevada governor blasts Trump for indoor rally against state rules," *Washington Post*, September 14, 2020, https://www.washingtonpost.com/nation/2020/09/14/trump-nevada-rally-coronavirus-sisolak/; Teo Armus, "A GOP county chair asked Trump to wear a mask to his rally. Instead, Trump mocked pandemic restrictions," *Washington Post*, September 9, 2020, https://www.washingtonpost.com/nation/2020/09/09/trump-rally-masks-nc/.

16 Jess Bidgood, "'If he believes he doesn't need a mask, good for him': Despite Trump's illness, supporters still aren't sure about masks," *Boston Globe*, October 4, 2020, https://www.bostonglobe.com/2020/10/04/nation/trumps-positive-covid-test-doesnt-change-views-some-supporters-wearing-masks/.

17 Alexis Madrigal, "Fauci to a Meddling HHS Official: 'Take a Hike'," *The Atlantic*, September 23, 2020, https://www.theatlantic.com/health/archive/2020/09/fauci-caputo-alexander-cdc-fda/616436/; Aaron Rupar, "Dr. Fauci and Dr. Birx detail how Trump's coronavirus response was even worse than we thought," *Vox*, January 25, 2021, https://www.vox.com/2021/1/25/22249050/fauci-birx-interviews-trump-coronavirus-response.

in October 2020.[18] The President refused to authorize the provision of stockpiled supplies like personal protective equipment (PPE) to states, although the federal government is responsible for doing so,[19] forcing states to purchase and distribute PPE in competition with both FEMA and other states.[20] And, the President opposed the Obama-era health reform law called the *Patient Protection and Affordable Care Act* (ACA), so he refused to open a special enrollment period on the federal health insurance exchange (or, the "Marketplace") to make it possible for more people to buy commercial insurance coverage with federal tax credits outside of the annual enrollment period that occurs only at year-end.[21] As the pandemic progressed, the White House undermined evidence and downplayed containment orders but pressured states to curb the outbreak.[22] These actions increased risks associated with novel coronavirus and forced state officials to act in ways meant to be avoided by federal laws that centralize disaster resources, such as having a national stockpile and emergency authority under the *Defense Production Act* to ramp up production of necessary supplies.[23]

The Operation Warp Speed vaccine development effort led by the White House both contrasts with and evidences leadership challenges. This program

---

18 Whether the President tested positive before October 2, 2020, when his COVID status was reported, is uncertain, as the White House issued differing timelines regarding positive status for the President and his advisors. Michael. C. Bender and Rebecca Ballhaus, "Trump Didn't Disclose First Positive Covid-19 Test While Awaiting a Second Test on Thursday," *Wall Street Journal*, October 4, 2020, https://www.wsj.com/articles/trump-didnt-disclose-first-positive-covid-19-test-while-awaiting-a-second-test-on-thursday-11601844813.

19 Federal Emergency Management Agency, "Bringing Resources to State, Local, Tribal & Territorial Governments," https://www.fema.gov/disasters/coronavirus/governments.

20 Quint Forgey, "'We're not a shipping clerk': Trump tells governors to step up efforts to get medical supplies," *Politico*, March 19, 2020, https://www.politico.com/news/2020/03/19/trump-governors-coronavirus-medical-supplies-137658; Jordan Fabian, "Trump Told Governors to Buy Own Virus Supplies, Then Outbid Them," *Bloomberg*, March 19, 2020, https://www.bloomberg.com/news/articles/2020-03-19/trump-told-governors-to-buy-own-virus-supplies-then-outbid-them; Olivia Ruben et al., "Despite Trump claim, 13 states say some orders for coronavirus supplies still unfilled," *ABC News*, July 23, 2020, https://abcnews.go.com/Health/trump-claim-12-states-orders-coronavirus-supplies-unfilled/story?id=71946598.

21 Susannah Luthi, "Trump rejects Obamacare special enrollment period amid pandemic," *Politico*, March 31, 2020, https://www.politico.com/news/2020/03/31/trump-obamacare-coronavirus-157788.

22 President Trump tweeted "liberate Michigan," which inspired a plot to kidnap the governor. Lauren de Valle, "Man pleads guilty in plot to kidnap Michigan Gov. Gretchen Whitmer," *CNN*, January 27, 2021, https://www.cnn.com/2021/01/27/politics/gretchen-whitmer-kidnapping-plot/index.html.

23 Defense Production Reauthorization Act of 2009, Pub. L. 111–67 (reauthorizing and amending Defense Production Act of 1950).

supplied substantial federal support for vaccine researchers and was deemed a success for generating vaccines ready for FDA emergency use approval within the calendar year 2020.[24] Vaccine distribution, on the other hand, suffered from many of the same flaws as other aspects of the pandemic response, such as a lack of centralized decision-making and marginal guidance to state public health officials. Vaccine distribution began with high variability across states, though little data was collected by most states so precise numbers are hard to come by.[25]

Overall, HHS exercised its emergency powers in a more predictable manner. HHS Secretary Alex Azar declared a PHE effective on January 27, 2020, shortly after SARS-CoV-2 reached U.S. borders.[26] This activated HHS' special authority to issue grants responding to the PHE, enter into contracts, access emergency funds, and temporarily increase state regulatory flexibility.[27] Once the President declared an emergency, the national emergency and PHE declarations together permitted the Secretary to issue emergency-related waivers to states. These waivers allowed certain Medicaid rules to be modified so officials could secure healthcare access, for example, waiving licensure requirements for out of state health care providers. Secretary Azar renewed the PHE declaration throughout 2020, issuing his last declaration on January 7, 2021 so the PHE continued through the start of the Biden administration.

The President's avoidance of emergency authority and responsibility unexpectedly thwarted longstanding national public health emergency architecture. Federal laws assume a federalism governance structure will work for emergencies – and in normal times – and do not address the possibility that the President would not take up special power to enact public health protections or that governors would follow his lead in failing to take action. Yet, both occurred throughout 2020 and into 2021 after the Biden administration took office facing the ongoing emergency of the pandemic. President Biden ran a campaign that promised an effective, coordinated approach to combatting COVID-19, and the

---

24 Dan Diamond, "The crash landing of 'Operation Warp Speed'," *Politico*, January 17, 2021, https://www.politico.com/news/2021/01/17/crash-landing-of-operation-warp-speed-459892.
25 Alejandro de la Garza and Chris Wilson, "Many States Don't Know Who's Getting COVID-19 Vaccines. That's a Huge Problem for Equity," *Time*, January 28, 2021, https://time.com/5934095/covid-vaccine-data/.
26 Secretary Alex M. Azar II, "Determination that a Public Health Emergency Exists," https://www.phe.gov/emergency/news/healthactions/phe/Pages/2019-nCoV.aspx.
27 42 U.S.C. § 247d(a).

common account is that President Biden's election reflected dissatisfaction and distrust with the Trump administration's erratic pandemic response.[28]

State Response

As previously noted, at the national level, CDC performs research, data collection, and surveillance, and can influence state and local actions with policy guidance and money but has little authority to compel uniform state or local action. As such, short-term federal emergency response builds on states' public health capacity. In other words, because state and local public health departments are frontline actors in day-to-day public health activities,[29] and state health policies impact neighbor states' and national public health efforts, state and local public health choices affect response to a national or global PHE.[30]

The pandemic hit within the context that states had consistently reduced public health spending over the last decade.[31] Such reductions diminished public health departments' ability to respond to public health events, and staffing dropped correspondingly. Defunded health departments faced a colossal containment task and vaccine rollout effort without staff or other resources adequate for such work.[32] States historically were responsible for and regulated public health, safety, and welfare by exercising their plenary police power; but, over

---

28 Ashley Parker et al., "How Trump's erratic behavior and failure on coronavirus doomed his reelection," *Washington Post*, November 7, 2020, https://www.washingtonpost.com/elections/interactive/2020/trump-pandemic-coronavirus-election/.

29 Centers for Disease Control and Prevention, "Health Department Governance: State and Local Health Department Governance Classification Map," accessed May 10, 2020, https://www.cdc.gov/publichealthgateway/sitesgovernance/index.html; Wendy M. Mariner et al., *Public Health Law* 18–20, 63–194 (3d ed. 2019).

30 David Holtz et al., *Interdependence and the Cost of Uncoordinated Responses to COVID-19*, May 22, 2020, https://osf.io/b9psy/.

31 Jennifer Haberkorn, "The Prevention and Public Health Fund Policy Brief," *Health Affairs* (2012), https://www.healthaffairs.org/do/10.1377/hpb20120223.98342/full/healthpolicybrief_63.pdf; "Hollowed-Out Public Health System Faces More Cuts Amid Virus," *Kaiser Health News* (July 1, 2020), https://khn.org/news/us-public-health-system-underfunded-under-threat-faces-more-cuts-amid-covid-pandemic/.

32 President Trump's appointees reportedly resisted giving more money to states for vaccine rollout. Nicholas Florko, "Trump officials actively lobbied to deny states money for vaccine rollout last fall," *STAT News*, February 1, 2021, https://www.statnews.com/2021/01/31/trump-officials-lobbied-to-deny-states-money-for-vaccine-rollout/?utm_source=STAT+Newsletters&utm_campaign=a94a277bf9-MR_COPY_14&utm_medium=email&utm_term=0_8cab1d7961-a94a277bf9-150488781.

time, federal power and responsibility have grown significantly, responding in part to state and local public health programs relying heavily on federal funding.

Yet, the vacuum of federal leadership boosted state responsibility for a disease outbreak greater than any public health challenge in recent history. Unsurprisingly, without more centralized federal direction, and political tensions running high, state leaders responded to the pandemic in a highly irregular fashion. Governors found themselves on the frontline, and many used emergency authority to swiftly contain the outbreak. But, some governors followed President Trump's model in resisting stringent containment measures recommended by CDC or other federal public health experts, which then left containment to mayors, education leaders, and other local officials.[33] In some states, such as Mississippi[34] and South Carolina,[35] governors superseded or limited local officials' stay-at-home and related containment orders and undermined their authority for issuing such rules, adding a micro-federalism dimension of intra-state conflict.[36] In 2021, a handful of state legislatures have enacted limits on gubernatorial emergency powers, which often parallel presidential emergency powers but are more extensive, in response to more stringent containment actions.[37] For example, Idaho enacted a law limiting gubernatorial power during emergencies, increasing legislative oversight of emergencies and limiting the containment measures that can be implemented in emergencies.[38] Arkansas enacted a law limiting containment measures but then experienced severe Delta variant out-

---

33 Jim Salter, "Missouri's COVID-19 Response in Spotlight at Governor Forum," *U.S. News*, October 9, 2020, https://www.usnews.com/news/best-states/missouri/articles/2020-10-09/missouris-covid-19-response-in-spotlight-at-governor-forum.

34 Mississippi Governor Tate Reeves Exec. Order 1463 (March 24, 2020).

35 Laurel Mallory, "S.C. attorney general says local governments cannot issue stay-at-home orders," *wbtv.com*, March 27, 2020, https://www.wbtv.com/2020/03/27/sc-attorney-general-says-local-governments-cannot-issue-stay-at-home-orders/.

36 Adam Gabbatt, "Which states have done the least to contain coronavirus?," *The Guardian*, April 3, 2020, https://www.theguardian.com/world/2020/apr/03/coronavirus-states-response-who-has-done-least-alabama-oklahoma-missouri.

37 David A. Lieb, "State lawmakers are pushing to curb governors' virus powers," *Associated Press*, January 28, 2021, https://apnews.com/article/state-lawmakers-governor-coronavirus-7d5710f2d8aa4e659c0ec68400ad3d3c?utm_source=Sailthru&utm_medium=email&utm_campaign=AP%20Morning%20Wire&utm_term=Morning%20Wire%20Subscribers; "Legislative Oversight of Emergency Executive Powers," National Conference of State Legislatures (2021), https://www.ncsl.org/research/about-state-legislatures/legislative-oversight-of-executive-orders.aspx#Emergency%20Powers%20Bills.

38 Idaho S.B. 1217, enacted May 10, 2021, https://custom.statenet.com/public/resources.cgi?id=ID:bill:ID2021000S1217&ciq=ncsl&client_md=2763280a02f529e8c9506c252a005b41&mode=current_text.

breaks in 2021, leading the governor to publicly express regret for signing the law.

Non-pharmaceutical interventions (NPI) were the primary tool for controlling the spread of novel coronavirus throughout 2020 and into early 2021.[39] CDC's NPI recommendations included mask-wearing, frequent hand and surface sanitizing, community measures such as physical distance and restricted occupancy in public spaces, limited gathering size, stay in place orders (SIP), and business, church, and school closures. Some states swiftly implemented stringent NPIs, like Washington and California, while others like Texas responded in a more relaxed fashion, reopening quickly from the March/April SIP orders and resisting additional containment measures. South Dakota had a particularly serious outbreak after resisting NPI and then allowing an unmasked motorcycle rally that led to outbreaks that bypassed state borders.[40] Texas continued the pattern when Governor Abbott decided to end executive orders requiring mask wearing and other NPI in the first week of March 2021, which Mississippi also did, despite President Biden's warnings to the contrary.[41]

Testing was not widely or consistently available in many places, and the federal government did not respond reliably to governor's requests for PPE, testing materials, and other supplies to deal with the pandemic due to political motivations combined with shortages in the federal stockpile of supplies. Data collection on infections, hospitalizations, and deaths due to COVID-19 were unreliable, even though states are obligated to collect certain kinds of demographic data within the Medicaid program that could have been extended to the pandemic context.

Studies show these heterogeneous containment policies affected infection and mortality rates, contributing to disproportionate health and economic im-

---

39 FDA Press Release, "FDA Takes Key Action in Fight Against COVID-19 by Issuing Emergency Use Authorization for First COVID-19 Vaccine," December 11, 2021, https://www.fda.gov/news-events/press-announcements/fda-takes-key-action-fight-against-covid-19-issuing-emergency-use-authorization-first-covid-19.

40 Rosalind J. Carter et al., CDC COVID-19 Response Team, "Widespread Severe Acute Respiratory Syndrome Coronavirus 2 Transmission Among Attendees at a Large Motorcycle Rally and their Contacts, 30 US Jurisdictions, August–September, 2020," 73 *Clinical Infectious Diseases*, S106–S109, Issue Supplement 1, July 15, 2021; Melanie J. Firestone et al., "COVID-19 Outbreak Associated with a 10-Day Motorcycle Rally in a Neighboring State – Minnesota, August–September 2020," 69 *Morb. Mortal. Wkly. Report* 1771, November 27, 2020, https://www.cdc.gov/mmwr/volumes/69/wr/mm6947e1.htm.

41 Marissa Martinez, "Texas no longer has a statewide mask mandate. But face coverings are still required in some businesses and public places," *The Texas Tribune*, March 10, 2021, https://www.texastribune.org/2021/03/10/texas-mask-mandate-coronavirus-restrictions/.

pacts across states. Researchers at Oxford University studied state containment policy differences, including types of NPI measures, stringency of rules, and duration of implementation. They have accumulated evidence with systematic data collection showing that more stringent state-level COVID-19 containment policies have correlated to lower outbreak severity.[42]

The novel coronavirus pandemic developed in parallel with the intensification of the Black Lives Matter movement in the wake of George Floyd's murder by a Minneapolis police officer on May 25, 2020. This spotlighted the fact that Black, Hispanic, and other populations of color were disproportionately infected and dying during the pandemic. Federalism in the United States historically has been more than a technical question of which level of government is best suited to perform certain functions but rather a compromise allowing states to maintain slavery, segregation, and other legal structures that explicitly or implicitly restrict access to resources for non-white populations.[43] Electoral systems in some states such as Mississippi and Alabama were designed so that the officials making policy decisions do not reflect or represent the populations they serve.[44] These approaches have continued even today, for example with Texas enacting a law in September 2021 that makes voting more difficult for low-income people, people of color, and people with disabilities.[45] Further, several states do not require state legislatures to implement laws that are passed by a majority of voters via ballot initiative. In states like Utah and Missouri, this feature delayed the implementation of Medicaid expansion.

National death rates from COVID-19 among Black, Hispanic, and Indigenous patients were 2–2.4 times higher than among White patients.[46] Studies indicate

---

42 Coronavirus Government Response Tracker, University of Oxford Blavatnik School of Government, https://www.bsg.ox.ac.uk/research/research-projects/coronavirus-government-response-tracker; "Variation in US states' responses to COVID-19," Version 2.0 published December 2020, https://www.bsg.ox.ac.uk/sites/default/files/2020-12/BSG-WP-2020-034-v2_0.pdf.

43 Daniel E. Dawes, *The Political Determinants of Health* (Baltimore: Johns Hopkins Press, 2020), 21; John A. Ferejohn and Barry R. Weingast, "Introduction," *The New Federalism: Can the States Be Trusted?* (Stanford: Stanford University Press, 1997), ix.

44 David. K. Jones, "Political Participation in the Least Healthy Place in America: Examining the Political Determinants of Health in the Mississippi Delta," *Journal of Health Politics, Policy and Law* 44, no. 3 (2019): 505–31.

45 Texas Senate Bill 1 (September 7, 2021), https://capitol.texas.gov/BillLookup/History.aspx?LegSess=872&Bill=SB1.

46 U.S. Centers for Disease Control and Prevention, "COVID-19 cases, data, and surveillance: hospitalization and death by race/ethnicity," accessed October 12, 2020, https://www-cdc-gov.ezproxy.bu.edu/coronavirus/2019-ncov/covid-data/investigations-discovery/hospitalization-death-by-race-ethnicity.html.

that people of color who are low-income and face high exposure suffered the most in every state,[47] but especially in states with less stringent NPI and low vaccination rates, many of which also are resistant to the full implementation of social welfare programs.[48] These states' short-term PHE response exacerbated long-term patterns of health disparities by race, ethnicity, and income.

Federalism, Healthcare, and Social Programs

COVID-19 has tested the limits of federalism in healthcare and social welfare programs, which, like public health systems, operate within a federalist governance structure. An example of this dynamic exists in Medicaid, the primary source of health insurance for low-income Americans and a federal program that provides money and rules to states, which have considerable flexibility within the program through exercising statutory options and seeking federal waivers to further the purpose of the program in new ways. Medicaid is not only an important source of public health insurance, it is also a key tool in public health emergencies. Like Medicaid, other social programs such as housing support, unemployment benefits, minimum hourly wage standards, and food assistance all vary at the state level within federal rules. Also, given that nursing homes were a primary source of COVID-19 infections and deaths, it is notable that the responsibility for quality assurance in nursing homes is shared between the federal government and states. The federal government issues standards related to the safety and quality of care delivered in nursing homes but regular inspection activities are conducted by local authorities. Here, Medicaid provides an example of the importance of long-term state choices in a short-term emergency response.

Congress enacted the ACA to improve access to healthcare by crafting near-universal health insurance coverage cobbled together through commercial and public insurance mechanisms.[49] The ACA offered federal money to states to

---

47 Erin K. Stokes et al., "Coronavirus Disease 2019 Case Surveillance – United States, January 22–May 30, 2020," 69 *Morb. Mortal. Wkly. Rep.* 759 (2020); Marie E. Killerby et al., "Characteristics Associated with Hospitalization Among Patients with COVID-19 – Metropolitan Atlanta, Georgia, March–April 2020," *Morb. Mortal. Wkly. Rep. ePub: 17 June 2020*; Sebastian D. Romano et al., "Trends in Racial and Ethnic Disparities in COVID-19 Hospitalizations, by Region – United States, March–December 2020," 70 *Morb. Mortal. Wkly. Rep.* 560, April 16, 2021.
48 Health Equity Considerations and Racial and Ethnic Minority Groups. Centers for Disease Control and Prevention (2021), https://www.cdc.gov/coronavirus/2019-ncov/community/health-equity/race-ethnicity.html.
49 Paul Starr, *Remedy and Reaction: The Peculiar American Struggle over Health Care Reform* (New Haven: Yale University Press, 2011).

establish health insurance exchanges ("Exchanges" or "Marketplaces") to sell "qualified health plans." HHS runs a national Exchange if states have not established their own, ensuring that an exchange exists in every state regardless of state leadership choices. However, if a state does not expand Medicaid eligibility under the ACA, a key feature of the ACA's expansion of insurance coverage, no federal backup exists. In Medicaid non-expansion states, people earning less than 100% of the federal poverty level do not qualify for insurance subsidies on the Exchange and cannot enroll in Medicaid, creating a coverage gap for over two million people that is concentrated in Deep South and central Midwestern states.[50] Approximately 28 million individuals were uninsured when novel coronavirus emerged, almost half of whom are eligible for Medicaid or for federal tax subsidies to purchase insurance on an Exchange.[51] Some four million people became eligible for Medicaid in 2020 due to recession-related job loss and other financial hardships accompanying the pandemic, a 6.2% increase.[52]

Before the pandemic reordered political priorities, the Trump administration was hostile to the ACA, directing federal agencies by Executive Order to avoid implementing and enforcing the law.[53] The administration took many actions to undermine the ACA when Congress did not repeal it, such as blocking federal payments to insurance companies for high-cost insurance subscribers,[54] ending cost-sharing reduction payments for low-income subscribers,[55] and reducing Marketplace outreach funding and open enrollment periods that help people

---

50 Medicaid non-expansion states are Texas, Tennessee, Florida, Georgia, South Carolina, North Carolina, Wyoming, Wisconsin, Alabama, Kansas, Mississippi, and South Dakota. Oklahoma and Missouri each had a successful ballot initiative to expand Medicaid in the summer of 2020, but expansion has not begun. Rachel Garfield et al., "The Coverage Gap," *Kaiser Family Foundation*, January 2020, https://www.kff.org/medicaid/issue-brief/the-coverage-gap-uninsured-poor-adults-in-states-that-do-not-expand-medicaid/.

51 Munira Z. Gunja and Sara R. Collins, "Who Are the Remaining Uninsured, and Why Do They Lack Coverage?," *Commonwealth Fund*, August 28, 2019, https://www.commonwealthfund.org/publications/issue-briefs/2019/aug/who-are-remaining-uninsured-and-why-do-they-lack-coverage.

52 Centers for Medicare & Medicaid Services, "CMS Releases Medicaid and CHIP Enrolment Trends Snapshot Showing COVID-19 Impact on Enrollment," September 30, 2020, https://www.cms.gov/newsroom/press-releases/cms-releases-medicaid-and-chip-enrollment-trends-snapshot-showing-covid-19-impact-enrollment?utm_campaign=wp_the_health_202&utm_medium=email&utm_source=newsletter&wpisrc=nl_health202.

53 Executive Order No. 13765, 82 Federal Register 8351 (January 20, 2017).

54 Maine Community Health Options v. United States, U.S., Docket No. 18–1023 (2020).

55 Sanford Health Plan v. United States, 2019–1290, 2019–1302 (D.C. Circuit Court of Appeals, August 14, 2020); Community Health Choice, Inc. v. United States, 2019–1633 (D.C. Circuit Court of Appeals, August 14, 2020).

find and enroll in coverage. To undercut Medicaid expansion, the administration crafted novel polices that required beneficiaries to work or engage in work-related activities to maintain Medicaid coverage,[56] which were never approved by Congress and no prior administration allowed. These policies had the predictable effect of disenrolling Medicaid beneficiaries by creating confusing paperwork and other administrative burdens.[57] Insurance rates declined due to these policies, with un-insurance rates especially high in non-expansion states. Ninety percent of people in the coverage gap lived in the eight Southern states that did not expand Medicaid, with Texas, Florida, and Georgia accounting for three-quarters of the uninsured.[58] These states' choices were crucial for people of color, who were disproportionately infected and dying from COVID-19, especially if they were also low income and in high-exposure jobs.[59]

Fourteen states had not implemented the ACA's Medicaid eligibility expansion by the time the pandemic began, to the detriment of low-income residents, healthcare providers, and state budgets. Non-expansion states already experienced economic inequality, parsimonious unemployment benefits, lower rates of employer-sponsored insurance coverage, and higher chronic disease incidence. These states' leaders, largely for political reasons, ignored the evidence from more than 400 studies that Medicaid expansion produces positive outcomes for individual and public health, increasing health insurance coverage and reducing health disparities by increasing access for minority populations, individuals with low educational attainment, and low-income workers.[60] These

56 Letter to State Medicaid Directors, SMD 18–002, Center for Medicare & Medicaid Services (January 11, 2018), https://www.medicaid.gov/federal-policy-guidance/downloads/smd18002. pdf; Healthy Adult Opportunity Fact Sheet, Center for Medicare & Medicaid Services (January 30, 2020), https://www.cms.gov/newsroom/fact-sheets/healthy-adult-opportunity-fact-sheet (federal policy guidance inviting block grant proposals from states for expansion population).

57 Ben Sommers et al., "Medicaid Work Requirements – Results from the First Year in Arkansas," New England Journal of Medicine 381, no. 1073 (2019).

58 Rachel Garfield, Kendal Orgera, and Anthony Damico, "The Coverage Gap: Uninsured Poor Adults in States that Do Not Expand Medicaid," *Kaiser Family Foundation* (2020), https://www. kff.org/medicaid/issue-brief/the-coverage-gap-uninsured-poor-adults-in-states-that-do-not-ex pand-medicaid/.

59 Richard A. Oppel et al., "The Fullest Look Yet at the Racial Inequity of Coronavirus," *New York Times*, https://www.nytimes.com/interactive/2020/07/05/us/coronavirus-latinos-afri can-americans-cdc-data.html.

60 Madeline Guth et al., "The Effects of Medicaid Expansion under the ACA: Updated Findings from a Literature Review," *Kaiser Family Foundation*, March 20, 2020, https://www.kff.org/ medicaid/report/the-effects-of-medicaid-expansion-under-the-aca-updated-findings-from-a-liter ature-review/.

Leadership Matters

The Institute of Medicine defined public health as "fulfilling society's interest in assuring conditions in which people can be healthy" and argued for greater attention to public health needs more than 30 years ago.[67] Instead, public health was deprioritized both fiscally and as a policy matter for years before the pandemic.[68] A government that does not fund public health will not have a healthy public, evidenced by declines in life expectancy even before COVID-19.[69] Decreased funding for public health and decentralizing public health responsibility have weakened the public's health in the U.S. and made already vulnerable populations less resilient in the face of an emergency, contributing to a 1.5 year decline in life expectancy in 2020.[70]

Public health federalism may operationalize a public health emergency response but also contributed to structural troubles that became so apparent during the PHE. Federalism in health laws occurs for a number of reasons. One is path dependence[71] combined with an instinct for incrementalism in health reform – public health emergency laws and the ACA both are examples of this tendency for past decisions to constrain the options that seem feasible in the future.[72] Another reason is that Congress may find it politically expedient to include states in public health laws so that the nationalization of state-based rules seems less threatening to state autonomy – health insurance exchange structure provides an example, where Congress invited states to continue using their decades of insurance regulation experience to guide a new insurance

---

67 Committee for the Study of the Future of Public Health, "The Future of Public Health," *Institute of Medicine* 19 (1988).

68 Karen B. DeSalvo et al., "Public Health 3.0: A Call to Action for Public Health to Meet the Challenges of the 21st Century," *National Academy of Medicine* (2017), https://nam.edu/public-health-3-0-call-action-public-health-meet-challenges-21st-century/.

69 Sherry L. Murphy et al., "Mortality in the United States, 2017," *National Center for Health Statistics Data Brief No. 328*, November 2018, https://www.cdc.gov/nchs/data/databriefs/db328-h.pdf.

70 Elizabeth Arias et al., "Provisional Life Expectancy Estimates for 2020," *NVSS Vital Statistics Rapid Release Report No. 15*, July 2021, https://www.cdc.gov/nchs/data/vsrr/vsrr015-508.pdf.

71 "Path dependence" describes the idea that history may prescribe policy choices, making any given decision less deliberate than it might have been without the initial set of decisions, often attributed to Professor Paul David, who framed the idea within the example of the inefficient QWERTY keyboard. Paul A. David, "Clio and the Economics of QWERTY," *Am. Econ. Rev. 75*, no. 332 (1985).

72 Abbe R. Gluck and Nicole Huberfeld, "What Is Federalism in Healthcare For?," *Stanford Law Review* 70, no. 1689 (2018): 1703–19.

product. Sometimes, Congress decides states must adhere to new federal baselines because state policy choices have failed, as with expanding Medicaid eligibility to childless adults under the ACA. Sometimes Congress takes over, especially when states or markets have failed in a health policy function, as with Medicare or current proposals for a public option for health insurance,[73] but this is less common.[74]

A crisis that exposes deep health disparities may clarify the weaknesses of federalism as a health governance approach, especially in a public health emergency. So, what are the lessons we can draw from the first year of the pandemic when it comes to the challenges that federalism is currently facing?

National leadership matters. The Trump administration's coronavirus response created a leadership vacuum that included delaying the national emergency declaration, inconsistent communication regarding the severity of the outbreak to the public, funding and supply delays, uneven assistance to states, and insufficient and botched testing.[75] The vaccine development encouraged by Operation Warp Speed was important, but pharmaceutical companies had been developing the technology for such mRNA vaccines for more than a decade before novel coronavirus. Many deaths were preventable and many people will be "long haulers" who face debilitating effects from COVID-19 for years to come. In constitutional law, the President has the most power when the Constitution and Congress agree that the President can act, which is the case in a PHE. This makes Trump's reluctance to lead all the more confounding.

On the other hand, the Biden administration entered office prioritizing expedient policy action and effective management. Vaccine distribution, strengthening the healthcare safety net, appointing experienced government officials, deference to science and evidence, and health equity were all articulated through early executive orders and swift regulatory actions. The Biden administration used existing laws to change the federal government's response to the pandemic. Leadership is important, but it is not the entire story, because state partnership

---

73 Medicare X Choice Senate bill available at https://www.bennet.senate.gov/public/index.cfm/press-releases?id=5D307D1A-B91B-465D-8D0B-6EE62C4E99D8.

74 See Gluck and Huberfeld, supra note 64, at 1716 – 19.

75 "'It Is Roiling Him': Reporter Maggie Haberman Unpacks Trump's Refusal To Admit He Lost," *Fresh Air*, December 10, 2020, https://www.npr.org/2020/12/10/944935318/it-is-roiling-him-nyts-maggie-haberman-unpacks-trumps-refusal-to-admit-he-lost; Michael Shear et al., "Inside Trump's Failure: The Rush to Abandon Leadership Role on the Virus," *New York Times*, July 18, 2020, https://www.nytimes.com/2020/07/18/us/politics/trump-coronavirus-response-failure-leadership.html.

and uptake of federal funding and guidance is still central to the public health system and especially a PHE.

The federal government is limited in its ability to mandate centralized action or to force states or localities to act, irrespective of leadership. The federal government typically is a backstop for states, though in the first year of the pandemic some states filled in the gaps and backed the federal government. History demonstrates that states cannot respond to a public health emergency alone. Public health emergencies require effective federal leadership and federal funding as well as coordinated state, local, and tribal implementation. Without coherent federal leadership, state policy heterogeneity made it so that state outbreaks were worse depending on short-term measures and so that millions of people were falling through preexisting holes in the safety net due to longer term state policy preferences.

Long-term planning for future public health crises must recognize that federalism is often a choice rooted in history and policy preference and not always a constitutional requirement. Congress could enact health reform that is purely national, in the model of Medicare for example, and this would be constitutionally more straightforward than including states. Other nations have decentralized policymaking through a federalist structure, but American federalism is different for the degree to which states control policy even when the federal government has power to offer national solutions. State and local leaders who do not favor policies such as spending on public health often argue that states have the "right" to control these policies, not the federal government. The U.S. Supreme Court decided long ago that Congress has authority to create social programs that are purely national.[76] If federalism governance structures are not constitutionally required, then using federalism for structuring social programs and policies raises important questions regarding whether, how, and when responses to national health needs should involve states. It also raises the question of whether states will predictably accept the invitation to engage.[77]

Though federalism is not required in laws governing social and public health programs, it is enshrined in American policymaking. For this reason, complete

---

76 United States v. South-Eastern Underwriters Association, 322 U.S. 533 (1944) (Congress has commerce clause authority to regulate national insurance markets); Helvering v. Davis, 301 U.S. 619 (1937) (old age benefits) and Steward Machine Co. v. Davis, 301 U.S. 548 (1937) (unemployment insurance) (both part of the Social Security Act). The Supreme Court rejected arguments that providing welfare to the elderly was reserved for states. Helvering, 640–45.

77 Robert F. Rich and William D. White, "Health Care Policy and the American States: Issues of Federalism," in *Health Policy, Federalism, and the American States* (England: Urban Institute Press, 1997).

centralization of public health policy is unlikely. Centralization of public health efforts also may not be the most efficient restructuring for response to public health crises. Federalism can be a rational policy choice, but public health federalism should be a purposeful choice that maximizes the nation's health with an understanding of the capacity that states and localities build or ignore within the federalist structure.

The evidence from novel coronavirus so far indicates that federalism's divided governance complicated the response to an infectious disease outbreak. Public health has largely been addressed at the whim of state budgets, politics, and policymaking, even when some uniform policy is more desirable, making states even less capable of responding to a public health emergency alone. Will we be ready for the next public health crisis? The system needs to be resilient enough to withstand an unpredictable leadership vacuum as well as the predictable variability of public health federalism.

The flexibility offered by public health federalism must have a floor, meaning federal rules for basic levels of support through social programs. Inequity is inherent to federalism's variability without such rules, which foreseeably results in different health outcomes that have been worse for vulnerable populations.

Increased spending is necessary for staffing public health at federal, state, tribal, and local levels. The Biden administration proposed creating a public health workforce in this regard, and that would be a fine start.[78] But the ACA promised public health funding to states, and Congress rolled it back. This policy idea should be renewed. A retrospective analysis of existing gaps and weaknesses in the public health infrastructure must occur to be prepared when the next emergency strikes.

Universal health insurance coverage must become the norm, whether building on the current patchwork or not. Eleven years after the ACA was enacted, millions of people remain in a coverage gap that left them and others unnecessarily exposed during an emergency. This would also help to improve other features of the safety net's infrastructure, such as community health centers and safety net hospitals, which rely heavily on Medicaid in their patient mix.

Consistent data collection is important for addressing the next public health emergency through better coordination and evidence-based action. State and local data collection is necessary given inconsistencies revealed during the pan-

---

78 Fact Sheet: Biden-Harris Administration to Invest $7 Billion from American Rescue Plan to Hire and Train Public Health Workers in Response to COVID-19, *The White House*, May 13, 2021, https://www.whitehouse.gov/briefing-room/statements-releases/2021/05/13/fact-sheet-biden-har ris-administration-to-invest-7-billion-from-american-rescue-plan-to-hire-and-train-public-health-workers-in-response-to-covid-19/.

demic that complicated the response to the emergency as well as the understanding of its impacts. Congress could choose to condition some portion of federal Medicaid spending on specific state health department data collection. A model for this already exists under ACA section 4302, which demands state and local collection and reporting of racial and ethnic data, and is a provision that could be enforced more consistently.[79] Data regarding race, ethnicity, socio-economic status, and other key identifying characteristics should be prioritized.

If federalism is to remain in the public health picture – and it seems like it will – then its policy heterogeneity must be recognized as both a possible challenge and a possible good. Federalism contributes to fragmentation in American public health and healthcare, even within laws that demand states meet federal requirements. Combined with underfunding of public health, previous policy choices, and a lack of coordination between federal and state leaders, it is no wonder that the U.S. had such poor results in addressing the pandemic.

Conclusion

American healthcare delivers shorter life expectancy, costs more than other wealthy nations, spends less on prevention, and perpetuates disparities for Black, indigenous, and people of color as well as low-income individuals within and across states.[80] All of these factors came into play as the pandemic hit U.S. soil.[81] Rather than focus on such long-term issues, many commentators have blamed leadership failures. While we believe this was an important factor in the failed U.S. response, we must also take a hard look at the governance choices that enabled such unnecessary disaster.[82]

---

79 Pub. L. No. 111–148 sec. 4302.

80 Steven H. Woolf and Heidi Schoomaker, "Life Expectancy and Mortality Rates in the United States," 1959–2017, 322 *JAMA* (2019): 1996, https://jamanetwork.com/journals/jama/article-abstract/2756187; Organization for Economic Cooperation & Development, "Health at a Glance 2019: OECD Indicators" (2019), https://www.oecd-ilibrary.org/docserver/4dd50c09-en.pdf?expires=1589998199&id=id&accname=guest &checksum=AC4537397D75ACC7E8AC3F3DCC07B31B.

81 Brian M. Rosenthal et al., "Why Surviving the Virus May Come Down to Which Hospital Admits You," *New York Times*, July 1, 2020, https://www.nytimes.com/2020/07/01/nyregion/Coronavirus-hospitals.html?referringSource=articleShare.

82 Michael D. Sparer and Lawrence D. Brown, "States and the Health Care Crisis: The Limits and Lessons of Laboratory Federalism," in *Health Policy, Federalism, and the American States* (England: Urban Institute Press, 1997).

Federalism is entrenched in the governance architecture of public health, reflecting historical, political, and policy choices, but not always constitutional requirements. The novel coronavirus pandemic highlighted the costs of this structure, paid in rates of infection and mortality, especially in places where the health and economic stability of people of color have long been disproportionately harmed by state policies. Pushing states and localities to the frontline slowed response times, fostered variability where commonality would have been more effective, and exacerbated existing health and economic inequalities. Bolstering resiliency ahead of the next pandemic requires enacting a national floor with respect to public health preparedness and social welfare programs so that when tested again, the flexibility of the federalist system bows but does not break.

Charles Breton and Paisley Sim

2 A Pandemic in a Highly Decentralized Federation

Variation, Innovation, and Coordination in Canada

Introduction

For many Canadians, the COVID-19 pandemic has been a crash-course on the workings of the federation. The public health restrictions and other measures introduced to curtail the spread of COVID and its economic and social consequences – ranging from mask mandates, school closures, paid sick leave, unemployment benefits, and the terms of mandatory self-isolation periods, for example – were not introduced or managed by a single government, but were a mix of directives from provincial governments and the federal government, with local measures from public health authorities and school boards.

To implement and manage these new policies, many traditional processes of intergovernmental negotiation were supplanted by close, and often ad hoc, intergovernmental cooperation.[1] Operating under conditions of imperfect knowledge, the pandemic has called on all orders of government to adapt and turn to a more coordinated and collaborative approach. Such modes have challenged existing norms and venues of intergovernmental relations (IGR), which in Canada are poorly institutionalized.[2] But did these arrangements curtail Canada's response to the pandemic?

Some have argued that federalism complicated the response to the pandemic by creating a "fragmented and disjointed response."[3] But no two federations are

---

1 André Lecours et al., "The COVID-19 Crisis and Canadian Federalism," *Forum of the Federations* 48 (2020): 1–20, http://www.forumfed.org/publications/the-covid-19-crisis-and-canadian-federalism-number-48/.
2 Mireille Paquet and Robert Schertzer, "COVID-19 as a Complex Intergovernmental Problem," *Canadian Journal of Political Science*, no. 53 (2020): 343–47, 10.1017/S0008423920000281.
3 For the United States see: Nicole Huberfeld, Sarah H. Gordon, and David K. Jones, "Federalism complicates the response to the COVID-19 health and economic crisis: What can be done?," *Journal of health politics, policy and law* 45, no. 6 (2020): 951–65, DOI: 10.1215/03616878–8641493.

Charles Breton, Executive Director, Institute for Research on Public Policy (IRPP).
Paisley Sim, Research Associate, Institute for Research on Public Policy (IRPP).

https://doi.org/10.1515/9783110745085-003

exactly alike, and some institutional features will make some federations better equipped to respond to a crisis than others. For instance, some institutional factors have made Canada's pandemic response more cooperative and less acrimonious compared to that of the United States.[4] Canada has low levels of integration between federal and provincial political parties, with no integration between conservative parties. This creates less rigid territorial partisan alignment, freeing political actors from the need to oppose government decisions, which may increase collaboration.[5] In addition, the mechanism of confidence in the Canadian parliament and flexible election timing may reduce partisanship and increase cooperation.

In conjunction with institutional factors that foster collaboration, federalism empowers sub-national units to act in response to their own context, a feature that will affect a country's overall response in times of crisis. In theory at least, federalism makes it possible for sub-national units to tailor policy responses using better on-the-ground knowledge and data. This is even more likely in federations where decentralization has led sub-national units to have important institutional capacity and infrastructure. Similarly, sub-national units can innovate as they respond to their specific context, creating the possibility for policy diffusion across jurisdictions.

There is a large body of research internationally that documents policy diffusion and mechanisms through which it occurs.[6] In Canada, instances of policy diffusion have also been documented and showed that diffusion can occur through various mechanisms such as learning, competition, copying, convergence or even coercion from the federal government.[7]

In this paper, we explore these potential advantages of federalism by looking at the Canadian response to the COVID-19 pandemic. We find that after a largely standardized response in the first pandemic wave, the decentralized nature of the Canadian federation allowed Provinces and territories to forge divergent paths. Provinces combined high institutional capacity, particularly in the

---

4 Mary J. Rozell and Clyde Wilcox, "Federalism in a time of plague: How federal systems cope with pandemic," *American Review of Public Administration* 50, no. 6–7 (2020): 519–25, https://doi.org/10.1177/0275074020941695.

5 André Lecours et al., "Explaining Intergovernmental Conflict in the COVID-19 Crisis: The United States, Canada, and Australia," *The Journal of Federalism* (2021): 513–36, https://doi.org/10.1093/publius/pjab010.

6 See for instance a review for the United States in Berry, Stokes, and Berry, "Innovations and Diffusion Models in Policy Research," in *Theories of the Policy Process*, edited by Christopher Weible and Paul Sabatier, 253–97 (Boulder, CO: Westview Press, 2018).

7 For recent examples see Brendan Boyd and Andrea Olive, *Provincial Policy Laboratories: Policy Diffusion and Transfer in Canada's Federal System* (Toronto: University of Toronto Press, 2021).

realm of healthcare delivery and public health, with the exceptional powers to curtail everyday life during a declared state of emergency and tailor their response to varied contexts and rates of viral transmission. We show how these policies varied with a unique dataset that tracks 12 different public health measures enacted by Provinces in the period between the onset of the pandemic in March 2020 and until the end of August 2021.[8] Focusing on two of these measures, we then show how even in a highly decentralized federation, innovation and policy diffusion was fairly limited.

Where one sees a disjointed response, another may see an appropriately tailored one. Yet, there is no question that high decentralization also created issues that were particularly acute for specific aspects of the pandemic response. The absence of centralized decision-making in Canada meant that high levels of coordination were required to handle policies that had cross-jurisdictional components. One such example is inter-provincial travel restrictions and control of internal borders. We highlight the difficulties of coordination in the realm of inter-provincial travel by describing one specific case: the Atlantic Travel Bubble. Covering four deeply interdependent Provinces on the east coast, the Bubble, as it went on to be known, was an example of highly coordinated, interjurisdictional travel restrictions and control of internal borders. The creation of this travel zone permitted an enviable level of normalcy during some of the highest periods of viral transmission and pandemic restrictions in Canada, and we explore its creation, impacts, and ultimate dissolution here.

Some Elements of Context about the Canadian Federation

Institutional

Canada is a bilingual, multinational federation defined by its colonial and Indigenous past. Unlike other federations such as Australia and the United States that have grown increasingly centralized over time, Canada has experienced a cumulative decentralization in the legislative, administrative, and fiscal policy spheres. There is considerable variation across policy fields, with educa-

---

8 Charles Breton and Paisley Sim, "*COVID-19 Canadian Provinces Measures Dataset,*" *Centre of Excellence on the Canadian Federation Institute for Research on Public Policy* (2021), https://centre.irpp.org/data/covid-19-provincial-policies/.

tion, law enforcement, and environmental protections being the most decentralized.[9] The result has been growing policy asymmetry and a dense arrangement of bureaucratic and often informal political networks across Provinces.

The post-World War II period was marked by an era of cooperative federalism highly influenced by federal priorities. Subsequent periods were defined by more competitive federalism, such as conflict over energy resource extraction royalties or Quebec's place as a majority French-speaking nation within the majority English-speaking federation.[10] Today, intergovernmental relations (IGR) operate under what can best be described as executive federalism, with negotiation processes dominated by First Ministers (provincial and territorial Premiers and the federal Prime Minister).

Canadian mechanisms for IGR are poorly institutionalized. At the highest level, First Ministers meetings are usually held annually at the behest of the Prime Minister who also controls the agenda. The main forum for horizontal IGR is the Council of the Federation, but it is mostly a vehicle for First Ministers to try to set the agenda for federal-provincial relations rather than a policy-focused coordinating body.[11] Many important decisions, such as adjustments to federal transfer payments, are made unilaterally by the federal government with little public or sub-national consultation. The sustained and substantial workhorses of IGR are found at the sectoral level, with dedicated tables led by ministers, supported by deputy ministers, to achieve degrees of coordination in areas such as immigration, the labor market, healthcare, and the environment.

Sectoral conferences are numerous. For instance, the government of Quebec states that they participate in approximately 80 forums annually.[12] One such working table is the Forum of Ministers Responsible for Immigration (FMRI) which has decision-making tables at the Ministerial, Deputy Minister, and Assistant Deputy Minister level. The FMRI in 2020 approved a three-year strategic plan that planned levels of immigration based on labor market needs and re-affirmed

9 Paolo Dardanelli et al., "Dynamic De/Centralization in Federations: Comparative Conclusions," *Publius: The Journal of Federalism* 49, no. 1 (Winter 2019): 194–219, https://doi.org/10.1093/publius/pjy037.

10 David Cameron and Richard Simeon, "Intergovernmental Relations in Canada: The Emergence of Collaborative Federalism," *Publius: The Journal of Federalism* 32, no. 2 (Spring 2002): 49–71, http://www.jstor.org/stable/3330945.

11 Jennifer Wallner, "Ideas and intergovernmental relations in Canada," *PS: Political Science & Politics* 50, no. 3 (2017): 717–22, https://doi.org/10.1017/S1049096517000488.

12 Secrétarait du Québec aux relations canadiennes, "Canadian Intergovernmental Conferences," septembre 8, 2021, https://www.sqrc.gouv.qc.ca/relations-canadiennes/relations-intergouvernementales/conferences-intergouvernementales-en.asp.

the desire to work collaboratively.[13] Another long-established forum is The Council of Ministers of the Environment (CCME) which since 1964 has been the main intergovernmental body addressing issues of national concern. Recently, the CCME has advocated to implement a Canada-wide strategy to reduce plastic waste and has focused on achieving net-zero emissions by 2050.[14]

Faced with a common perception of an emergency, patterns of elite negotiation can trigger high levels of cooperation and unity of intent that quickly upend traditional processes.[15] One example is that since March 2020 the Prime Minister and all 13 First Ministers have held over 33 calls to discuss their shared response to the pandemic, a frequency unheard of outside of this crisis period.[16]

In Canada, the public health sector has largely avoided the establishment of dedicated IGR venues, in favor of *ad hoc* arrangements which have impacted the pandemic response.[17] Healthcare is primarily a provincial responsibility, as Provinces license physicians and manage public healthcare systems. The federal government is responsible for imposing quarantine periods on international travelers and delivers some elements of healthcare to First Nations people. In the area of public health, provincial Chief Medical Officers of Health are responsible for sanitation and disease prevention, and the federal Public Health Agency of Canada is responsible for overarching health guidance, and national and international aspects of emergency management.

The day-to-day work of delivering healthcare services is mostly devolved by Provinces to local public health authorities. This adds another layer of coordination to an already complex sphere. Local authorities act as on-the-ground policy implementers that relay context to provincial operators and further tailor service delivery.

Canadian Provinces used their autonomy to forge distinct policy paths throughout the pandemic, but a variety of coordination mechanisms were used to share knowledge mostly behind closed doors. This includes the Council of

---

13 Forum of Ministers Responsible for Immigration, "Newsroom," July 28, 2021, https://www.fmri.ca/newsroom.
14 Government of Canada, "2020 Meeting of the Canadian Council of Ministers of the Environment," July 11, 2021, https://www.canada.ca/en/services/environment/weather/climatechange/pan-canadian-framework/canadian-council-ministers-environment.html.
15 Andrea Riccardo Migone, "Trust, but customize: federalism's impact on the Canadian COVID-19 response," *Policy and Society* 39, no. 3 (2020): 382–402, https://doi.org/10.1080/14494035.2020.1783788.
16 Government of Canada, "Prime Minister Justin Trudeau holds 33rd call with premiers on COVID-19 response," July 15, 2021, https://pm.gc.ca/en/news/readouts/2021/07/15/prime-minister-justin-trudeau-holds-33rd-call-premiers-covid-19-response.
17 Paquet and Schertzer 2020.

the Federation which issued a collective declaration opposing the invocation of the federal *Emergency Management Act* and called for increases to the federal health transfer. The Federation of Canadian Municipalities Big City Mayors' Caucus worked directly with the federal government to appeal for an increase to the gas tax fund, a direct federal-municipal transfer that was doubled in August 2020. The Pan-Canadian Health Network Council of Chief Medical Officers of Health brought together provincial Chief Medical Officers and Public Health Officers to share knowledge and provide unified recommendations, when possible, on issues such as masking, personal protective equipment, and variant transmission.[18]

Political Context

Under a minority Liberal government, the pandemic presented Prime Minister Justin Trudeau's government with incentives to reduce intergovernmental conflict, chief among them the urgent need to act and be seen acting.[19] It also provided the opportunity to prolong the minority government and set the stage for the September 20 federal election. At the end of August 2021 then, the federal response generally demonstrated respect for sub-national autonomy.

An example of this is the federal government's decision not to invoke the *Emergency Management Act*. Under s. 5 of the Act, the pandemic met the definition of a public welfare emergency, given that every Province had registered cases of COVID-19. Pursuant to s. 8(1), declaring a public welfare emergency would have granted the federal Cabinet the authority to exercise extraordinary powers, many of which are constitutionally reserved to the Provinces and would have infringed on civil liberties such as the right to inter-provincial mobility. Invoking the Act would also have allowed the federal government to regulate or distribute essential goods and services, regulate or prohibit travel, render persons or services essential, and evacuate or remove persons from a region.[20]

Invoking the Act requires consultation with each Province and territory, and on April 9, 2020, provincial Premiers collectively told Prime Minister Trudeau

---

18 Pan-Canadian Public Health Network, "About the Network," May 20, 2020, http://www.phn-rsp.ca/network-eng.php.
19 Lecours et al. 2020.
20 Shaun Fluker, "COVID-19 and the *Emergencies Act* (Canada)," *ABlawg*, March 27, 2020, https://ablawg.ca/2020/03/27/covid-19-and-the-emergencies-act-canada/.

that declaring a public welfare emergency was unnecessary.[21] Not invoking exceptional federal authority balances the importance of respecting provincial autonomy, while acknowledging that mobility restrictions and widespread closures imposed by Provinces met most of the aims of the Act.

Consequently, since the beginning of the pandemic and through the summer of 2021, the federal government focused on responsibilities that fall within its purview including international travel restrictions, healthcare funding, economic stimulus, employment insurance, and vaccine procurement. Provinces led the healthcare and public health response, and introduced restrictions designed to meet local circumstances. These included restrictions on public gatherings, school and business closures, mask requirements, and intra–and inter-jurisdictional travel restrictions.

Variation

COVID-19 has been enormously challenging for all levels of government but experienced differently across diverse regions and segments of society. The first presumptive case reported on January 25, 2020 was a man in Toronto, Ontario who had recently travelled in Wuhan, China. Subsequent cases were associated with travel to China and Iran.[22] On March 18, 2020, Canada banned international flights into the country, and from that point on, local transmission was deemed the primary source of viral spread. By March 22, 2020, all Provinces had declared a state of emergency.

By August 2021, Canada had reported over 26,850 COVID-related deaths.[23] Compared to other G7 nations, Canada's pandemic experience was somewhat less intense, with lower reported excess mortality rates than five of seven nations.[24] While Canada ranks thirteenth highest for pandemic death rate amongst the 38 OECD nations, the death rate per 100,000 people is in the bottom third of OECD countries. During the first wave of the pandemic (March to August 2020) it

---

21 The Council of the Federation, "Letter from Canada's Premier's to Prime Minister Justin Trudeau," April 14, 2020, https://www.canadaspremiers.ca/wp-content/uploads/2020/04/Letter_to_PM_from_Canadas_Premiers_Apr_14_2020.pdf.
22 The Canadian Press, "Timeline of COVID-19 cases across Canada," *CBC News*, March 13, 2020, https://www.cbc.ca/news/health/canada-coronavirus-timeline-1.5482310.
23 Ritchie et al. 2021.
24 OECD, "Data on Canada," 2021, https://www.oecd.org/canada/.

is estimated that 80% of deaths were concentrated among elderly residents of institutional care settings, double the OECD peer-average of 40%.[25]

Like many other Western nations, most of Canada experienced three distinct pandemic waves but the start and end dates of these waves varied greatly. The first wave began in March 2020 and eased in June 2020, concentrated in Ontario and Quebec, the country's most populous Provinces. A second, much more severe wave was linked to the return to school in September 2020, and receded in some parts of the country, but not entirely, by February 2021. A third wave took shape in March 2021 and with population-wide vaccination efforts declined significantly by July 2021. By the end of August 2021, many Provinces were either experiencing or nearing a fourth wave.

The primary tool to fight the spread of the virus prior to vaccine development was public health restrictions. As a result of the ebb and flow of viral transmission and differing governmental priorities, provincial governments demonstrated significant heterogeneity in their approach to public health restrictions.

To compare government responses in a systematic way and show how they varied, we evaluated 12 different sub-national measures and combined them in an overall index. The results provide a snapshot of provincial policy stringency at a given point in time. The index captures measures within Provinces' control such as gathering restrictions, mask mandates, school closures, restaurants closures, inter-provincial travel limitations, intra-provincial travel limitations, curfews, and long-term care home visitation. Ultimately, we coded 12 of these public health measures for all 13 Provinces and territories.[26] Figure 1 shows how provincial responses varied in terms of measures adopted, timing, and overall stringency.

Figure 1 also highlights how Provinces adapted to different contexts. For example, Yukon and the Northwest Territories had very few cases for much of the second and third waves and were able to maintain relatively low levels of strin-

---

25 Developing research highlights that Canada's delayed death-reporting procedures and flawed cause of death attribution practices may have led to approximately 6,000 underreported COVID-related deaths, see: Tara Moriarty et al., "Excess All-Cause Mortality During the COVID-19 Epidemic in Canada," *Royal Society of Canada* (2021): 1–54, https://rsc-src.ca/sites/default/files/EM%20PB_EN.pdf; Canadian Institute for Health Information, "Pandemic Experience in the Long-Term Care Sector: How Does Canada Compare with Other Countries?," June 2020, https://www.cihi.ca/sites/default/files/document/covid-19-rapid-response-long-term-care-snap shot-en.pdf.

26 For more on the methodology behind the coding of each measure and the calculation of the index itself, see: Emily Cameron-Blake et al., "Variation in the Canadian Provincial and Territorial responses to COVID-19," *Blavatnik School of Government Working Paper* (2021): 1–43, www.bsg.ox.ac.uk/covidtracker.

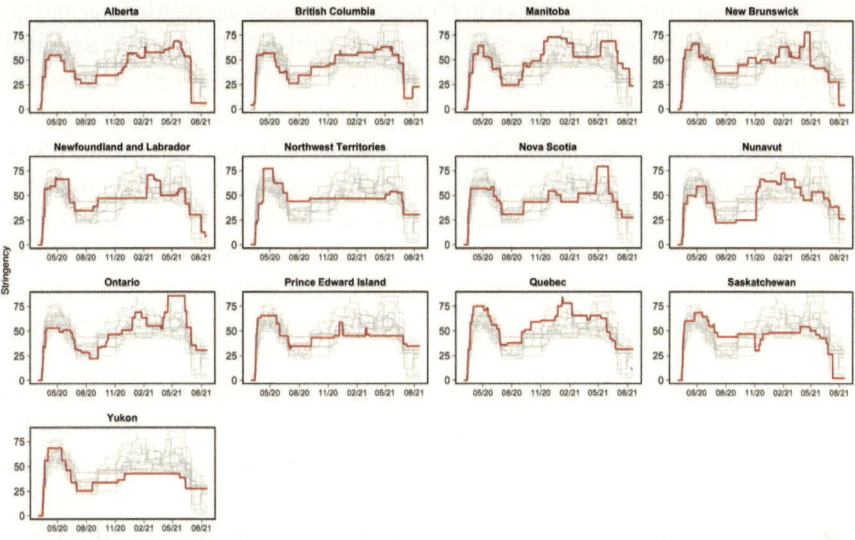

Figure 1: Variation in stringency of Canadian provinces and territories' COVID-19 measures (March 2020-August 2021).

gency of public health measures. Nunavut, the third northern territory, stands in stark contrast because cases flared up during the winter and consequently policy stringency grew.

We can identify three general approaches to public health measures designed to counter the pandemic. Most Provinces increased the stringency of measures when cases were going up and relaxed measures when cases were going down (e.g., Quebec, Ontario, Manitoba). Other Provinces introduced new measures when cases went up but kept many in place even as cases were very low (e.g. most of the Atlantic Provinces). Finally, two Provinces stand out for how they kept stringency at a minimum, even when cases were increasing: Alberta and Saskatchewan.

A look at Alberta illustrates this different approach. Restrictions in Alberta were more limited compared to the other Provinces during the first wave and many were lifted as early as May 15, 2020. Policy stringency only ramped back up over the December 2020 holiday when the Province faced rapidly increasing case numbers. Remaining restrictions began to be lifted on May 29, 2021, and all restrictions were gone, including mask mandates, as of July 1, 2021, Canada Day, when the government proclaimed that it was "open for good."[27]

---

27 Dylan Short, "'We will be open for good': all restrictions lifted on Canada Day, says Kenney,"

Alberta was the first Province in Canada to withdraw all restrictions and declare a return to normal. While the Provinces of British Columbia and Saskatchewan removed mask mandates at the same time, they continued to recommend their use in certain settings. The government of Alberta moved away from advising the public on masks entirely, and mask mandates became at the discretion of local authorities. At the end of August 2021, Alberta had the highest number of cases per capita in the country while also being the second least stringent Province. Importantly, the approach taken by Alberta is not due to a difference in institutional capacity or financial situation. Alberta has the same tools and powers as the other Provinces and is also the richest Province in the country. These were thus political choices.

The aggregate stringency index highlights how stringency varied from one Province to another at the same point in time. What it does not show however, is which measures were or were not adopted by a given Province. We found that there was variation in the timing of measures, but little variation in the nature of the measures. For example, of the 12 measures we captured, ten of them were adopted by all Provinces, at least for a time. We now turn to one measure that was highly variable in its application.

Intra-provincial Travel

Restricting intra-provincial travel – where one can go within one's own Province – is a policy area in which Provinces' approaches varied widely. Limiting freedom of movement is also, arguably, one of the most stringent measures a Province can put in place because it conflicts with the *Canadian Charter of Rights and Freedoms* right to inter-provincial mobility. Section 6(1) states that "every citizen of Canada has the right to enter, remain in and leave Canada."[28] Violations of section 6 may be deemed constitutional because they are justified by section 1 of the Charter, which guarantees the rights and freedoms set out in the Charter only to such reasonable limits prescribed by law as can be demonstrably justified in a free and democratic society.[29]

Calgary Herald, June 18, 2021, https://calgaryherald.com/news/local-news/we-will-be-open-for-good-nearly-all-restrictions-to-be-lifted-on-canada-day-says-kenney.

28 Government of Canada, "The Canadian Charter of Rights and Freedoms," 2018, https://www.justice.gc.ca/eng/csj-sjc/rfc-dlc/ccrf-ccdl/rfcp-cdlp.html.

29 Yves Faguy, "What is a reasonable limit on our right to travel?," *The Canadian Bar Association*, January 26, 2021, https://www.nationalmagazine.ca/en-ca/articles/law/in-depth/2020/what-is-a-reasonable-limit-on-our-right-to-travel.

Perhaps as a result, Provinces were reluctant to restrict travel within their territories even if it was a means to limit viral transmission. This also explains why the use of vague and indefinite language such as recommend, advise, discourage, and urge caution was so widely used in this realm. Examples include the Prince Edward Island Chief Medical Officer of Health stating that she "recommends [that] all Islanders who are self-isolating must now remain on their own property when outside," and in Saskatchewan where "public health officials are discouraging recreational travel to and from Saskatchewan," without accompanying enforcement.[30] As a result, most Provinces strongly recommended residents stay home and limit travel, but very few backed up mobility restrictions with meaningful enforcement. Only a few Provinces, generally those who took a more restrictive, stringent approach to public health measures, ultimately enforced travel restrictions with road closures and checkpoints.

For example, on March 24, 2020, Quebec shut down and residents were ordered to stay at home. Checkpoints were erected within eight regions of Quebec to limit the number of people entering and leaving these zones.[31] These restrictions were gradually lifted beginning on May 4, 2020. Checkpoints remained in place for the northern areas of Nunavik and the Cree Territory of James Bay, with government stating that the police may be present to validate the appropriateness of a person's travel.[32] Outside these areas, residents were generally discouraged from travelling between regions that were at different levels of pandemic restrictions such as "yellow" and "red zones," but enforcement was much less systematized.

Manitoba also restricted movement within its territory. Beginning on September 4, 2020, intra-provincial travel north of the fifty-third parallel for nonessential reasons was banned for anyone who did not live north of that point.[33] Citing rising case numbers, the ban was introduced to accommodate re-

---

30 Prince Edward Island, "Prince Edward Island tightens restrictions on self-isolating," March 25, 2020, https://www.princeedwardisland.ca/en/news/prince-edward-island-tightens-re strictions-on-self-isolating; Saskatchewan, "COVID-19 Update: Ten New Cases, Two in Hospital, Three More Recoveries," September 3, 2020, https://www.saskatchewan.ca/government/news-and-media/2020/september/03/covid-19-update-september-3.

31 Patrice Bergeron, "Des barrages policiers bloquent l'accès à l'Est et le Nord du Québec," *La Presse Canadienne*, mars 28, 2020, https://www.lesoleil.com/actualite/covid-19/des-barrages-po liciers-bloquent-lacces-a-lest-et-le-nord-du-quebec-0be6b6727f5a3f0168125a331cd8464c.

32 Gouvernement du Québec, "Déplacements entre les regions et les villes dans le contexte de la COVID-19," juin 25, 2021, https://www.quebec.ca/sante/problemes-de-sante/a-z/coronavirus-2019/deplacements-regions-villes-covid19.

33 Government of Manitoba, "Essential items for retail sale – detailed list," November 21, 2020, https://manitoba.ca/asset_library/en/covid/covid-essential-retail-items.pdf.

mote healthcare realities where around 90,000 people are spread out over 438.5 km², an area larger than the state of California.

On the west coast, the residents of British Columbia were not subject to targeted orders limiting travel until November 19, 2020, but this remained a recommendation, backed up with limited enforcement. During the summer of 2020, travel into the Haida Gwaii archipelago was restricted to non-residents, due to limited healthcare capacity in the remote region.[34] This order was relaxed in September 2020 for travelers who could provide a negative coronavirus test. On April 23, 2021, British Columbia restricted non-essential travel between three regional zones, and road checkpoints enforced by the Royal Canadian Mounted Police (RCMP) were put in place on May 6.[35] Most restrictions in the Province were lifted as of July 1, 2021, but at the end of August 2021 travel between regions was still discouraged.

Innovation and Coordination

As shown in previous sections, Canadian Provinces varied greatly in their application of public health measures. In addition to enabling a more tailored pandemic response, the decentralized nature of the Canadian federation should have created the opportunity for inter-jurisdictional innovation and policy diffusion through learning. Though we find that Provinces responded to their own context and that the timing of public health restrictions varied accordingly, restrictions were often highly similar. Because there were very few innovations, opportunities for policy-learning across Provinces was also limited. The following discussion highlights one clear example of inter-jurisdictional policy diffusion: Manitoba's "essential goods" list, and one example of a policy innovation that was effective, but not adopted elsewhere: Quebec's nightly curfew.

Manitoba's "Essential Goods" list

The central Province of Manitoba stands out for limiting residents' in-store retail purchases in COVID hotspots to a list of essential goods beginning on November 20, 2020. At the time, Manitoba had the second highest caseload per

---

34 British Columbia, "Province restricts travel to Haida Gwaii to protect communities," July 30, 2020, https://news.gov.bc.ca/releases/2020PSSG0041-001429.

35 Royal Canadian Mounted Police, "BC RCMP to increase travel checks," May 19, 2021, https://bc-cb.rcmp-grc.gc.ca/ViewPage.action?siteNodeId=2087&languageId=1&contentId=69561.

100,000 people in Canada and the highest level of policy stringency. The Province's Chief Medical Officer of Health was frustrated with growing caseloads and introduced an "Essential Item for Retail" list to limit in-store shopping and encourage curbside pick-up or delivery. The list included food, clothing, and household goods. When introduced, it was not uncommon to see magazine or paperback novels sold in pharmacies or grocery stores shielded behind yellow caution tape, the justification being that selling these items in stores deemed essential when speciality magazine or bookstores were closed would unfairly privilege one retailer over another, a move that was met with public criticism. The essentials list was gradually expanded to include seasonal items, gift cards, and greater personal care products that had been initially overlooked.[36] Second-hand stores were initially deemed non-essential but permitted to open following pressure from low-income advocacy groups.[37]

On February 1, 2021, the essential items list was suspended for northern Manitoba because people living under a higher level of policy stringency in communities north of the fifty-third parallel were travelling south where restrictions were relaxed, and they had greater variety in retail.[38] Travel from north to south was unintentionally increasing the likelihood of viral transmission in remote communities with precarious and limited healthcare resources.[39]

In late December 2020, the Province of Quebec followed Manitoba's lead and introduced an essentials list, with the accompanying caution tape and store section closures, when the Province went into lockdown. But Quebec learned from Manitoba's experience, and the essentials list was adapted in such a way that it did not lead to the similar unintended consequence of travel between regions, or the need to add items to the list because they had initially been overlooked. The essential goods list is a clear example of inter-jurisdictional policy diffusion, though Quebec officials did not officially credit Manitoba for this policy innovation.

---

36 CBC News, "Cosmetics now an essential item in Manitoba public health orders," *CBC News*, December 23, 2020, https://www.cbc.ca/news/canada/manitoba/cosmetics-essential-manitoba-public-health-orders-1.5851572.

37 Peggy Lam, "Winnipeg's thrift shops experience surge of customers in first days of reopening," *CBC News*, December 15, 2020, https://www.cbc.ca/news/canada/manitoba/winnipeg-s-thrift-stores-reopening-covid-december-1.5841425.

38 Rachel Bergen, "Manitoba's 3rd lockdown another 'brutal' hit for small businesses," *CBC News*, May 9, 2021, https://www.cbc.ca/news/canada/manitoba/covid-19-manitoba-lockdown-1.6019734.

39 Kayla Rosen, "Province lifts non-essential item restrictions for northern Manitoba," *CTV News*, February 2, 2021, https://winnipeg.ctvnews.ca/province-lifts-non-essential-item-restrictions-for-northern-manitoba-1.5291928.

Quebec's Nightly Curfew

Perhaps one of the most striking pandemic policy innovations is Quebec's curfew. Beginning on January 9, 2021, over eight million residents were not permitted to leave their homes between 8:00 p.m. and 5:00 a.m., and this restriction was met with significantly increased enforcement by police on the ground. It is estimated that Quebec issued $28 million in fines from April 1, 2020 to May 31, 2021, related to quarantine and curfew violations.[40] Nightly curfew hours were pushed to between 9:30 p.m. and 5:00 a.m. in some regions as of February 26, 2021, and in total some form of nightly curfew remained in effect in the Province until it was suspended on May 28, 2021.

While under curfew, Quebec had the highest, or second highest, level of policy stringency anywhere in Canada throughout the pandemic. Despite having comparable or even higher caseloads, no other Province followed in Quebec's footsteps by introducing a curfew. The closest was when on April 16, 2021, in the thick of the third wave, Ontario Premier Doug Ford introduced a severe state of lockdown that closed public parks, empowered police to conduct street checks if people were outside of their homes, and severely restricted outdoor recreation. Measures to restrict outdoor activities were immediately criticized by the public and public health advocates because they contradicted guidance that suggested outdoor transmission was significantly lower than indoor transmission.[41] Similarly, the scope of new police powers was highly criticized, and the result was that within two days the more severe features of this proposed lockdown had been rescinded. What's more, in April 2021, citing rising viral transmission, the Province of Alberta threatened to introduce a nightly curfew should case numbers reach a designated threshold in certain areas, but it ultimately did not progress beyond a threat.[42]

The effect of Quebec's curfew can't be easily disentangled from the other measures in place at the time, but it did greatly reduce mobility and publicly sig-

---

40 Isaac Olson, "More than $28M in fines issued in Quebec during lockdown," *CBC News*, June 7, 2021, https://www.cbc.ca/news/canada/montreal/quebec-fines-court-public-health-mea sures-1.6054546.
41 David Lao, "Ontario's new COVID-19 restrictions have science 'absolutely upside-down,' experts say," *Global News*, April 16, 2021, https://globalnews.ca/news/7765156/ontario-covid-19-re strictions-ford-david-fisman/.
42 Bill Kaufmann, "Alberta sets daily, active COVID case records as government tightens restrictions, threatens curfews," *Calgary Herald*, April 29, 2021, https://calgaryherald.com/news/local-news/alberta-sets-daily-active-covid-case-records-as-government-tightens-restrictions-threatens-curfews.

nal that the trajectory of the pandemic was going in the wrong direction. Following nearly five-months under a nightly curfew, Quebec's viral transmission rate had significantly declined compared to neighboring Ontario, and the third wave was declared over before many other regions in the country. Acknowledging that there are multiple factors at play, we believe that the nightly curfew positively contributed to Quebec's very low transmission rates relative to population and the end of the third wave. What is surprising is that despite other Provinces threatening to introduce a curfew or policing powers that would mirror its effects, Quebec is the only Province to have introduced such a policy.

While it is difficult to offer general explanations as to why other Provinces did not follow suit, there are various factors that can explain Quebec's decision to introduce the curfew. First, on the policy itself, Quebec's politicians tend to follow more closely what is happening in Europe and in France especially. Some French cities, for instance, had been under a curfew in the fall of 2020 which might have been the motivation for Quebec to use this policy tool. But once the policy was proposed, how can we explain the public's support for it? First, Quebec was the hardest hit Province during the first wave and although most of the deaths occurred in long-term care homes, the population might have been more willing to accept more drastic measures having gone through such a crisis in spring 2020. Second, as of the end of August 2021, Quebec's Premier François Legault had benefitted from some of the strongest approval ratings among all provincial Premiers,[43] allowing him to introduce more stringent measures as well.[44]

---

43 The polling firm Angus Reid has been tracking provincial Premiers' approval ratings throughout the pandemic. In March 2021, coming out of the curfew period, Legault had an approval of 62% of Quebecers, second to British Columbia Premier John Horgan at 66%. In comparison, Doug Ford in Ontario was at 50% and Jason Kenney in Alberta at 39%. When asked in June of 2021 whether their Premier had done a good job handling the pandemic, 74% of Quebecers agreed compared to 34% in Ontario and 33% in Alberta.

44 We do not stipulate here on the direction of the causal relationship between approval ratings and stringent measures but just suggest that they are linked. Arguably, the introduction of stringent measures might have contributed to Legault's approval ratings which in turn might have made it possible for him to introduce even more stringent measures.

Inter-provincial Travel Restrictions: When Coordination across Jurisdictions becomes Essential

As we documented, few Provinces restricted freedom of movement within their territory. The same is true for travel between Provinces. Here, the Province of Ontario stands out. Ontario did not issue intra-provincial travel restrictions despite enforcing prolonged stay-at-home orders but did restrict inter-provincial travel during the challenging third wave. Beginning on April 19, 2021, the borders with the neighboring Provinces of Manitoba and Quebec were closed to non-essential travelers and did not reopen until June 16, 2021.[45] Quebec also closed its borders with Ontario in the spring of 2020.[46]

Inter-provincial travel is one area where the Federal government could have played a central, coordinating role, but here again opted to let Provinces manage it. As a result, in the example described above, Quebec and Ontario appear to have only loose coordination with their neighbors.

But some Provinces did manage to extensively coordinate inter-provincial travel. The Atlantic Provinces – New Brunswick, Newfoundland and Labrador, Nova Scotia, and Prince Edward Island (PEI) – experienced relative normalcy over the course of the pandemic compared to the rest of Canada. With a combined population of just over 1.8 million people, the Atlantic Provinces' response was considerably more coordinated than elsewhere in Canada, with a greater emphasis on epidemiological contact tracing.

The Council of Atlantic Premiers, composed of leaders from the four Provinces, stands out from other decision-maker groups for working closely across jurisdictions to coordinate pandemic restrictions, and create the Atlantic Travel Bubble. The Bubble illustrates what coordination across jurisdiction can achieve, but also illustrates how difficult this level of cooperation can be to sustain. It shows how Provinces were able to coordinate horizontally, with the federal government playing absolutely no role in the process.

---

45 Lucas Powers, "Ontario to reopen borders with Quebec, Manitoba as 2nd dose bookings open in delta hot spot," *CBC News*, June 14, 2021, https://www.cbc.ca/news/canada/toronto/covid-19-ontario-june-14-2021-delta-sports-framework-1.6064793.
46 Daniel Leblanc, "Quebec re-opens border to Ontario cottagers and other non-essential travellers," *The Globe and Mail*, May 15, 2020, https://www.theglobeandmail.com/politics/article-quebec-re-opens-border-to-ontario-cottagers-and-other-non-essential/.

Initial stay-at-home orders and local mobility restrictions were uncoordinated in the Atlantic region. Beginning with the declaration of state of emergencies in Spring 2020, Nova Scotia, New Brunswick, and Newfoundland all issued a stay-at-home requirement for residents, while PEI only ever issued a strong recommendation. Lockdowns began to ease on May 1, 2020, and by June 5 staying at home was no longer mentioned in most public health updates. Citing low case numbers across the region, on June 24, 2020 the Council of Atlantic Premiers announced the creation of an inter-provincial travel zone that did not require residents to self-isolate.[47] The Council noted that the decision to ease travel restrictions was done in consultation with Chief Medical Officers of Health in each Province and would be monitored closely.[48]

Beginning on July 3, 2020, the Atlantic Travel Bubble allowed the residents of the region to travel freely without the requirement to self-isolate if they had already been in one of the four Provinces in the previous 14 days. In the rest of Canada at the time, inter-provincial travel required two-weeks of self-isolation and in many cases was enforced through check-ins by law enforcement.

Travelers from outside of the Atlantic Provinces were not permitted to enter the Bubble without explicit permission, and upon entry were required to self-isolate for 14 days, at their own expense. Within the Bubble, residents of the Atlantic Provinces experienced fewer pandemic restrictions compared to the rest of the country. Restaurant and bar capacity was higher, larger outdoor gatherings were permitted, more retail and services were open and at greater capacities, and more cultural venues were open.

The Bubble was in place from July 3 to November 24, 2020, when PEI left in response to increased cases in New Brunswick and Nova Scotia. Newfoundland and Labrador left the Bubble on November 25 and New Brunswick on November 27, 2020. Nova Scotia never officially left the travel Bubble and did not reinstate 14-day quarantine requirements for travelers until April 19 2021.[49]

The Council of Atlantic Premiers twice delayed reopening inter-provincial travel due to variant-driven outbreaks. But towards the tail end of a third wave, Atlantic residents were permitted to travel within the region without self-isolating, be-

---

47 The Council of Atlantic Premiers, "Atlantic Provinces Form Travel Bubble," June 24, 2020, https://cap-cpma.ca/wp-content/uploads/2021/04/CAP-Release-AP-Form-Travel-Bubble-June-24-2020.pdf.

48 The Council of Atlantic Premiers, "Atlantic Provinces Form Travel Bubble," June 24, 2020, https://immediac.blob.core.windows.net/cap-cmha/images/Newsroom/Draft%20news%20release%20(v7).pdf.

49 CBC News, "N.S. limits travel in and out of province to essential trips only," April 20, 2021, https://www.cbc.ca/news/canada/nova-scotia/covid-19-update-april-20-2021-1.5994280.

ginning on June 23 in Newfoundland and Labrador, June 26 in PEI, and June 30, 2021 for Nova Scotia and New Brunswick.[50]

The Atlantic Travel Bubble is Canada's only example of coordinated travel restrictions that increased mobility while maintaining very low relative case-loads. Similar models were not adopted elsewhere, and inter-jurisdictional travel varied greatly from Province to Province. The economies of the Atlantic Provinces are deeply interlinked and dependent on seasonal resource development, tourism, and free movement between Provinces. While Canada's decentralized system engages in multiple policy fields and often looks like "institutionalized ambivalence" where cooperation and order can be difficult to discern, the Atlantic Travel Bubble is the country's leading example of a highly coordinated and institutionalized pandemic response. By opting to act together, the pandemic mitigated historical and political conditions that had previously hindered the Council of Atlantic Premiers and resulted in the creation of a highly successful policy innovation that met public health and political objectives.

Population demographics are also key to understanding the creation of the Bubble. Outbreak dynamic research has shown that especially for smaller Provinces, tight border control is often easier and more effective than quarantine, and that partial reopening, for example within local travel bubbles, can be an effective compromise and reasonable first steps towards lifting all mobility restrictions.[51] Unlike inter-jurisdictional travel restrictions introduced by Ontario and Quebec, the Atlantic Travel Bubble was frequently discussed publicly by Premiers with stakeholders from the public health, business, and tourism sectors implicated in discussions and decisions that impacted the region. The success of the Bubble, though not particularly long-lasting, stands out amongst pandemic policy innovations for not only ensuring a high level of freedom of movement, but very low viral transmission and case growth.

Conclusion

The COVID-19 pandemic has been enormously challenging for all levels of government. And the pandemic response is made even more challenging when different levels of government have different priorities, tools, and resources. In this

---

50 Allan April, "Most of Atlantic Canada to reopen to regional travel on June 23," *CTV News Atlantic*, June 15, 2021, https://atlantic.ctvnews.ca/most-of-atlantic-canada-to-reopen-to-regional-travel-on-june-23-1.5471172.
51 Kevin Linka et al., "Is it safe to life COVID-19 travel bans? The Newfoundland story," *National Institutes of Health – Preprint* (2020), 10.1101/2020.07.16.20155614.

chapter, we investigated how federalism has influenced the pandemic response in Canada and among Canadian Provinces specifically.

Early in the pandemic, the federal government stayed within its own jurisdiction, a decision that demonstrated respect for Provinces' autonomy. In a highly decentralized federation like Canada, where Provinces control many of the policy levers needed to respond to a pandemic, but where the federal government has more financial capacity, this has meant that Provinces enacted much of the public health restrictions and on-the-ground management. The federal government managed much of the income support for individuals but also transferred more than $29 billion to Provinces. Up until September 2021, direct federal spending had amounted to $336 billion. With Provinces committing an additional $57 billion in spending, the federal government covered approximately 86% of all pandemic expenditures.[52]

The separation of powers and the fact that the ground level operations were managed by the Provinces led to significant variation in policy response timing. It also highlighted the importance of policy coordination. At the highest level, the provincial Premiers and the Prime Minister met weekly for most of the pandemic, an intensity in IGR never seen before. However, this form of executive federalism did not necessarily lead to a more coordinated response.

In this chapter, we demonstrated that from March 2020 to the end of August 2021, policy restrictions across 13 Canadian Provinces and territories varied greatly in their timing but also, to a limited extent, in their nature.

The pandemic is a complex intergovernmental problem because it challenged existing norms and venues of IGR.[53] Yet, its urgency upended typically slow-moving processes. While the factors that influence cross-jurisdictional policy coordination may vary, a fast-evolving pandemic situation and nearly constant flows of new information and public health advice makes dedicating the resources and necessary time to study, coordinate, and implement cross-jurisdictional policy responses challenging. There is also the question of whether the political will exists to engage in cross jurisdictional coordination, or, if as many Provinces ultimately chose, it was better to go it alone.

While best practices and public health information were shared amongst Provinces throughout the pandemic, we found that innovations test-driven in one Province were rarely adopted in another. We described one such example: the adoption of a non-essential items list. The list, originally introduced by Man-

52 David Macdonald, "Still picking up the tab: Federal and provincial government COVID-19 spending," *Canadian Centre for Policy Alternatives* (2021): 1–50, https://www.policyalternatives.ca/publications/reports/still-picking-tab.
53 Paquet and Schertzer 2020.

itoba to curtail the public's in-person shopping, was later adopted by Quebec. By learning from the pitfalls Manitoba struggled through, Quebec's non-essentials list was introduced more seamlessly.

On the other hand, Quebec's successful nightly curfew that required residents to stay at home between 8:00 p.m. and 5:00 a.m. over a period of five months was not adopted by other Provinces. The curfew greatly reduced internal movement and likely contributed to low-case levels in Quebec by the end of the third wave. Despite this success, no other Province introduced a curfew, but some did publicly toy with introducing a curfew to increase restriction compliance. Overall, Quebec's handling of the pandemic offers an interesting avenue for future research. Factors such as a first wave that marked Quebecers by its deadliness, high approval ratings for the Premier, and a greater attention to measures enacted in Europe seem to have contributed to the imposition and acceptance of more stringent measures in the Province (i.e. curfew, internal travel restrictions). The direction of the causal relationship between stringency and approval ratings in itself represents an interesting future research question.

It might be too early to adjudicate between the mechanisms that could explain policy diffusion, or lack thereof, during the pandemic – whether it was learning, competition, copying or simply convergence. What is clear however is that the diffusion of policies that did occur across Provinces was not due to coercion from the federal government, which decided very early on to stay out of provincial jurisdictions and public health measures.

Our clearest example of innovative policy coordination is the creation of the Atlantic Travel Bubble. Reducing internal mobility has been shown to be a highly effective measure to manage pandemic outbreak dynamics, but it does not come without strong social and economic constraints. For the duration of the Bubble, Atlantic Canadians had high levels of mobility, low case growth, and a sense of relative normalcy compared to the rest of the country. In lieu of similar regional bubbles, well-established systems to test, trace, and isolate suspected COVID-19 cases should remain in use to reduce quarantine time and encourage inter-provincial travel and trade.

Despite heightened federal-provincial diplomacy, we find that the benefits of federalism have been unevenly leveraged in managing the outcomes of the pandemic. Apart from the four Atlantic Provinces, in the end, most Provinces opted to go it alone. At the same time, the federal government chose not to play a coordinating role, opting instead to focus solely on its field of jurisdiction while providing Provinces with financial assistance.

As Canadian Prime Minister William Lyon Mackenzie King once said, "it is what we prevent, rather than what we do that counts most in government." As Canadian Provinces chart a post-pandemic future, the effect of decentralization will continue to be felt in the deconfinement phase with some Provinces reducing restrictions long before others. And on this front, the clear division of responsibility of the Canadian response to the pandemic might at least make it easier for citizens to hold governments accountable. One thing remains clear, however; many governments' failure to prevent the worst outcomes of the COVID-19 pandemic will continue to echo in our public policy sphere for years to come.

Birte Wassenberg

3 Cooperative Federalism or *Flickenteppich* (Patchwork)?

Crisis Management during the COVID-19 Pandemic in the Federal Republic of Germany, a Comparative Approach with Regard to France

Introduction

"Nous sommes en guerre!" (We are at war!)[1] – this was President Emmanuel Macron's key expression during his speech to the French people on March 15 2020 when the first wave of the COVID-19 pandemic hit the European continent. Three days later, on March 18, German Chancellor Angela Merkel addressed the German people. She started by saying she was sorry that German grandparents could no longer see their grandchildren, as it was too dangerous; and she then kindly asked the German people to be reasonable and to stay home: *"Bitte bleiben Sie zu Hause!"*[2] The two speeches by the heads of State and Government of France and Germany could not have been more different, and they indeed reflect two different political cultures: German cooperative federalism versus French centralism. It is therefore not surprising either to observe, from the very start of the pandemic, two diametrically opposed sets of measures applied to combat the virus: while Emmanuel Macron announced a generalized and immediate "confinement" (lockdown) for the whole territory of France, in Germany, each *Land* applied its own

---

1 "Nous sommes en guerre: le verbatim du discours d'Emmanuel Macron," *Le Monde*, March 16, 2020, https://www.lemonde.fr/politique/article/2020/03/16/nous-sommes-en-guerre-retrouvez-le-discours-de-macron-pour-lutter-contre-le-coronavirus_6033314_823448.html, accessed July 1, 2021.
2 "Address to the nation by Angela Merkel," March 18, 2020, https://www.bundesregierung.de/breg-de/themen/coronavirus/-this-is-a-historic-task-and-it-can-only-be-mastered-if-we-face-it-together-1732476, accessed July 1, 2021.

Birte Wassenberg, Professor in Contemporary History at the Institute for Political Studies (Sciences Po) of the University of Strasbourg and member of the Research Unit Dynamiques européennes (UMR).

https://doi.org/10.1515/9783110745085-004

rules ranging from no restriction at all to a complete lockdown.[3] But, In the end, at each stage of the pandemic, which political system proved to be better equipped for its management and what were the consequences of these two diametrically opposed approaches for the German and French border regions, which find themselves at the junction between the two state systems?

This chapter examines whether the federal state structure of Germany, with its tools of decentered management, was indeed an advantage in the fight against the pandemic or, on the contrary, was rather an obstacle by causing incoherence and uncertainty. It retraces the multiple set of different solutions applied at the same time in Germany, which stand in deep contrast with the more homogenous and centralized measures taken by the French public authorities. By analyzing the measures taken by the German authorities during the first wave of COVID-19 in the spring of 2020 until the third wave in the spring of 2021 and by evaluating their impact on French-German border regions, this chapter also illustrates how German federalism first translated into a non-coordinated patchwork of *Länder*'s decisions used for political purposes by a certain number of Minister-presidents. It then shows how this progressively converged towards a system of multi-level governance between the *Bund* and the *Länder* orchestrated by Chancellor Angela Merkel, which quickly revealed important shortcomings and limits, thus questioning German cooperative federalism as a model during the pandemic.

A Diametrically Opposed Management of the COVID-19 Crisis in the Federal Republic of Germany and France: From a Non-coordinated Patchwork to a System of Multi-level Governance at the French-German border (March–May 2020)

The pandemic came as a shock to all member states of the European Union (EU) and, due to a lack of competences at the community level in terms of health issues, the immediate reactions were mostly national ones and they were neither

---

3 Birte Wassenberg, "'The return of mental borders': A Diary of the COVID19 crisis experienced at the Franco-German border between Kehl and Strasbourg (March-June 2020)," *Borders in Globalization Review* 1, no. 3 (2020): 114–20.

coordinated nor harmonized between the different member states.[4] Indeed, the pandemic did not hit them at the same time nor to the same extent, so that measures were not being taken in parallel, but successively, depending on the impact of the pandemic. If we consider France and Germany, there was a clear imbalance between measures from the start, as the pandemic spread from the region of Alsace, where a religious congregation had caused a hotspot in Mulhouse in early March 2020. This resulted in a very high degree of contamination in this French region, which then quickly affected the whole of France (with a total number of 120,753 COVID-19 cases and 24,352 deaths in April 2020).[5] If Germany also counted many COVID-19 infections by April 2020 (163,009 in total), it still stayed rather unaffected during the first wave of the pandemic because of the extremely low death rate (only 6,623 deaths were counted in Germany in April 2020, i.e. 2.3 per million inhabitants per day as compared to 10.2 in France.[6] This was probably one of the reasons why Emmanuel Macron announced the immediate and total lockdown of the French population on March 16, 2020, whereas in Germany, the measures taken at that time were much softer, largely avoiding an overall lockdown.[7] However, in Germany, the different approaches to the pandemic were also a result of the character of the German Federal State, which, as a system of cooperative federalism, much depended on a decentralized, negotiated, and bottom-up method for the definition and implementation of measures to combat COVID-19. "Cooperative federalism" in Germany is indeed often highlighted as a model of democratic functioning, a "coming together federalism," with a decentralized decision-making process negotiated between the *Bund* and the *Länder,* creating an overall beneficial and consensual system of mutual political interconnection, the so-called *"Politikverflechtung"* identified by political scientist Fritz W. Scharpf.[8]

---

4 Frédérique Berrod and Pierrick Bruyas, "Union Européenne: La Frontière Comme Antidote à l'épidémie?," *The Conversation,* March 29, 2020, https://theconversation.com/union-europeen ne-la-frontiere-comme-antidote-a-lepidemie-134844, accessed July 1, 2021.
5 Cf. https://www.data.gouv.fr/fr/reuses/statistiques-sur-la-pandemie-de-coronavirus-covid-19-rapportees-au-nombre-dhabitants-par-pays/, accessed October 20, 2021.
6 Ibid., cf. also Frédérique Berrod, Morgane Chovet, and Birte Wassenberg, "La frontière franco-allemande au temps du COVID-19: la fin d'un espace commun," *Bordering in Pandemic Times, Insights into the COVID-19 Lockdown,* Special Issue, UniGR-CBS, June 30, 2020, 39 – 43.
7 "Robert Koch-Institut, COVID-19-Dashboard Germany," August 3, 2020, https://experience. arcgis.com/experience/478220a4c454480e823b17327b2bf1d4, accessed July 14, 2021.
8 Fritz W. Scharpf, Bernd Reissert, and Fritz Schnabel, *Politikverflechtung. Theorie und Empirie des kooperativen Föderalismus in der Bundesrepublik Deutschland* (Kronberg: Scriptor Verlag, 1976).

Indeed, in comparison to the centralized state of France, where health crisis management is under the control of the central executive power in Paris (the French president and his government), in Germany, the competences for health policy measures are delegated to the 16 *Länder* which defined and implemented the so-called Corona-rules (Corona-*Verordnungen*) during the pandemic. It is therefore the Fundamental Law (*Grundgesetz*) more than the political federal culture in Germany which sets the framework for a privileged *Länder* action in the matter.[9] The central government in Berlin mainly has a coordinating function outlined in the federal framework law for health protection (*Bundesinfektionsgesetz*).[10] The only other "central" authority for the pandemic is the Robert Koch Research Institute in Berlin, which acted as a scientific advisor for the government by announcing the rates of COVID-19 infections (seven-day incidence) and the number of deaths daily. The Institute is a national public health authority with a long history (it was created in 1891),[11] but during the pandemic, based on its statistical evidence, it mainly classed regions and states as "high risk" areas and therefore determined when and for whom restrictive measures should apply.[12] This is important, as many Corona-rules also relied on this classification for a differentiated approach to opening or closing measures (schooling, travels, etc.) employed by the Minister-presidents of the 16 German *Länder*.

However, the system of cooperative federalism is still a challenge to the fight against COVID-19, as there is no central power allocation in Germany, as opposed to France, which could make quick and binding decisions for the whole of the country at once.[13] These types of decisions are however indispensable during a pandemic, especially when the spread of the virus follows an exponential logic, not leaving much time for hesitation. Thus, although many praise cooperative federalism as a democratic multi-level-governance process respecting the principle of subsidiarity, its fallbacks, during the pandemic, were certainly foreseeable. On the one hand, in France, the rapid specific decisions taken by Pres-

---

9 Art. 73–75 GG: see Eibe Riedel and Ulrich Derpa, *Überblick ber die Verteilung der Bundes-und Länderkompetenzen im Gesundheitswesen* (Heidelberg: Springer, 2002).
10 BGBI, Gesetz zur Verhütung und Bekämpfung von Infektionskrankheiten beim Menschen (IfSG), July 20, 2000, p. 1174.
11 See for example: Marion Hulverscheidt, *Infektion und Institution: Zur Wissenschaftsgeschichte des Robert Koch-Instituts im Nationalsozialismus* (Göttingen: Wallstein Verlag, 2009).
12 Cf. https://www.rki.de/EN/Home/homepage_node.html, accessed July 14, 2021; and for the high risk areas: https://www.travelbook.de/service/corona-risikogebiete-rki, accessed July 14, 2021.
13 For a comparison of the French and German political and administrative system see: Yves Mény, Andrew Knapp, and Janet Lloyd, *Government and Politics in Western Europe. Britain, France, Italy, Germany* (Oxford: Oxford University Press, 1993).

ident Macron were felt as arbitrary and lockdown measures took the French population completely by surprise. On the other hand, in Germany, the slow decision-making process and the adoption of different rules in each *Land* led to costly delays in the fight against the virus – the German decisions to impose lockdowns generally lagged behind the French ones – and to a process of internal bordering resulting in a patchwork of different rules in the 16 *Länder* of the Federal Republic.[14] Internal bordering thereby mainly referred to the introduction of different administrative or legislative regulations in the *Länder*, which could adopt their individual *Corona-Verordnungen* (Corona-laws) concerning, for example, the obligation to wear masks or not, the number of people who were allowed to assemble, the functioning of schooling, etc. However, sometimes internal bordering also led to the physical closure of *Länder* borders, forbidding travels from and to certain *Länder*, as it was for instance the case in the spring of 2020, when Mecklenburg-Vorpommern introduced a general *Einreiseverbot* (entry stop) to prevent massive tourist flows coming in from Berlin. When it comes to external bordering during the pandemic, the decisions were more centralized in Germany. Indeed, it was the *Bund*, i. e. the Minister of Internal Affairs (Horst Seehofer), who had the authority to determine the introduction of border controls and to decide rapidly on a border closure with Germany's neighbors, without consulting the *Länder* that were affected in the border regions.[15] Without following a cooperative federalism approach to external bordering, there was therefore a risk of non-consideration of the specific situation of border regions and this led to significant problems during the first lockdown of the pandemic in March 2020, especially in the case of the French-German border. However, central decision-making for external bordering did not necessarily mean that there was a homogenous approach to external bordering: thus, for example, the border between Germany and the Netherlands stayed open during the first wave of the pandemic in the spring of 2020, whereas the border with France was immediately closed.

At the outbreak of the pandemic, whilst France decided to apply strict lockdown measures from March 16 onwards, with a complete closure of schools, shops, and a standstill of nearly all public life on the entire French territory, in Germany, there were two different schools of thought. The first school of thought advocated a "soft lockdown" under the leadership of the Minister-pres-

---

14 Nathalie Behnke, "Föderalismus in der (Corona-)Krise? Föderale Funktionen, Kompetenzen und Entscheidungsprozesse," Bundeszentrale für politische Bildung, August 21, 2020, accessed July 14, 2021, https://www.bpb.de/apuz/314343/foederalismus-in-der-corona-krise.
15 Andreas Knorr and Wolfgang Stölzle, "Dossier: Die Verheerungen geschlossener Grenzen," *Achgut.*, April 6, 2021, accessed July 14, 2021, https://www.achgut.com/artikel/dossier_die_ver heerungen_geschlossener_grenzen.

ident of North-Rhine-Westphalia, Armin Laschet, who, based on evidence collected by epidemiologist Hendrik Streek from the University of Bonn in the city of Heinsberg, favored minimal measures of restrictions or no restrictions at all for the population.[16] Contrarily, the second school of thought, represented by the Minister-president of Bavaria, Markus Söder, favored a hard lockdown similar to the one implemented in France.[17] These two clashing views were not only based on different opinions about how to combat the pandemic, but were intrinsically linked to the political battle about who would become the successor of Angela Merkel as the official Chancellor candidate for the Christian Democratic Party (CDU) and its Bavarian sister party, the Christian Social Union (CSU).[18] Thus, the candidate of the CDU, Armin Laschet, presented himself as flexible, open-minded, and close to the citizens, trying to keep a normal life going during the pandemic, whereas Markus Söder, from the CSU, conveyed the image of a hardliner and authoritarian COVID-19 manager. He would save the German population with strict rules guided only by the final objective of national health security.[19] These two schools divided the Federal Republic of Germany into two opposing types of rules during the first wave of the pandemic. Following the speech given by Angela Merkel on March 18 urging the German population to stay at home, but not imposing any rules on a national scale, it was indeed in the hands of the Minister-presidents to determine the Corona-rules. Each Minister-president therefore adopted his/her own set of restrictions according to the affiliation with one or the other of the two Corona-schools of thought. Thus, there was a progressive and regionally differentiated lockdown between mid-March and mid-April 2020 with specific rules for each *Land* concerning the closure of shops, schooling, quarantines, etc.[20] In Bavaria, the situation was close to a total lockdown, whereas in North-Rhine Westphalia, there was no restriction to free movement at all. In between these two extremes, anything was possible in the 16 German *Länder:* it was forbidden to assemble, with limits

---

16 Heinsberg-Studie, published by the Unviersity of Bonn on May 4, 2020, cf. also Hendrik Streeck et al., "Infection fatality rate of SARS-CoV2 in a super-spreading event in Germany," *Nat Commun* 11, no. 5829 (2020).
17 Holger Dambeck et al., "Bayern und Nordrhein-Westfalen im Vergleich Söder oder Laschet – wessen Corona-Strategie ist erfolgreicher?," *Der Spiegel* 43 (2020).
18 Christian Wernicke, "CDU/CSU: Laschet und Söder behindern eine sinnvolle Corona-Politik," *Süddeutsche Zeitung*, April 8, 2021, accessed July 12, 2021, https://www.sueddeutsche.de/mei nung/kanzlerkandidatur-union-laschet-soeder-1.5258624.
19 "Söder verteidigt Corona-Strategie – Schutz von Leben steht ganz oben," *PNP*, September 26, 2020, accessed July 12, 2021, https://www.pnp.de/nachrichten/bayern/Soeder-im-Livestream-Co rona-ist-Naturkatastrophe-und-Pruefung-3796245.html.
20 Birte Wassenberg, "'The return of mental borders'", 115.

ranging from two up to five people depending on which *Land* was concerned, and nobody really understood anything. The German media unanimously denounced a non-coordinated German federal *"Flickenteppich"* (Patchwork). After a week, the federal Government ended up deciding that social distancing (*Kontaktsperre*) was to be generalized across Germany.[21] At the same time, in centralized France, the general lockdown was already well in place (until May 11) for all French people, whether they lived in the much-affected regions of Alsace and Ile-de-France or in the almost completely COVID-free region of Bretagne.[22] Just like the two addresses to the nation, the measures in Germany and France to combat the pandemic could not have been more different either.

In contrast to this internal patchwork of *Länder* measures, the federal authorities of Germany imposed an almost uniform external bordering policy, without any coordination with the neighboring countries.[23] The only exception was the border between Germany and the Netherlands, which remained open during the first wave of the pandemic, thanks to the personal intervention of Armin Laschet. At the French-German border, however, the decision made by the German Ministry of Interior to unilaterally shut down the border on March 16, under the pretext of the high COVID-19 incidence rate in the Grand Est region, which was experienced as a real trauma by the local and regional actors in the border regions.[24] There was an immediate standstill of cross-border mobility, with all border crossings – by train, tramway, road, etc. – being blocked and systematic controls being performed by the German authorities at the border.[25] The only flow that was initially authorized was that of trucks transporting goods so as not to block the functioning of the EU internal market. However, the immediate consequence for the German *Länder* at the French border (Rhineland-Pfalz, Baden-

---

21 Jürgen Overhoff, "Hemmschuh "Flickenteppich"?: Ein Wortgespenst geht um in Deutschland," *FAZ*, May 12, 2020.

22 Frédérique Berrod, Morgane Chovet, and Birte Wassenberg, "La frontière franco-allemande au temps du COVID-19," 40.

23 "Deutschland schließt Grenzen zu Frankreich, Österreich und der Schweiz," *Spiegel online*, March 15, 2020, accessed July 12, 2021, https://www.spiegel.de/politik/deutschland/coronavirus-deutschland-schliesst-grenzen-zu-frankreich-oesterreich-und-der-schweiz-a-9910fb81-f635-4be5-8138-bcbcbfd491d4.

24 Reports by Joachim Beck and Birte Wassenberg, in "Eprouver les frontières au temps de la COVID19," webinar of the Franco-German Jean Monnet excellence Center in Strasbourg, July 17, 2020, accessed July 12, 2021, https://centre-jean-monnet.unistra.fr/2020/07/17/webinaire-eprouver-les-frontieres-au-temps-de-la-covid19/.

25 Pierre Haski, "COVID-19: les frontières sont de retour en Europe," *France Inter*, March 17, 2020.

Wurttemberg, and Saarland) was a total disruption of the regional economy.[26] Indeed, the border regions largely depend on cross-border workers, with a significant proportion of French employees working in Germany (e. g. 22,700 Alsatians in Baden-Wurttemberg, 33,200 in Rhineland-Pfalz, and 18,000 in Saarland).[27] Thus, during the week of March 16, under the pressure of the Minister-presidents of the three aforementioned German *Länder*, exemptions were quickly adopted, allowing these workers to continue to cross the border in order to reach their workplaces.[28] This was the first collective action taken by these Minister-presidents in order to adapt a central decision taken by Berlin to the territorial reality at the French border. It was also an example of ingenious coordination of regional governance by the *Länder*, which shared the specificity of border territories. Their common interest in keeping the mobility function at the border urged them to create a horizontal network and defend their standpoint together with regard to the central authorities in Berlin and to the other *Länder*. This then led to an effective lobbying action on the part of this new league of Minister-presidents in order to coordinate measures, not only with the federal authorities in Berlin, but also with the neighboring state of France.

The federal structure of Germany hereby proved to be an asset for developing innovative cross-border cooperation in order to combat the pandemic together. Indeed, the centralized approach in France had rather absurd implications for the French border regions, as attempts to transfer patients from the highly affected Grand Est region did not take into account the fact that, in the neighboring German regions, there were empty hospital beds available for them.[29] Indeed, in March 2020, in Mulhouse, the French army started a complex and costly operation of flying out patients by helicopter to Toulon and Marseille.[30] On March 27, from Strasbourg, a TGV (high-speed train) transported 48 COVID-19 patients to Mar-

---

26 Frédérique Berrod, Morgane Chovet, and Birte Wassenberg, "La frontière franco-allemande au temps du COVID-19," 40.

27 Rachid Belkacem and Estelle Evrard, "Travail frontalier et fermeture des frontières: l'exemple de la Grande Région Sarre-Lor-Lux," Borderobs, June 8, 2020, accessed July 12, 2021, http://cbs.uni-gr.eu/fr/ressources/borderobs; *Atlas historique du Rhin supérieur*, map "Flux des travailleurs frontaliers" (Strasbourg: PUS, 2020).

28 Sébastien Lumet and Jacques Enaudeau, "Organisation du territoire européen en temps de Covid-19, entre coopération et repli," *Le Grand Continent*, April 1, 2020.

29 For intercultural learning between French and German political and administrative systems in a cross-border context see: Joachim, Beck, and Franz Thedieck (eds.), *The European dimension of administrative culture* (Baden-Baden: Nomos, 2008).

30 "Coronavirus à Mulhouse: Des patients évacués par l'armée vers Toulon et Marseille," *20 minutes*, March 18, 2020, accessed July 13, 2021, https://www.20minutes.fr/sante/2742771-20200318-coronavirus-mulhouse-patients-evacues-armee-vers-toulon-marseille.

seille, which is 1,000 kilometers away, even though in the neighboring regions, the German partners were willing to welcome French patients.[31] Facing this paradoxical situation, the Minster-presidents of Baden-Wurttemberg, Winfried Kretschmann, Rhineland-Pfalz, Malu Dreyer, and Saarland, Tobias Hans, contacted the president of the Grand Est region, Jean Rottner, and decided to create an ad hoc working group, which associated stakeholders from the regional political level and the national level in Berlin and Paris.[32] It was, *de facto*, a practical implementation of the new bilateral French-German Treaty, which had been signed on January 22, 2019 in Aachen and whose Chapter IV on cross-border cooperation provided for the setting-up of a "joint coordination committee" reuniting governance institutions on local, regional, and national levels.[33] Thanks to the *ad hoc* group, on March 21, the first patients from the French border region of Alsace were transported to a hospital in Freiburg, near the border. For centralized France, this multi-level governance approach was a novelty and it allowed, for the first time, the implementation of regionalized and decentralized solutions for the COVID-19 crisis.

However, all in all, during the first stage of the pandemic from March to May 2020, Germany turned out not to be a model in terms of measures to combat the pandemic. The crisis had rather led to a patchwork of multiple internal measures of more or less strict lockdowns. This changed when discussions started to emerge on how to coordinate scaling-down measures, when the rate of COVID-19 cases began to decrease.

Decentralized Scaling-down Strategies: German Cooperative Federalism as a Model for France? (May-October 2020)

The distribution of competences for health measures in Germany clearly favors the *Länder* level as opposed to the *Bund*. However, in the spring of 2020, the pop-

---

31 "Coronavirus: 48 malades du Grand Est évacués en train vers le Sud-Ouest ce week-end," *Le Parisien*, March 27, 2020, accessed July 13, 2021, https://www.leparisien.fr/societe/sante/corona virus-48-malades-du-grand-est-evacues-en-train-vers-le-sud-ouest-ce-week-end-27-03-2020-8289546.php.
32 "Ministerpräsident Tobias Hans: in der Grenzregion geschlossen gegen COVID handeln!," Declaration on March 15, 2020, accessed July 13, 2021, saarland.de.
33 See report by Jean-Baptiste Cuzin, administrator for cross-border cooperation at the Region Grand Est, in "Eprouver les frontières au temps de la COVID19."

ulation increasingly criticized the patchwork of individual *Länder* measures during the first wave of the pandemic, as the lack of coordination between the *Länder* and the *Bund* had led to a lot of confusion regarding what was allowed or not during the lockdown period.[34]

This continued in May 2020, when the *Länder* announced the first scaling-down measures. Again, there were different rules and schedules in the 16 *Länder* regarding the strategies for opening shops, schools, and resuming travelling. Regarding the reference criteria for the *Länder* being the incidence rate (*Inzidenzrate*) in a given territory, there were even different measures inside each *Land*. For example, in North-Rhine-Westphalia, 45 different Corona regulations were adopted between May and October 2020. Not only did some critics actually describe the situation as a non-coordinated federal patchwork, but they also pointed out a splintering of Law (*Rechtszersplitterung*), i.e. the breaking down of German Law into millions of different regulations, which were no longer linked by a common logic, with the image they used being that of a glass which had broken into a thousand of shards.[35] The confusion among the population was at its highest by the end of May, as there was no uniform approach at the national level and internal bordering, de-bordering, and re-bordering practices/policies between the different *Länder* were the general rule at that time. In this respect, the Federal Republic of Germany represented in no way a model for centralized France, where the scaling-down measures were taken for the whole of the country by the so-called Defense Council (*Conseil de defense sanitaire*) in Paris.[36] They were centrally announced, either by President Emmanuel Macron himself, by his Prime Minister, Jean Castex,[37] or by the Minister of Health, Olivier Véran.

At the federal level in Germany, Chancellor Angela Merkel realized that new mechanisms of *Bund-Länder* coordination were needed in order to better harmonize the different approaches of the Minister-presidents, who were already called

---

34 "Beratungen über Corona-Maßnahmen-Spahn: Flickenteppich schafft Verwirrung," *ZDFheute*, May 6, 2020, accessed July 13, 2021, https://www.zdf.de/nachrichten/politik/coronavirus-massnahmen-lockerungen-spahn-100.html/.

35 Nathalie Behnke, "Föderalismus in der (Corona-)Krise?"

36 Arthur Berdah, François-Xavier Bourmaud, and Marcelo Wesfreid, "Le Conseil de défense, lieu favori d'Emmanuel Macron pour des arbitrages en série", *lefigaro*, May 19, 2020, accessed July 13, 2021, https://www.lefigaro.fr/politique/le-conseil-de-defense-lieu-favori-d-emmanuel-macron-pour-des-arbitrages-en-serie-20200519.

37 On July 3, 2020, Jean Castex replaced Edouard Philippe as Prime Minster following the decision by President Emmanuel Macron to reshuffle his government.

ironically the "regional Dukes" (*Länderfürsten*).[38] One solution was the progressive institutionalization of the meetings between the *Bund* and the *Länder* in Berlin on the state of the pandemic. In the course of the year 2020, they thus became periodic discussion forums for the evaluation of the Corona measures and their adaptation[39]: Angela Merkel invited all Minister-presidents (partially online and partially in person) every two to three weeks in order to ensure a minimum coordination of scaling-down measures for the summer. Not only was this institutionalization of the *Bund-Länder* conferences the first response to growing criticism coming from public opinion, but it was also a possibility for Angela Merkel to try and impose her own view on how to combat the virus. Indeed, from the start, she had been rather in favor of the school represented by Markus Söder who advocated a hard lockdown and who was cautious about quick and all-englobing scaling-down measures. Although Söder was not part of Angela Merkel's political party (CDU) – but of the small Bavarian "sister" party, CSU – Angela Merkel still fervently defended the maintaining of restrictions. It was also probably due to the fact, that, as a physical scientist, she knew well about the exponential spreading threat of COVID-19.[40] Nonetheless, the *Bund-Länder* conferences turned out to be a platform for cooperative decision-making in the form of compromises between the position of the *Kanzleramt* represented by the General Secretary of the Chancellor, Helge Braun, and the 16 Minister-presidents. The criteria for reaching this compromise were fixed on the basis of scientific evidence from the Robert Koch Institute and a few research advisors, who were epidemiologists, were invited to these meetings.[41] In the end, this led to a rather efficient coordination between the *Länder* and the *Bund* insofar as they established a general framework for scaling-down measures depending on the number of COVID-19 cases/per capita in each specific geographic area. Contrary to France, where measures were still put in place for the entire territory of France, this approach

---

38 "Merkels Corona-Ringen mit den eigenwilligen Landesfürsten," *Saarbrückener Zeitung*, October 15, 2020, accessed July 13, 2021, https://www.saarbruecker-zeitung.de/nachrichten/politik/merkels-corona-ringen-mit-den-eigenwilligen-landesfuersten_aid-54068741.
39 Cf. "Kurzinformation: Bund-Länder Konferenzen zur Corona-Pandemie," February 8, 2021, accessed July 13, 2021, https://www.bundestag.de/resource/blob/828932/f901ae2c63048b60a12b1839928d6688/WD-3-031-21-pdf-data.pdf.
40 "Corona-Debakel in Bayern: Merkel stützt Söder – und bekommt nun selbst Breitseite," *Merkur*, July 14, 2020, accessed July 13, 2021, https://www.merkur.de/politik/angela-merkel-markus-soeder-coronavirus-bayern-test-kritik-staatsversagen-lauterbach-berlin-zr-90023923.html.
41 The new aspect is here the vertical coordination between Bund and Länder, as the horizontal coordination between Länder is an integral part of the functioning of cooperative federalism, cf. Yvonne Hegele and Nathalie Behnke, "Horizontal Coordination in Cooperative Federalism: The Purpose of Ministerial Conferences in Germany," *Regional & Federal Studies* 5 (2017): 529–48.

allowed for differentiated regional measures according to diverging territorial infection rates within the Federal Republic of Germany. This territorial differentiation was further reinforced by the decision of the *Bund-Länder* conference on May 6, 2020 to introduce the possibility of decentralized decisions for health protection (*Infektionsschutz*) on the *Landkreis*-level (county), i.e. below the *Land*. The multi-level governance of COVID-19, which was already operational on a cross-border level, was now also functioning internally, on the *Bund-Länder* level.[42]

The federal structure of Germany was well suited for this regionalized approach to addressing the COVID-19 crisis and it was rapidly identified as a best-practice model in Europe.[43] This was also the case for centralized France: indeed, during the scaling-down stage between May and June 2020, the French media praised the German federal model as a much more suitable way to define COVID-19 rules than the uniform set of measures, which was proclaimed every three to six weeks by the central authorities in Paris. The German model was certainly also appealing insofar as the infection rates throughout Germany overall remained largely beneath the ones in France, despite the much more stringent lockdown that had been imposed there until May 2020. It was therefore not surprising to see the French government taking measures inspired by the German decentralized model. Thus, a map was produced which divided the French territory into regions depending on their incidence rate, differentiating between low "green," medium "orange," and high risk "red" areas, with each area being allocated a set of different rules of more or less stringent restrictions concerning scaling-down measures. However, if these measures were now applied locally or regionally in France, they were still taken by the central state authorities, i.e. by the Prefects of Regions or Departments representing the central State of Paris in the "Province" and not by the local and regional authorities, for example by the Presidents of the Regional Councils. The role of the latter, although elected by the citizens, was often reduced to logistical tasks, for example the distribution of masks or, later on, the organization of the vaccination. Also, when it eventually came to progression of the lockdown (*déconfinement*) in France, the method of a regional differentiated approach to scaling-down measures was

---

42 "Ein ausgewogener Beschluss," May 6, 2020, accessed July 13, 2021, https://www.bundesre gierung.de/breg-de/aktuelles/merkel-bund-laender-gespraeche-1751020.
43 Philip Oltermann, "Germany's Devolved Logic Is Helping It Win the Coronavirus Race," *The Guardian*, April 5, 2020, accessed July 13, 2021, http://www.theguardian.com/world/2020/apr/05/ germanys-devolved-logic-is-helping-it-win-the-coronavirus-race; Guy Chazan, "How Germany Got Coronavirus Right," *Financial Times*, June 4, 2020, accessed July 13, 2021, http://www.ft. com/content/cc1f650a-91c0-4e1f-b990-ee8ceb5339ea.

not implemented and it was again central rules for the whole country which were applied.

However, in Spring 2020, the maps illustrating the regional distribution of COVID-19 cases in France resembled those regularly published by the Robert Koch Institute for the 16 German *Länder*. But compared to the Federal Republic of Germany, it was still the central government in Paris who decided on the regional measures and not, for example, the Presidents of Regions who represent the decentralized territorial political authorities.[44] A multi-level governance system similar to the one which existed between *Bund* and *Länder* in Germany was therefore not adopted in France.At the same time, horizontal multi-level governance continued to function in the French-German border regions. Thus, the French-German *ad hoc* group managed to negotiate a coordinated re-opening of the border on June 15, 2020. In contrast to the unilateral bordering policy that was imposed in March, external de-bordering thus took place after bilateral consultation and in a concerted manner.[45] This cross-border coordination regarding the scaling-down measures was also encouraged by the European Commission, which, in May 2020, had advocated a progressive scaling-down of restrictive measures throughout the European Union (EU) by privileging cross-border areas and by respecting the rules of social distancing.[46] The Commission advocated a general progressive removal of physical barriers to exchanges, but also an immediate removal of border controls "for those regions, zones and member states, which present a favorable and sufficiently equivalent epidemical situation."[47] Such a removal of barriers in specific areas was seen as a positive measure for the people living in the French-German border regions, who had experienced border restrictions in a much more traumatic way than those located in "internal" regions. The Commission also tried to smoothen the crossing of borders by proposing a protocol on the principle of mutual recognition of contact tracing

---

44 Vincent Hoffmann-Martinot and Hellmut Wollmann, eds., *State and Local Government Reforms in France and Germany. Divergence and Convergence* (Wiesbaden: Verlag für Sozialwissenschaften, 2006).

45 Common Declaration by Richard Ferrand and Wolfgang Schäuble, "La France et l'Allemagne, ensemble dans la crise du Coronavirus pour une nouvelle dynamique en Europe," May 26, 2020, accessed July 13, 2021, https://www.assemblee-nationale.fr/dyn/actualites-accueil-hub/la-france-et-l-allemagne-ensemble-dans-la-crise-du-coronavirus-pour-une-nouvelle-dynamique-en-europe.

46 Communication from the Commission, "Towards a phased and coordinated approach for restoring freedom of movement and lifting internal border controls – COVID-19," *Official Journal of the EU*, no. 169, May 15, 2020.

47 Communication from the Commission, 30.

applications so that they could be operational on a cross-border level.[48] However-er, a multi-level-governance model that implied perfect coordination between the European, bi-national, and regional level was not really in place by the end of the summer of 2020. Indeed, national scaling-down measures in France still largely differed from the largely differentiated ones applied by the 16 *Länder* in the Federal Republic of Germany.[49]

Besides, whereas the *Bund-Länder* conferences had resulted in some sort of federal coordination in Germany, not all Minister-presidents always respected the framework decisions adopted during these meetings. In the end, the competence for the Corona-rules still remained in the hands of the *Länder* executives who interpreted the framework decisions according to their own political priorities – which were not always in favor of the re-introduction of restrictions when a cluster of infection was identified in one of their *Landkreise*. Finally, there were some policy areas which were resistant to any attempt at coordination on the federal level. For example, measures concerning schooling were mostly not successful in the *Bund-Länder* discussions, as the Minister-presidents insisted that these are "exclusive" *Länder* competences, according to the *Grundgesetz* (Fundamental Law),[50] and that the federal level had no right to intervene.[51] Germany's federal model, if partially adopted by the French central authorities in the form of a more regionalized approach to scaling-down measures, was also used as an example for applying a decentralized approach to schooling in France. Thus, even if it was always the Ministry of Education in Paris who adopted the general rules for primary and secondary schools, the decentralized powers of the central state in the regions, i.e. the Rectorates, could now introduce some regional differentiation, as could the Regional Health Agencies (ARS) as far as health security plans are concerned.[52]

---

48 European Commission, press release on a common approach for safe and efficient mobile tracing apps across the EU, May 13, 2020.

49 "Coronavirus: 11 mai, 2 juin, 10 juillet… les grandes dates du déconfinement, *Le Parisien*, May 7, 2020, accessed July 13, 2021, https://www.leparisien.fr/societe/coronavirus-11-mai-2-juin-10-juillet-voici-les-grandes-dates-du-deconfinement-07-05-2020-8312667.php.

50 Art. 30, GG, see also: Manfred G. Schmidt, *Das Politische System Deutschlands, Institutionen, Willensbilder und Politikfelder* (Munich: Beck, 2021).

51 "Bund-Länder-Beratungen: Vorerst kein Beschluss zu schärferen Corona-Auflagen für Schulen," Deutsche Presse-Agentur, headtopics, November 16, 2020, accessed July 13, 2021, https://headtopics.com/de/bund-lander-beratungen-vorerst-kein-beschluss-zu-scharferen-corona-auflagen-fur-schulen-16881413.

52 Cf. website of the French government, accessed July 13, 2021: https://www.education.gouv.fr/covid19-mesures-pour-les-ecoles-colleges-et-lycees-modalites-pratiques-continuite-pedagogique-et-305467.

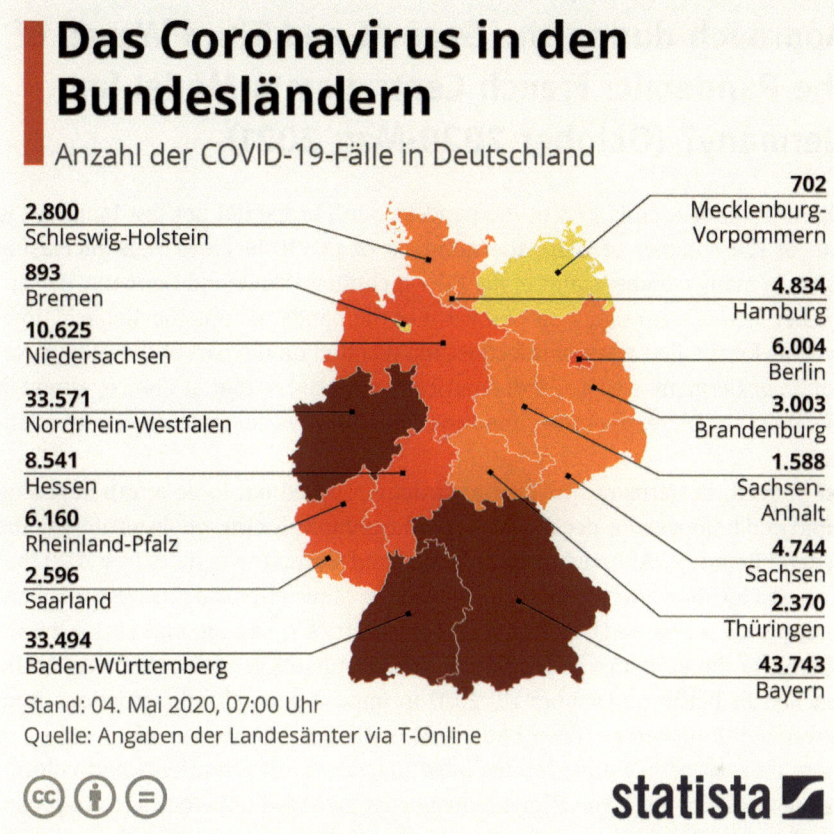

Das Coronavirus in den Bundesländern
Anzahl der COVID-19-Fälle in Deutschland

2.800
Schleswig-Holstein

893
Bremen

10.625
Niedersachsen

33.571
Nordrhein-Westfalen

8.541
Hessen

6.160
Rheinland-Pfalz

2.596
Saarland

33.494
Baden-Württemberg

702
Mecklenburg-
Vorpommern

4.834
Hamburg

6.004
Berlin

3.003
Brandenburg

1.588
Sachsen-
Anhalt

4.744
Sachsen

2.370
Thüringen

43.743
Bayern

Stand: 04. Mai 2020, 07:00 Uhr
Quelle: Angaben der Landesämter via T-Online

statista

Map 1: Map of the situation of the COVID-19 Epidemic in Germany: low-risk areas in yellow; medium-risk areas in orange; high-risk areas in red; very high-risk areas in dark red (May 2020). Source: Robert-Koch Institute, Berlin, Statista, May 2020.

Finally, the model of the Federal Republic of Germany on how to control the virus was not without flaws and shortcomings, which became more and more visible, when the second and third waves of the pandemic hit Europe from October 2020 onwards. This time, the German infection rates were increasing just as rapidly as the French ones and, in order to stop the exponential spread of the virus, there were now voices in Germany calling for a more centralized management of COVID-19.

The Shortcomings of the German Federalist Approach during the Second and Third Waves of the Pandemic: French Centralism a Model for Germany? (October 2020-May 2021)

The illusion of a rapid end of the pandemic in Europe did not last long: at the end of the summer of 2020, the numbers of COVID-19 cases were increasing again in many member states of the EU – including France and Germany. By September, it was clear that a second wave of the pandemic was inevitable.[53] However, as for the first wave of infection, the reaction on the part of the Federal Republic of Germany was again diametrically opposed to that of France, although this time, the increase of the virus contamination was comparable in both countries.

Indeed, in Germany, the federal structure turned out to be a trap impeding rapid and homogenous decisions on new restrictions for the whole territory of the Federal Republic. Although Angela Merkel had warned as early as July 2020 that a second lockdown would be unavoidable, the Minister-presidents were reluctant to agree on a renewed shutdown of the country's economic and social lives.[54] Thanks to the existence of the *Bund-Länder* conferences, a decision was finally reached in Berlin on October 28, 2020 to impose generalized restrictions from November 2 onwards. These had to do with the interdiction of meetings of more than 10 people and also included the closure of restaurants and cultural venues in Germany.[55] The Minister-presidents managed nonetheless to negotiate a rather "soft" lockdown, as for example hairdressers, shops, schools, and play-schools were allowed to remain open. As was the case during the first lockdown,

---

53 "Wie schlimm wird die zweite Corona-Welle?," *Spiegel online*, September 22, 2020, accessed July 13, 2021, https://www.spiegel.de/panorama/wie-schlimm-wird-die-zweite-corona-welle-hohe-infektionszahlen-leere-intensivbetten-a-29bb39fe-92f4-4ab0-806a-a1915b037fd3; Hans van Leeuwen, "Europe faces up to pandemic's second wave," *Financial Review*, September 11, 2020, accessed July 13, 2021, https://www.afr.com/world/europe/europe-faces-up-to-pandemic-s-second-wave-20200910-p55ujh.

54 "Sommer-PK: Angela Merkel warnt vor Corona-Herbst – und spricht über Schreckensszenario, zweiter Lockdown, *Merkur*," July 14, 2020, accessed July 13, 2021, https://www.merkur.de/politik/merkel-coronavirus-warnung-deutschland-sommer-pk-lockdown-herbst-berlin-trump-soeder-zr-90032100.html.

55 "Bund-Länder-Beratungen. Einschränkungen schon ab Montag geplant," *tagessschau*, October 28, 2020, accessed July 13, 2021, https://www.tagesschau.de/inland/corona-bund-laender-107.html.

each *Land* could then determine, more individually, which specific restrictions it would impose on its population.[56] Depending on the evolution of the infection rate, this also included travel restrictions within the Federal Republic. Thus, whereas, for example, in Thüringen, there was no limitation to travel from and into the *Land*, Mecklenburg-Vorpommern imposed a general obligation of quarantine. The only more or less homogenous measure was that most *Länder* introduced a so-called "*Beherbergungsverbot*" (interdiction of lodging) which made it impossible for hotels and B&Bs to welcome any guests. Despite the general will of *Bund-Länder* coordination, the situation of restrictions in each German *Land* was therefore again very different, questioning the relevance of the cooperative federalist model. Some critics humorously spoke of a German "*Föderallala*" (chaotic federalism).[57] The main problem for Germany was that the negotiations in Berlin seemed to converge towards only minimal restrictive measures as a rule for the general framework, which – against all advice from competent epidemiologists – did not help stop the exponential spread of the virus.

Indeed, with regard to decisions made to combat the pandemic, the centralist French state now seemed better equipped, as it could make the rapid, top-down, albeit unpopular, decision to lock down the country. Thus, on October 28, Emmanuel Macron announced a second general lockdown until December 15, which imposed hard and immediate restrictions on the entire French population.[58] Proclaimed as a general decision of the Health Defense Council (*Conseil de défense sanitaire*), it implied the closure of most private and public institutions (shops, hairdressers, theatres, etc.) and the passage towards online teaching at universities and hybrid teaching in secondary schools. Not only did the government impose restrictions on the free circulation of people with the lockdown but it also limited the number of social interactions that were allowed outside at the end of the lockdown. There was also a general curfew set at 6 p.m.,[59] a measure, which was unthinkable in Germany, where any prospect of a curfew im-

---

56 "Lockdown "light" ab 02. November 2020 – Bund-Länder-Beschluss vom 28. Oktober 2020," *anwalt*, November 30, 2020, accessed July 13, 2021, https://www.anwalt.de/rechtstipps/lockdown-light-ab-02-november-2020-bund-laender-beschluss-vom-28-oktober-2020_181602.html.
57 ZDF, *Heute-Show*, May 15, 2020, accessed July 13, 2021, http://www.zdf.de/comedy/heute-show/heute-show-vom-15-mai-2020-100.html.
58 Speech by Emmanuel Macron announcing a new confinement for three months minimum in order to fight against the COVID19 pandemic, October 29, 2020, accessed July 13, 2021, https://www.vie-publique.fr/discours/276951-emmanuel-macron-28102020-covid-19.
59 This measure had in fact already been put in place before the lockdown and was therefore simply being continued.

mediately stimulated debates on the infringement on individual freedom, reviving the memories of repression during Nazi-Germany.[60]

The diametrically opposed measures imposed by Germany and France continued in the course of the second and third waves of the pandemic, until March 2021. Indeed, in Germany, the reluctance to introduce a new hard lockdown quickly led to a catastrophic increase in COVID-19 cases to the point that, for the first time, in some German *Länder*, there had been a shortage of reanimation beds – although Germany had a much higher number of beds per capita than France. The exponential spread of the virus therefore forced the convening of an emergency *Bund-Länder* conference on December 16, 2020, during which a hard(er) lockdown was announced, now including the closure of hairdressers and all non-essential shops.[61] Most Minister-presidents also decided to close schools and move to 100 percent online schooling. In contrast, at the same time, the hard lockdown measures imposed in France showed their positive results with the COVID-19 incidence rate decreasing so that Emmanuel Macron could announce a softening of restrictive measures.[62] As a consequence, while in Germany, shops and hairdressers were now closed, they started reopening in France during the first two weeks of December. Besides, Emmanuel Macron announced a general scaling-down strategy, depending on the evolution of the spread of the virus, but at the same time he maintained the general curfew at 6 p.m., whereas in Germany there was no curfew, but the announcement of a harder lockdown rather than a scaling-down strategy.

From mid-December 2020 onwards, France and Germany regularly prolonged these measures, when the spread of the new British variant of the virus resulted in an ever more rapid increase of COVID-19 cases in both states, in spite of all the restrictions that were in place.[63] While in France this situation

---

60 "Warum sich Deutschland mit Ausgangssperre so schwertut," *Focus online*, March 10, 2020, accessed July 13, 2021, https://www.focus.de/politik/deutschland/soeder-prescht-voran-merkel-deutete-sie-nur-an-warum-sich-deutschland-mit-ausgangssperre-so-schwertut_id_11789268.html.

61 "Entscheidung gefallen: Bund und Länder beschließen harten Lockdown ab dem 16. Dezember," *Saarbrücker Zeitung*, December 13, 2020, accessed July 13, 2021, https://www.saarbruecker-zeitung.de/nachrichten/politik/inland/bund-und-laender-beschliessen-harten-lockdown-ab-dem-16-dezember_aid-55169879.

62 "Déconfinement: les nouvelles mesures en vigueur le 15 décembre," *franceinfo*, December 10, 2020, accessed July 13, 2021, https://www.francetvinfo.fr/sante/maladie/coronavirus/deconfinement-les-nouvelles-mesures-en-vigueur-le-15-decembre_4214805.html.

63 "Merkel sieht Deutschland in "dritter Welle," *Spiegel online*, February 23, 2021, accessed July 13, 2021, https://www.spiegel.de/ausland/coronavirus-angela-merkel-sieht-deutschland-in-dritter-welle-a-2e8dc0f6-88db-44aa-8432-1cc8c687dbfa/.

did not provoke a panic reaction in Paris, in Germany, at the federal level, Angela Merkel was extremely alarmed and called for a new *Bund-Länder* conference on March 22 in order to take immediate measures against the British variant. During a long night session, Merkel ended up imposing a nationwide hard lockdown for Easter, a decision which was not shared by many Minister-presidents, including Armin Laschet.[64] However, this "forced" decision proved inapplicable in practice so that Angela Merkel, under the pressure of many lobbying groups from different economic sectors, cancelled the decision on March 24 and publicly apologized to the German nation – something which had never happened before in the history of the Federal Republic.[65] Although the hard lockdown was not yet implemented, several Minster-presidents took advantage of this situation in order to bypass the general framework of restrictions that everyone had agreed upon beforehand. Thus, Tobias Hans, the Minister-president of Saarland, presented a scaling-down model based on a test strategy and Armin Laschet announced a scaling-down strategy for schools in North-Rhine Westphalia.[66] The cooperative federalist model seemed to be in a deadlock, as proved by the criticism Angela Merkel aimed openly at the Minister-presidents and their scaling-down strategies in an interview with Anne Will on television on March 28, 2021.[67]

The *Bund-Länder* conference also seemed inefficient in comparison with the French *Conseil de défence*, which could make rapid, binding, and uniform decisions for the whole of France. The French centralized state therefore now acted as a model for Germany, especially for Angela Merkel, who wished to increase the federal competence in the fight against the pandemic. In order to do so, on April 23, 2021, a new *Infektionschutzgesetz* (Law on the protection against in-

---

64 "Kein Urlaub, keine Lockerungen: Merkel rechtfertigt knallharten Oster-Lockdown," *focus online*, March 23, 2021, accessed July 13, 2021, https://www.focus.de/politik/deutschland/coro na-gipfel-im-news-ticker-merkel-beschliesst-knallharten-oster-lockdown-ohne-urlaub-und-lock erungen_id.

65 "Merkel stoppt die Osterruhe und entschuldigt sich," *Merkur*, March 24, 2021, accessed July 13, 2021, https://www.merkur.de/politik/merkel-stoppt-die-osterruhe-und-entschuldigt-sich-zr-90259135.html.

66 "Hans will im Saarland bald neue Corona-Politik," *Saarbrücker Zeitung*, March 24, 2021, accessed July 13, 2021, https://www.saarbruecker-zeitung.de/saarland/landespolitik/lockdown-an-ostern-tobias-hans-will-neue-corona-politik-im-saarland_aid-56974915; "Noch vor dem Corona-Gipfel: Laschet verkündet erste Entscheidungen für NRW," *Ruhr24*, March 23, 2021, accessed July 13, 2021, https://www.ruhr24.de/nrw/corona-gipfel-nrw-armin-laschet-lockerungen-22-maerz-bund-laender-oeffnungen-gastronomie-kultur-90253881.html.

67 Interview with Angela Merkel by Anne Will, ARD, March 28, 2021, accessed July 13, 2021, https://www.youtube.com/watch?v=UpEPnbgPkm0&ab_channel=DACHMedien.

fections) came into force.[68] It introduced a principle of a *Notbremse* (emergency break) allowing for the implementation of the same restrictions for all *Länder* defined on the federal level when the COVID-19 situation required such measures. The criteria for the implementation of these restrictions was an incidence rate of more than 100 new infections in seven days per 100,000 inhabitants.[69] The introduction of a more centralized management following the example of France did however not alter the main multi-level governance approach to the pandemic in the Federal Republic of Germany – even if it must be underlined that there was also much criticism in Germany during the pandemic that the Parliaments at federal and state levels were generally bypassed in the decision-making process. Thus, for example, at the same time as the new federal Law was adopted, there were experiments of COVID-19 measures at the local level, which circulated as "best-practice" models for Germany. For example, the mayor of Tübingen, Boris Palmer, presented a scaling-down strategy for his town based on the systematic and massive use of PCR tests as a condition for entry into shops, cafés, etc.[70] In centralized France, local initiatives of massive testing also existed – for example in January 2021 in Roubaix – but the use of such models for the introduction of a nationwide applied rule did not seem likely. What's more, the cooperative federalist model continued to function, even if the *Bund-Länder* conferences were replaced by the new *Infektionsschutzgesetz* (Protection Law against infection) on the federal level, on the one hand, and decisions by the Minister-presidents for each *Land* within the limits of this Law, on the other hand. The scaling-down strategies adopted by the 16 *Länder* from June 2021 indeed all led to a general normalization of public and economic life in the Federal Republic of Germany.

Despite the opposite measures implemented by France and Germany during the second and third waves of the pandemic, there was also a surprising shift in the border regions, where cross-border mobility was maintained and re-border-

---

68 Infektionsschutzgesetz §28b, Bundesgesetzblatt Teil 1, no. 18, 2021, accessed July 13, 2021, https://www.bundesgesundheitsministerium.de/fileadmin/Dateien/3_Downloads/Gesetze_und_Verordnungen/GuV/B/4_BevSchG_BGBL.pdf.
69 "Infektionsschutzgesetz. Das regelt die bundeseinheitliche Notbremse," accessed July 13, 2021, https://www.bundesregierung.de/breg-de/aktuelles/bundesweite-notbremse-1888982.
70 "Boris Palmer: Tübinger Modell gegen Lockdown," *Kommunal*, March 23, 2021, accessed July 13, 2021, https://kommunal.de/tuebinger-modell-boris-palmer-podcast; "Tübingen bleibt Modellstadt. So optimiert Boris Palmer das Corona-Projekt," *Stuttgarter Zeitung*, April 6, 2021, accessed July 13, 2021, https://www.stuttgarter-zeitung.de/inhalt.boris-palmer-optimiert-corona-projekt-tuebinger-modell-laeuft-unter-auflagen-weiter.1edf0f48-9347-48ce-8d72-2f9ec9dae6d7.html?reduced=true.

ing was largely avoided.[71] As a result of successful lobbying on the part of the French-German *ad hoc* working group and the cross-border governance institutions (mainly the Upper Rhine Conference and the Greater Region Summit) in the Upper Rhine Region and the Grand Est Region, the border regions could continue to function as integrated spaces. The regional authorities at the border managed to avoid a new closure of the border and a disruption of cross-border life in the border regions. The availability of tests made it possible to control the crossing of the border in function of sanitary criteria (COVID infected or not) instead of national criteria (national ID card or passport) and it was no longer the passport or identity card which was the magic key of entry to the neighboring state, but rather the scientific proof of non-infection.[72] This imparted to the border a new sanitary function, but it still represented a form of re-bordering, as people could only enter the neighboring state if they were in possession of a negative COVID test. However, specific rules were introduced for the borderlanders – both cross-border workers and families. At the French-German border, a 24-hour rule guaranteed the possibility for the border population to cross the border for a limited period of time in order to work, shop or visit relatives, whereas other French or German citizens had to be quarantined.[73] Even when the Robert Koch Institute declared France as a high-risk country on March 26, 2021, a separation of the border population was avoided by means of an arrangement between the German border *Länder* and the Region Grand Est. Thus, the crossing of the border was possible for families and cross-border workers on the condition they had a negative PCR test which had to be shown two or three times a week depending on the *Land* (Saarland, Baden-Wurttemberg or Rhineland-Pfalz).[74] Besides, in order to reassure the French neighbors, complementary testing stations were set up near the border, for example by the town of Kehl in the

---

71 "Keine Grenzschließungen zwischen Saarland und Frankreich," *Saarbrücker Zeitung*, February 22, 2022, accessed July 13, 2021, https://www.saarbruecker-zeitung.de/saarland/land espolitik/corona-keine-grenzschliessungen-zwischen-saarland-und-frankreich_aid-56396651.

72 "Hochinzidenzgebiet Frankreich: Niedrige Hürden gefordert," *Zeit online*, March 26, 2021, accessed July 13, 2021, https://www.zeit.de/news/2021-03/26/hochinzidenzgebiet-frankreich-nie drige-huerden-gefordert.

73 "Coronavirus: une dérogation de 24 heures pour aller faire ses courses en Allemagne," *France bleu*, October 16, 2020, accessed July 13, 2021, https://www.francebleu.fr/infos/societe/ la-regle-des-24h-entre-en-vigueur-des-samedi-pour-les-frontaliers-1602838098.

74 "COVID19 et santé aux frontières," webinar of the Franco-German Jean Monnet excellence Center in Strasbourg, May 17, 2021, accessed July 13, 2021, https://www.youtube.com/watch?v= j4Xxen1QIKg&ab_channel=Universit%C3%A9deStrasbourg.

Euro-district Strasbourg-Kehl Ortenau.[75] The local stakeholders on both sides of the border thus cooperated closely in order to maintain cross-border normality and to avoid a new traumatic experience of separation and the sentiment of dis-integration in the border region. This proves that, regardless of the state structure, federal or centralized, the crisis management of the pandemic also depended on the goodwill and the capacity of innovation of stakeholders in France and Germany, be it on national, regional or local levels.

Conclusion

When the COVID-19 pandemic started, it was a true challenge for the federal political structure of Germany. The system of cooperative federalism, praised by Fritz W. Scharpf as a model of democratic functioning and entanglement between the regional and central levels of government, proved both an advantage and an obstacle for the management of the crisis. On the one hand, as the competences for health policy are mostly in the hands of the 16 German *Länder*, as defined by the *Grundgesetz*, during the first phase of COVID-19 the lockdown measures were largely different in each *Land* and they led to an uncoordinated patchwork of rules throughout the territory of the Federal Republic. On the other hand, the focus on the *Länder* governance level also meant that they could adapt their decisions to the regional situation and to the incidence rate of COVID-19 in each *Landkreis* (district), thus avoiding a uniform implementation of restrictions everywhere, without any justification of infection.

The advantages of this decentralized approach to combatting the virus with, as a proof of success, low national infection rates during the first wave of the pandemic, led the French authorities to consider German federalism as a model and to adopt a more regionalized approach to the definition of restrictive measures. However, drawing a regional map of COVID-19 infections as a reference is one thing, but a multi-level governance approach to the fight against the pandemic is another. Even in Germany, the criticism against the uncoordinated patchwork of rules led to the reconsidering of the functioning of this governance approach during the course of the pandemic. With the gradual institutionalization of the *Bund-Länder* conferences as a forum for coordination between

---

75 "Ortenaukreis schafft Erleichterungen für Grenzpendler aus Hochinzidenzgebieten," February 19, 2021, accessed July 13, 2021, https://www.ortenaukreis.de/Landkreis-Verwaltung/Gesundheit-Sicherheit-/Corona/Ortenaukreis-schafft-Erleichterungen-f%C3%BCr-Grenzpendler-aus-Hochinzidenzgebieten.php?object=tx,3406.5.1&ModID=7&FID=3406.11166.1&NavID=3406. 117.

the federal and regional levels of governance, this governance model started to work better, leading to the determination of a framework on the national level and to decentralized implementation on the *Länder* level, but the functioning of this model remained fragile. When the second wave hit Germany in the fall of 2020, the concertation mechanism ended up in a deadlock, as the Minister-presidents did not favor a new hard lockdown, whereas Angela Merkel wanted the opposite, but did not have the power to impose her will. At that point, the French centralized model appeared as a solution, in that decisions, albeit unpopular, could be proclaimed by the French president without any need for negotiation with local or regional authorities. The remedy of a new Law for the protection against infections at the federal level in March 2021 did not however represent a transformation of the Federal Republic of Germany into a centralized state. It was a mere attempt to strike a better balance in the distribution of competences on health policy between the *Bund* and the *Länder*. Overall, the fragility of Germany's federal system during the pandemic did not so much stem from an imbalance of competences between the federal and regional levels, but rather from the misuse of the *Länder* competences by certain Minister-presidents for their own political purposes. The two opposed schools between a "soft" and a "hard" lockdown embodied respectively by Markus Söder and Armin Laschet did not help to develop a common approach to combatting the virus. Even if specific measures may diverge on the *Länder* level, the way they diverge has to be decided in function of the virus and not in function of who can win public support for an election as candidate for the succession of Angela Merkel.

After all, as far as the management of the COVID-19 crisis is concerned, it is questionable if German cooperative federalism can be used as a model for France, or conversely, the French centralized system as a model for Germany. For, the German population, with its federal political culture, would not accept an overall top-down centralized approach as upheld by Emmanuel Macron during the three waves of the pandemic. And in France, a transfer of competences to the regional territorial authorities for the definition of a health crisis which threatens the security of the French nation, and the implementation of measures to fight it, seems to be just as impossible, even if it may be embraced by some, for example the border regions and border towns which particularly suffered from the centralized decisions made in Paris without taking into account their cross-border situation. Mutual learning from each other's political system and a coordinated approach between France and Germany can however be necessary and useful, when it comes to the management of the crisis in border regions. Our European border regions have developed into integrated living spaces, which are located in-between different political systems and the application of purely national responses to the crisis – including the hermetic closure of borders – was not an adequate response to the COVID-19 pandemic in the EU. A coordinated approach between the Minister-presidents of the German *Länder* at the French border and the French Grand Est Region, together with the national authorities in Paris and Berlin, was therefore a salvation for cross-border regions. As a first practical application of the Treaty of Aachen, this multi-level governance helped to convert the traumatized border regions, which had been separated during the first wave of the pandemic, into innovative transnational spaces of cooperation during the second and third waves of the pandemic. Coupled with efforts by the EU to put into place an EU Health Union, this kind of cooperation may lead to a better management of future sanitary – and other – crises at European borders and to a multi-level governance that includes European, national, regional, and local policy levels.

Michelle Falkenbach
4 COVID-19: Austria's Fall From Grace

A Game of Credit and Blame

Introduction

February 25, 2020 marked the arrival of the first COVID-19 case in Austria. Within a few days, the trio made up of the Minister of Health, Anschober (Green), the Minister of Interior, Nehammer (new ÖVP)[1], and most importantly, Chancellor Kurz (new ÖVP) became the faces of the crisis management. These three men would be seen in almost daily press conferences setting new rules and announcing new measures that would accompany the country throughout the first wave of the pandemic.[2] During this first wave, the success of the national government can be attributed to two factors that go hand in hand: quick, decisive decisions that were well communicated and public support.

The trust citizens have in their government is an essential determining factor of their willingness to comply with, in this particular case, public health regulations and guidelines.[3] Public trust in a government's ability to manage crises, such as the COVID-19 pandemic, is critical, seeing that trust relates to the publics' willingness to follow rules during precarious times.[4] On the flip side, a sense of distrust can harm social cohesion as well as economic stability.[5]

---

1 New ÖVP – new Austrian People's Party.
2 Thomas Cyzpionka and Miriam Reiss, "Three Approaches to Handling the COVID-19 Crisis in Federal Countries Germany, Austria, and Switzerland," in *Coronavirus Politics The Comparative Politics and Policy of COVID-19*, ed. Scott L. Greer et al. (University of Michigan Press, 2021).
3 Olivier Bargain and Ulugbek Aminjonov, "Trust and Compliance to Public Health Policies in Times of COVID-19," *Journal of Public Economics* 192 (2020): 104316; Ziqiang Han, Xiaojiang Hu, and Joanne Nigg, "How Does Disaster Relief Works Affect the Trust in Local Government? A Study of the Wenchuan Earthquake," *Risk, Hazards & Crisis in Public Policy* 2, no. 4 (December 1, 2011): 1–20, https://doi.org/https://doi.org/10.2202/1944-4079.1092.
4 Sofie Marien and Marc Hooghe, "Does Political Trust Matter? An Empirical Investigation into the Relation between Political Trust and Support for Law Compliance," *European Journal of Political Research* 50, no. 2 (2011): 267–91; Daisy Fancourt, Andrew Steptoe, and Liam Wright, "The Cummings Effect: Politics, Trust, and Behaviours during the COVID-19 Pandemic," *The Lancet* 396, no. 10249 (2020): 464–65.

Michelle Falkenbach, PhD. Postdoctoral Associate, Cornell University, Ithaca, NY Department of Public Health.

https://doi.org/10.1515/9783110745085-005

In its most general sense, this chapter analyzes how the COVID-19 pandemic was approached from a political standpoint in Austria and how these approaches impacted public support. Specifically, this chapter seeks to understand when and why the national government moved from a centralized COVID-19 crisis management strategy that worked well during the first wave to a decentralized one that ended up leading to general confusion. By focusing on these levels of governance, the politics of credit and blame relating to decision-making and public support will be touched on. As mentioned, this chapter will look not only to the national government but also the subnational government as well as the involvement of opposition parties and the country's social partners within the decision-making process.

The chapter is divided into five main sections. The first section will describe some of the key and unique features of Austrian politics and the Austrian healthcare system. The main portion of the article will look specifically at the role and actions of the federal government concerning the management of the pandemic, the credit, and blame they claim and pass, and the impact these actions have on public opinion. To accomplish this, different waves of the pandemic and the governmental responses as well as public opinion data relating to those responses are used. The first wave (March to May 2020) nicely demonstrated the Austrian government's ability to work quickly and effectively with the support of all actors and opposition parties, garnering them much credit among voters and the international community alike. The summer months (June to August 2020) depict the slow unraveling of the unanimous governmental support from all actors and the public. Moving into the second wave (September 2020 to February 2021), the government's credibility continued to decline as it had to call out two additional lockdowns within a matter of weeks. By the third wave (March to May 2021), the public's confidence in the government hit an all-time low following the vaccine fiasco, the health minister's resignation, and corruption charges against the Chancellor and several of his closest allies.

Key Aspects of the Austrian Political System

Politically, Austria is a federal, parliamentary, representative democratic republic. Each of Austria's nine *Länder*, except for Vienna, is divided into administrative regions, which branch into local authorities. The federal legislative power is divided between the government and the two chambers of Parliament known as the nation-

---

5 Bargain and Aminjonov, "Trust and Compliance to Public Health Policies in Times of COVID-19."

al and federal councils. The judiciary system is solely federal, independent of the legislative and executive branches, meaning there are no state courts in Austria.

Since January 2020, Austria has been run by a coalition between the Conservative party (new ÖVP),[6] led by Chancellor Kurz, and the Green Party, which had never been in office. Given the new ÖVP's dominance in the 2019 national election with over 37% (71 seats in the National Council), it was natural that the party would lead more ministries.[7] The Greens were given five ministries, including the Ministry of Social, Health, Care, and Consumer Protection led by Rudolf Anshober. The new ÖVP, on the other hand, took control of nine ministries, including the Ministry of Finance (Gernot Blümel) and the Ministry of Interior (Karl Nehammer).

From a health systems perspective, Austrian health insurance makes up one part of the Austrian social insurance system. The system was founded on the Bismarckian principles, based on contributions from wages. The general difficulty within the Austrian healthcare system is that healthcare is represented by several different actors. Therefore the complexity of the setup often gets in the way of its efficiency.[8] While the bureaucratic circumstances were not optimal for a pandemic, the hospital capacity is well above the EU average, with 264 hospitals and 2,369 ICU beds.[9] The so-called "Influenza Pandemic Plan" in Austria was created in 2006 and last updated in 2009.[10] The plan included creating crisis management teams at both the federal and regional levels, a 24/7 emergency service, and states that the federal government should take the national response lead.

---

6 When Chancellor Kurz took over the ÖVP in May of 2017 he rebranded the Austrian People's Party (ÖVP) and created "The New Austrian People's Party," changing the party's color from black to turquoise and distancing himself from the Catholic Conservative ideology of the party by moving closer towards a radical right populist ideology. Michelle Falkenbach and Raffael Heiss, "The Austrian Freedom Party in Government: A Threat to Public Health?," in *The Populist Radical Right and Health: National Policies and Global Trends*, ed. Michelle Falkenbach and Scott L. Greer (Springer, 2021); Emily Schultheis, "A New Right-Wing Movement Rises in Austria," *The Atlantic*, 2017, accessed April 28, 2021, https://www.theatlantic.com/international/archive/2017/10/austria-immigration-sebastian-kurz/542964/.

7 The Green Party achieved almost 14% in the election translating into 26 seats, making them the fourth strongest party in the National Council.

8 Maria M Hofmarcher, "Das Österreichische Gesundheitssystem" (Berlin, 2013).

9 Jan Bauer et al., "Access to Intensive Care in 14 European Countries: A Spatial Analysis of Intensive Care Need and Capacity in the Light of COVID-19," *Intensive Care Medicine* 46, no. 11 (2020): 2026–34.

10 Katharina Habimana and Andreas Schmidt, "Austria: Governance," COVID-19 Health Systems Response Monitor, 2020, accessed May 21, 2021, https://www.covid19healthsystem.org/countries/austria/livinghit.aspx?Section=5. Governance&Type=Chapter.

As far as public health is concerned, as shown by Figure 1 below, the federal government, according to Austrian Federal Constitution (B-VG), possesses the power to pass and execute laws relating to public health including the management and prevention of epidemics and pandemics. The exception, under (Art. 10 par 1 n. 12 B-VG), is in dealing with the organization of hospitals and municipal sanitation, which is a *Länder* competency. While the governors of the *Länder* are bound to the legislations passed by the federal government and its ministries, the *Länder* governors have the power to implement these instructions. This makes for an interesting power dynamic as on the one hand the federal government can legally (Art. 20) make the governors follow orders, but on the other the orders can only be followed if the *Länder* possess the capacity and commitment to actually implement and enforce the orders.[11] What this implies in terms of the COVID-19 pandemic is that the federal government can say people need to be tested, vaccinated, and there has to be enough room in the hospitals for COVID-19 patients, but it is the *Länder* that decide how people will be tested, who will get vaccines at what time and where, and how sufficient capacities in hospitals can be maintained. In addition, the *Länder* must have or be given the resources (tests and vaccines) to fulfill the wishes of the federal government.

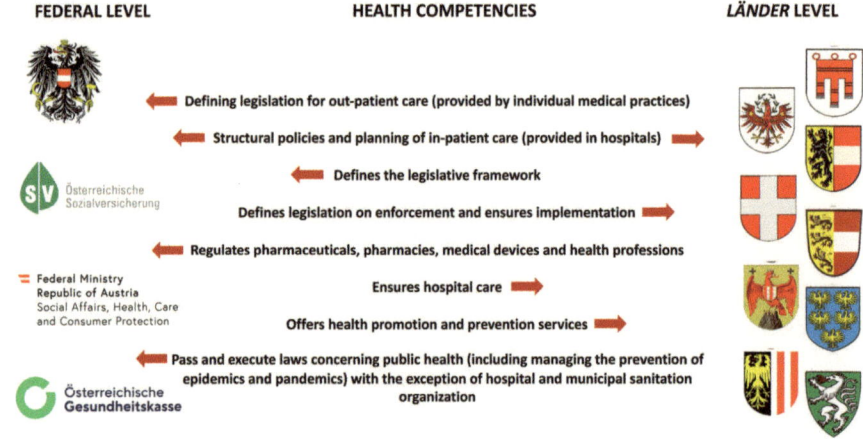

Figure 1: Healthcare competencies in Federal Austria. Source: author's own.

11 Peter Bußjäger, "COVID-19 Crisis Challenging Austria's Cooperative Federalism," foederalismus.at, 2020, accessed April 18, 2021, https://www.foederalismus.at/blog/covid-19-crisis-challenging-austria's-cooperative-federalism_235.php?&title=covid-19-crisis-challenging-austria's-cooperative-federalism&id=235.

First Wave (March – May 2020)

The first wave of the pandemic, beginning on February 25, 2020, with the arrival of the first COVID-19 case, showed a strong, united government (national and subnational) with the full support of the opposition and social partners. Proposals, communication, and containment measures came exclusively from the national government during this time, specifically by Chancellor Kurz, Health Minister Anschober, and Minister of Interior Nehammer.

By February 28, Health Minister Anschober made it clear that Austria would pass the same measures for all the *Länder* and that there would be no regional differences regarding contact points, testing strategies, and other containment measures.[12] Minister Nehammer, backed by the National Security Council, confirmed that they would support the Health Minister by getting all the experts together at one table to pass country-wide measures.

On March 5, Health Minister Anschober gave an interview stating that corona tests would be given to those patients who displayed symptoms and that the government worked well together. According to the Austrian confidence index[13] rating from March 2020, this "governmental collaboration resulted in the highest confidence values ever measured."[14] At this stage in the pandemic, the population was very motivated to follow the instructions of the political leaders to defeat the virus. While this type of behavior is typical during crises[15] it is very plausible that the Austrian government garnered extra support and trust due to their very effective communication strategy. The pervasive media presence among the trio of leaders garnered officials,[16] but especially Chancellor Kurz, led to particularly stark increases in confidence (see Figure 2).[17]

---

12 Birgit Baumann, Davina Brunnbauer, and Sebastian Fellner, "Coronavirus: Kurz Warnt Vor Panik Und Hamsterkäufen," der Standard, 2020, accessed June 3, 2021, https://www.der standard.at/story/2000115110169/anschober-erlaesst-bundesweit-einheitliche-vorgaben-fuer-um gang-mit-coronavirus.
13 This Index is created by OGM, a full-service market and opinion research institute founded in 1976 by Wolfgang Bachmeyer in Vienna, Austria. The company has its own online panel with 28,000 survey partners throughout Austria and also has its own call center located in Vienna.
14 Wolfgang Bachmeyer, "APA/OGM Vertrauensindex BundespolitikerInnen März/April 2020," OGM Research and Communication, 2020, accessed June 28, 2021, https://www.ogm.at/2020/04/ 01/apa-ogm-vertrauensindex-bundespolitikerinnen-marz-april-2020/.
15 Bargain and Aminjonov 2020; Han, Hu, and Nigg 2011.
16 Interior Minister Karl Nehammer went from minus four trust points in January to 29 points by April and Chancellor Kurz and Health Minister Anschober settled at 51 and 49 respectively, with over 30 point gains on Bachmeyer, "APA/OGM Vertrauensindex BundespolitikerInnen März/ April 2020."

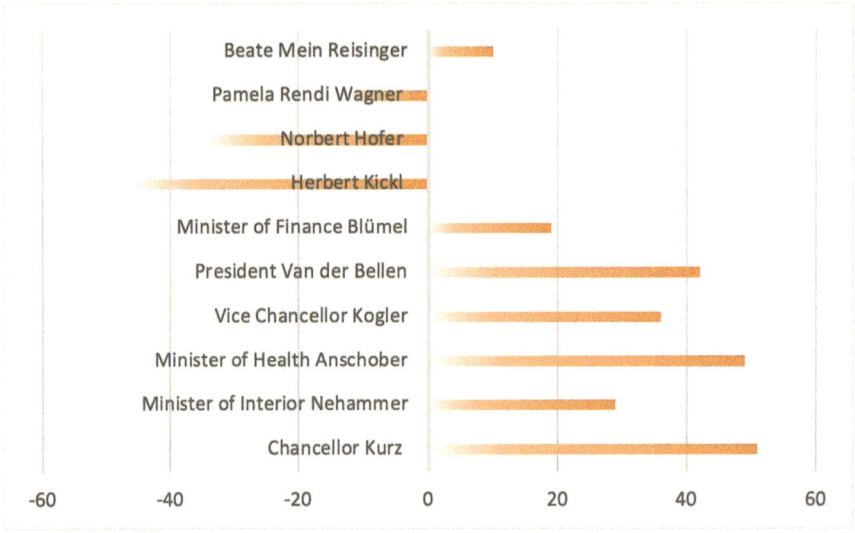

Figure 2: Confidence Rating Points March 2020. Source: Wolfgang Bachmeyer, "APA/OGM Vertrauensindex BundespolitikerInnen März/April 2020," OGM Research and Communication, 2020, accessed April 28, 2021, https://www.ogm.at/2020/04/01/apa-ogm-vertrauensindex-bundespolitikerinnen-marz-april-2020/.

The trio effectively decreased panic and confusion surrounding the first lock-down that went into effect on March 16. They communicated in small steps preparing the populace for more extensive changes, which were announced on March 13 and included school, store, and restaurant closures. One day after announcing the lockdown, the Parliament unanimously passed several COVID-19 laws that would go into effect in the coming weeks, including exit restrictions, economic aid measures, and additional security measures.[18]

Decisions were made on the national level for the entire country. An exception to this was the March 15 quarantine for the province of Tyrol, including traffic restrictions, restriction of movement, and a general call for confinement. This strict lockdown, one day before the general lockdown, was spurred due to complaints

---

17 Wolfgang Bachmeyer, "APA/OGM Vertrauensindex BundespolitikerInnen März/April 2020," OGM Research and Communication, 2020, accessed April 28, 2021, https://www.ogm.at/2020/04/01/apa-ogm-vertrauensindex-bundespolitikerinnen-marz-april-2020/.

18 Traar Christina and Claudia Gigler, "Coronavirus in ÖsterreichAusgangsbeschränkungen, Kontrollen Ab Montag, Zivil- Und Präsenzdienst Verlängert," Kleine Zeitung, 2020, accessed June 8, 2021, https://www.kleinezeitung.at/international/corona/5784852/Coronavirus-in-Oes terreich_Ausgang-in-ganz-Oesterreich-beschraenkt.

from Scandinavian countries that the ski mecca Ischgl had covered up a corona outbreak in late February, early March.[19] The hesitation of local authorities to report the Ischgl hotspot was likely linked with fears surrounding a shortened ski season in Austria.[20] After this scandal, other popular ski resorts were quicker to act. The Arlberg was quarantined on March 17, and three municipalities in Salzburg (Gasteintal, Großarltal, and Flauchau) were quarantined on March 18.

To counterbalance the lockdown measures, the government introduced a 38 billion euro aid package (more than 1% of the country's GDP). Chancellor Kurz introduced the package on March 18, stating that "no matter the cost, we will save jobs," and vice Chancellor Kogler assured that "no one will be left behind."[21] The interesting thing about this aid package was that it went against the Conservative approach to the welfare state, which favors savings plans and retrenchment[22] as opposed to increasing the deficit to help struggling businesses and workers.

The March 2020 polls revealed that these measures were successful, and Austrian public opinion was overwhelmingly (74%) in favor of the government's reaction to the pandemic.[23] This immense understanding and support for the restrictions of freedom the Austrian public had to endure was likely a result of the timely, relatively transparent, and well-communicated leadership of the national government on the one hand and the cooperation of the *Länder*, social partners, and relevant stakeholders on the other. On April 6, Chancellor Kurz, accompanied by vice Chancellor Kogler, announced the "start-up plan" that would take Austria out of its first Lockdown on April 14, wherein a step-by-step opening of stores would ensue. On April 14, Chancellor Kurz held another press conference where he stated that the government's plans for the following months were: "As much

---

19 Iceland declared Ischgl an area of risk on March 5, implying that the infections were already spreading before that time. Austrian officials in Tyrol did not confirm the outbreak until March 10 after almost a week of denial and inaction; Jakob Winter and Thomas Hoisl, "Causa Ischgl: Behörden Spielten Corona-Gefahr Herunter," Profil, 2020, accessed May 15, 2021, https://www.profil.at/oesterreich/causa-ischgl-behoerden-spielten-corona-gefahr-herunter/401058831.

20 Konrad Lachmayer, "Austria: Rule of Law Lacking in Times of Crisis," Verfassungsblog, accessed May 15, 2021, 2020, https://verfassungsblog.de/rule-of-law-lacking-in-times-of-crisis/.

21 Michael Bachner, "38 Milliarden Gegen Corona: Koste Es, Was Es Wolle," Kurier, 2020, accessed April 28, 2021, https://kurier.at/politik/inland/38-milliarden-gegen-corona-koste-es-was-es-wolle/400785833.

22 Michelle Falkenbach, M.P.M. Bekker, and S.L. Greer, "Do Political Parties Matter to Health?," *European Journal of Public Health* 29, no. Supplement_4 (2019): ckz185–781.

23 Evgenia Koptyug, "Opinions on Measures against the Coronavirus (COVID-19) in Austria in 2020," Statista, 2021, accessed May 5, 2021, https://www-statista-com.proxy.lib.umich.edu/statistics/1116220/measures-against-coronavirus-covid-19-opinion-austria/.

freedom as possible and as many restrictions as necessary."[24] By May 15, all restaurants and bars opened their doors, and on May 29, hotels and tourist attractions opened again, thereby putting an end to the first wave in Austria.

In summary, Austria presented itself well during the first wave. Even though Austria, among other countries (particularly Germany), is very rooted in a bureaucratic constitutional state *Rechststaat*, public administrations in Austria reacted quickly and unusually flexibly in their adjustment of laws and governance structures to combat the COVID-19 pandemic.[25] Orders from the National government were swiftly applied without discussion from the *Länder*, municipalities, social partners, or, surprisingly, opposition members. This, in turn, resulted in an increase in public support and compliance, which enforced the effectiveness of the measures.

Summer (June – August 2020)

The summer months can be divided into two parts. The first saw the government bask in praise, allowing them to claim credit for being one of the first countries to re-open and return to a new normal. The second half of the summer, moving into the fall, showed a different picture, namely the beginning of an unraveling government that was chasing the pandemic more than controlling it. Media attention from across the globe showered Austria and, specifically, Chancellor Kurz with compliments for their/his quick and decisive measures and subsequent early openings and relaxation measures.[26] However, while the government was enjoying international praise from abroad, the country's internal situation was changing. The *Länder*, specifically those led by SPÖ[27] governors, and

---

24 Austrian Press Agency, "Was Hat Die Regierung Gut Gemacht, Was Weniger Gut?," accessed April 30, 2021 (Die Presse, 2020), https://www.diepresse.com/5799961/was-hat-die-regierung-gut-gemacht-was-weniger-gut.

25 Rahel M Schomaker and Michael W Bauer, "Mild Hit, Flexible Response: How Local Administrations in Austria and Germany Confronted (First Wave) of the COVID-19 Pandemic," in *Good Public Governance in a Global Pandemic*, ed. Paul Joyce and Fabienne Maron (Brussels: IIAS Public Governance Series, 2020), 525.

26 Elisalex Henckel, "Der Grüne, Der Kurz Die Schau Stiehlt," Welt, 2020, https://www.welt.de/politik/ausland/article206477139/Oesterreichs-Umgang-mit-Corona-Der-Gruene-der-Kurz-die-Schau-stiehlt.html; Raffaela Lindorfer and Johanna Hager, "Deutsche Medien Zu Corona-Strategie: 'Österreich Ist Einen Schritt Voraus'" (Kurier, 2020), accessed May 15, 2021, https://kurier.at/politik/inland/deutsche-medien-zu-corona-oesterreich-ist-einen-schritt-voraus/400805138.

27 SPÖ – Social Democratic Party of Austria.

the country's three opposition parties (SPÖ, FPÖ,[28] and NEOS[29]) began voicing their disapproval with governmental measures. Complaints included being excluded from discussions, that suggestions were not being heard, and that there was no transparency in the measures passed. In addition, the general public's confidence in the government began to decrease, likely a result of the increased internal conflicts and lack of transparency. Four specific points of criticism likely sparked increasing resentment and discontent.

The first situation arose in May when Chancellor Kurz led a publicity endeavor in a little town in Tyrol. He did not uphold his own distance rules and engaged with crowds that should never have been allowed to form under the corona laws. In addition, neither the Chancellor nor his companions were wearing masks.[30] Criticism rained down even from the usually silent coalition partner, the Greens. Chancellor Kurz defended his visit, stating that he asked residents to keep their distance and finally said that certain things just couldn't be planned,[31] signifying that he was above his own laws.

The second point of criticism pertained to the preparation plans, or in this case, the lack thereof, for the autumn. By June, oppositional parties began criticizing the government for not presenting concrete data and for not having a detailed plan as to what the autumn would look like. Citizens and business owners joined the criticism when it came to the topic of aid distribution. Although the Austrian government was generous with their aid, many complaints surrounded the bureaucratic hoops businesses had to jump through compared with the neighboring countries of Germany and Switzerland.[32] The government negated these claims and stated that the added bureaucracy was put in place to prevent people from abusing the aid.[33]

---

28 FPÖ – Freedom Party of Austria.

29 NEOS – The New Austria and Liberal Forum.

30 Austrian Press Agency, "Kurz Über Besuch Im Kleinwalsertal: 'Bitte Um Verständnis,'" Salzburger Nachrichten, 2020, accessed May 1, 2021, https://www.sn.at/politik/innenpolitik/kurz-ueber-besuch-im-kleinwalsertal-bitte-um-verstaendnis-87524992.

31 Maria Jelenko-Benedikt, "Kurz Verteidigt Seinen Besuch Im Kleinwalsertal," meinbezirk.at, 2020, accessed May 8, 2021, https://www.meinbezirk.at/wieden/c-politik/kurz-verteidigt-seinen-besuch-im-kleinwalsertal_a4069164.

32 Zachary Desson et al., "Europe's Covid-19 Outliers: German, Austrian and Swiss Policy Responses during the Early Stages of the 2020 Pandemic," *Health Policy and Technology* (2020), https://doi.org/https://doi.org/10.1016/j.hlpt.2020.09.003.

33 Jörg Leichtfried, "Es Braucht Echte Hilfe Statt Leerer Versprechen – Das Versagen Der Kurz-Regierung Bei Der Bekämpfung Der Wirtschaftlichen Und Sozialen Krisen-Folgen" (Vienna, 2020), accessed April 28, 2021, https://www.parlament.gv.at/PAKT/VHG/XXVII/NRSITZ/NRSITZ_00032/A_-_15_00_31_00216316.html.

The third point of criticism surrounded several inopportune mistakes made by members of the national government. The first occurred during a budget meeting where the SPÖ discovered that Finance Minister Blümel (new ÖVP) forgot to add six zeros into the budget, thus showing that only €102,000 were used for corona measures. This displayed excessive carelessness and increased the doubt surrounding Blümel's role as Minister of Finance. To make matters worse, Minister Blümel, as well as Chancellor Kurz, had to take the stand in the Ibiza investigation.[34] While Austria follows the innocent until proven guilty rule, it was rather suspicious that both officials answered that they "could not remember"[35] details of their involvement when questioned by investigators. In fact, Minister Blümel said this 86 times during his investigation, and Chancellor Kurz mentioned his foggy memory 29 times. This occurrence also marked the first time that Chancellor Kurz and his new ÖVP actively criticized judicial proceedings, thereby attempting to divert attention from the actual trial.

Suspicion of corruption is not a new concept in Austria; in fact, it has always plagued the country, sometimes more, sometimes less (see Austria's Corruption Index).[36] The 2021 Council of Europe summarized the situation in Austria as "failing in its fight against corruption through insignificant progress."[37] It is not just corruption among governmental officials, but also the amount of bribery taking place amongst Austrian officials that remains particularly problematic in the country. Austria shows "above-average bribery rates when compared to West-

---

34 The "Ibiza scandal" was an Austrian political scandal that was triggered by the publication of a secretly recorded video in May of 2019. The scandal caused the ÖVP-FPÖ coalition to collapse when Chancellor Kurz was voted out of office (see Frederik Obermaier and Bastian Obermayer, *The Ibiza Affair* (Kiepenheuer and Witsch, 2019), https://bilder-kiwi.s3.eu-central-1.amazonaws.com/sampletranslations/obermaier_obermayer_ibiza_englishsample.pdf. for more information) and opened the door to several additional investigations of corruption and bribery including the "Casino Affair" where the Novomatic Gaming group made a significant donation to the ÖVP in return for tax aid in Italy Renate Graber, "Geplatzter Traum: Wie Novomatic Und Sazka Die Casinos Austria Aufteilen Wollten," der Standard, 2021, https://www.derstandard.at/story/2000126511730/geplatzter-traum-vom-glueck-wie-novomatic-undsazka-die-casinos-austria; Sam Jones, "Graft Probe Reaches into the Highest Levels of Austria's Government," Financial Times, 2021, accessed July 28, 2021, https://www.ft.com/content/40847df7-cc7a-42f0-8294-6e6de4e8997f.
35 Hans Rauscher, "Ein Akt Der Vergesslichkeit," der Standard, 2020, accessed April 20, 2021, https://www.derstandard.at/story/2000118352698/ein-akt-der-vergesslichkeit.
36 Trading Economics, "Austria Corruption Index," Trading Economics, 2021, accessed July 28, 2021, https://tradingeconomics.com/austria/corruption-index.
37 Euronews and AFP, "Austria Has Failed in Fight against Corruption, Says Council of Europe," Euronews, 2021, accessed July 28, 2021, https://www.euronews.com/2021/03/01/austria-has-failed-in-fight-against-corruption-says-council-of-europe.

ern European countries."[38] Looking beyond bribery, the calling in of favors or use of personal connection in Austria is one of the highest across Europe.[39]

The worrying aspect of these continued developments is threefold: 1) when considering COVID-19 management, accusations of corruption within the government impact trust. As previously mentioned, trust impacts compliance and acceptance of rules and restrictions during a pandemic. In addition, increased corruption leads to democratic backsliding and a decreased trust in institutions both of which have a negative impact on the country's welfare state, its connection with the European Union and the well-being of the general public; 2) Chancellor Kurz and Finance Minister Blümel did not admit to the accusations that were made, instead they chose tactics of deflection, avoidance and blame (see Table 1) resulting in no charges and no consequences (as of yet) for the officials; 3) even if new elections were to be called out due to these charges, there is little hope of improved progress in fighting corruption.

Table 1: Corruption scandals.

Scandal	Uncovered	Accused	Blame Avoidance
Ibiza Scandal	May 2019 hearings began June 2020, "Ibiza Committee Hearings"[40]	Former Vice Chancellor Strache	
"Casino Affair" aka Novomatic Scandal	August 2019 hearings within Ibiza Committee	Finance Minister Blümel	Criticize the Ibiza Committee; criticize the legal system – requested an independent state attorney[41] (backed by entire ÖVP and Chancellor Kurz)

---

38 Martinez B. Kukutschka 2021, 18.

39 Martinez B. Kukutschka 2021, 23.

40 The "Ibiza U-Ausschauss" or Committee of Inquiry into the alleged marketability of the turquoise-blue federal government (Ibiza Committee of Inquiry) began in January 2020. Within this committee the scandals surrounding Novomatic and ÖBAG were uncovered. The committee was forced to end its inquiries in July 2021 as the new ÖVP and Greens (together a majority in Parliament) voted against its continuation.

41 On February 15 the new ÖVP requested, for the first time in their history, an independent attorney general. This is pivotal for two reasons: 1) the request was made around the time that Gernot Blümel was accused of corruption involving the Novamatic scandal; and 2) requests for an independent attorney general have been made repeatedly by the opposition parties over the past decades. Currently, Austria's attorney general sits within the Ministry of Justice and is

Table 1: Corruption scandals. *(Continued)*

Scandal	Uncovered	Accused	Blame Avoidance
ÖBAG Scandal[42]	March 2021 hearings within Ibiza Committee	Chancellor Kurz & Finance Minister Blümel	Get rid of some ÖVP officials (Brandstetter, Schmid)[43]; re-focus on migration; announce corona relaxation measures

A final point of criticism involved the corona measures. On July 22, the Health Ministry's Corona ordinance was deemed illegal by the Austrian constitutional court[44] and thus 35,000 violations were void. Also, in July, the government started its test offense claiming to want to test over 30,000 people per week, and two days later, Minister Anschober (Greens) introduced the traffic light system to determine how dangerous the COVID-19 situation was in every Austrian district. Every Friday would be "traffic light day," wherein districts and cities would be assigned colors depending on various indicators. What the different colors actually meant[45] was not announced until September 14 where a law stated that

---

not independent of that house (generally controlled by the ÖVP), which increases polarization and party politics.

42 Chancellor Kurz and Finance Minister Blümel both allegedly helped civil servant Thomas Schmid secure the powerful position as head of the ÖBAG, a state holding that can be seen as a National Wealth Fund. Investigations into the claims have secured chat protocols suggesting that Schmid wrote the job description for which he later applied to and that Chancellor Kurz wrote that Schmid would "get everything (he) wants"; Matthew Karnitschnig, "The House of Kurz Scandal, Explained," Politico, 2021, accessed July 28, 2021, https://www.politico.eu/article/the-house-of-sebastian-kurz-scandal-explained-austria-chancellor-perjury-allegations/.

43 Wolgang Brandstetter (ÖVP) previously served as Minister of Justice (2013–2017) and was most recently a legal scholar serving as a member of the Austrian Constitutional Court (2018–2021). In 2021, Brandstetter resigned after a chat protocol that contained sexist and racist language became public. In addition, he is suspected of having passed on information about an investigation against the former politician Christoph Chorherr (Greens) to the entrepreneur Michael Tojner. Thomas Schmid (ÖVP) is under investigation for several wrongdoings, however the most popular is how Schmid became ÖBAG head. According to text messages exchanged between himself and Chancellor Kurz, he apparently had the job description tailored to himself and helped with the selection of the ÖBAG supervisory board, which would later appoint him.

44 Austrian Constitutional Court 2020.

45 See Kroisleitner, Mittelstaedt, and Scherndl 2020.

all measures would be the same across the country. Each province could increase the measures as they saw fit.[46]

While this "traffic light system" sounded logical, arguments between the districts and cities as well as between the federal government and the regions became louder. Complaints arose that it was not fair, for example, that Wiener Neustadt (new ÖVP governor), with an incidence rating of 44, was green, while Linz (SPÖ governor), with an incidence of only 26, was yellow. Arguments intensified when Governor Platter of Tyrol (new ÖVP) argued for increased regional diversification between communities and municipalities regarding the COVID-19 measures. Governor Luger of Linz (SPÖ) stated: "the color scheme was absolutely incomprehensible and had no relation to the reality in the city (Linz)."[47] As the month of September progressed, the "corona traffic light" was deemed chaotic by all opposition parties; even Chancellor Kurz stated that one had to discern between two things: "the traffic light and governmental decisions," signifying that both were not on the same page,[48] despite coming from the same offices.

The diverging agendas became apparent when Chancellor Kurz warned citizens of a second wave stating that "the virus comes by car."[49] As a result, 800 soldiers and 500 police officers were sent to the Southern borders of Carinthia and Tyrol. What ensued were horrendous waiting times (12 h) and very upset travelers as well as cross-border workers. While travel warnings were assigned through the Foreign Ministry (new ÖVP), the Health Ministry (Greens) designed these border regulations, forcing regional implementation. The outcome showed the province of Carinthia blaming the Health Ministry for the chaos and vice-versa. The blame for these chaotic regulations was passed between the *Länder* and the national government, with no one wanting to be responsible.

Given these points of criticism, the confidence index scores began to decline throughout the summer (Figure 3). By July, most politicians' scores had lost at least five percentage points from their all-time highs back in April (Kurz, Nehammer, Kogler, Blümel, Anschober). One explanation for this could be the reduced press conferences and the fact that the government's media presence in general

---

46 Health Committee, "Gesundheitsausschuss: 'Corona-Ampel-Gesetz' Mit Den Stimmen von ÖVP, Grünen Und SPÖ Angenommen," Austrian Parliament (Austria, 2020), accessed May 6, 2021, https://www.parlament.gv.at/PAKT/PR/JAHR_2020/PK0918/index.shtml#.
47 ORF, "Erste Ampelschaltung Erhitzt Gemüter," news ORF.at, 2020, accessed May 3, 2021, https://orf.at/stories/3180035/.
48 ORF, "Zeit Im Bild 15.09.20" (Austria: ORF, 2020).
49 Julia Wenzel, "'Virus Kommt Mit Dem Auto': Kontrollen Und Tests Für Heimkehrer," Die Presse, accessed April 28, 2021, 2020, https://www.diepresse.com/5853699/virus-kommt-mit-dem-auto-kontrollen-und-tests-fur-heimkehrer.

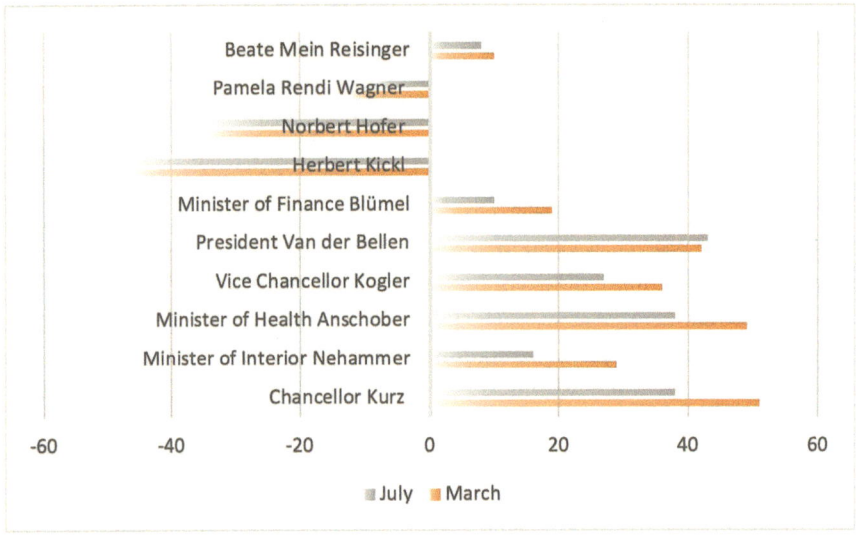

Figure 3: Confidence Rating Points March vs. July 2020. Wolfgang Bachmayer, "APA/OGM Vertrauensindex BundespolitikerInnen Juli 2020," OGM Research and Communication, 2020, accessed April 24, 2021, https://www.ogm.at/2020/07/13/apa-ogm-vertrauensindex-bundes politikerinnen-juli-2020/.

decreased.[50] Looking specifically at the decreases surrounding Chancellor Kurz and Finance Minister Blümel (-13 and -9 respectively), the corruption charges surrounding the Novomatic and ÖBAG scandals processed within the Ibiza hearings likely took a toll on their favorability. The blame avoidance strategies practiced by Kurz and Blümel to deflect attention from their accusations likely prevented their numbers from tanking. In terms of the pandemic, while the government, particularly Chancellor Kurz, claimed credit for having mastered the first wave of the pandemic, signs of discord amongst the government and other actors became apparent, building up to a tumultuous autumn. Specifically, the relations between the *Länder* and the national government became increasingly strained.

---

50 Wolfgang Bachmayer, "APA/OGM Vertrauensindex BundespolitikerInnen Juli 2020," OGM Research and Communication, 2020, accessed April 24, 2021, https://www.ogm.at/2020/07/13/ apa-ogm-vertrauensindex-bundespolitikerinnen-juli-2020/.

Second Wave (September 2020-February 2021)

The more or less relaxed summer months turned into a hectic autumn with numbers increasing and the government struggling to find acceptable solutions. It was during this wave that we saw Chancellor Kurz begin to share his spotlight with the social partners (Austria's most important form of civil society)[51] and the *Länder,* signifying that unpopular decisions (further lockdowns) had to be made and the governmental coalition needed support in communicating undesirable measures (see Table 2). This so-called "regionalization of the COVID-19 crisis management"[52] [53] led to considerable delays in implementing contact tracing and different vaccination strategies. These decisions and the governments' lack of preparation further decreased their confidence ratings and led to the passing of blame.

With the new corona laws[54] introduced at the end of September, the lockdowns now had a legal basis, and high fees could be charged for not wearing a mask in public. Two opposition parties, the FPÖ, and the NEOS, saw these changes as a massive invasion into people's right to freedom and voted against the laws increasing tensions between the government and opposition parties. With these laws, the *Länder* officially received more power to develop stricter measures to fight the pandemic. The consistent back and forth between who was making decisions (national government or *Länder*) and whether the corona laws were legally binding or not was likely a reason for the decrease in trust (although not as significant as one might have guessed) of governmental officials (see Figure 4).[55] This translated, as the section will demonstrate, into the public's reluctance to adhere to recommendations, their unwillingness to participate in the mass testing strategy, and an initial vaccination scepsis.

---

51 Scott L. Greer and Michelle Falkenbach, "Social Partnership, Civil Society and Health Care," in *Civil Society and Health: Contributions and Potential* (Copenhagen: WHO, 2017), 141–59.

52 While the first wave of the pandemic saw the national government take control of measures and decisions, the second wave saw the reigns of the COVID-19 management being passed to the regions.

53 Maria M. Hofmarcher and Christopher Singhuber, "Föderalismus Im GesundheitswesenSchwächen Des COVID-19 Krisenmanagements" (Vienna, 2021), accessed July 17, 2021, http://www.healthsystemintelligence.eu/docs/HSI_PolicyBrief_Foederalismus_06_2021_final.pdf.

54 Ministry of Health, "Coronavirus – Rechtliches," Bundesministerium für Soziales Gesundheit Pflege und Konsumentenschutz, 2020, accessed April 28, 2021, https://www.sozialministerium.at/Informationen-zum-Coronavirus/Coronavirus--Rechtliches.html.

55 Wolfgang Bachmeyer, "Vertrauensindex Bundespolitiker November 2020," OGM Research and Communication, 2020, accessed April 24, 2021, https://www.ogm.at/2020/11/20/apa-ogm-vertrauensindex-bundespolitiker-november-2020/.

Table 2: Credit and blame.

Time Period	Decision Makers	Credit	Blame
First wave (March–May 2020)	Chancellor Kurz Minister Nehammer Minister Anschober	Quick action and adjustment of laws to combat COVID-19	
Summer (June–August 2020)	Chancellor Kurz Minister Anschober	Early re-opening of stores, restaurants, hotels, etc.	
Second wave (Sept 2020–Feb 2021)	Government *Länder* Social Partners	Vaccination Press	*Länder*, Technology
Third Wave (March–May 2021)	Government *Länder* Social Partners Opposition	Race to announce the end of the lockdown	EU/Health Minister/ Vaccine Production

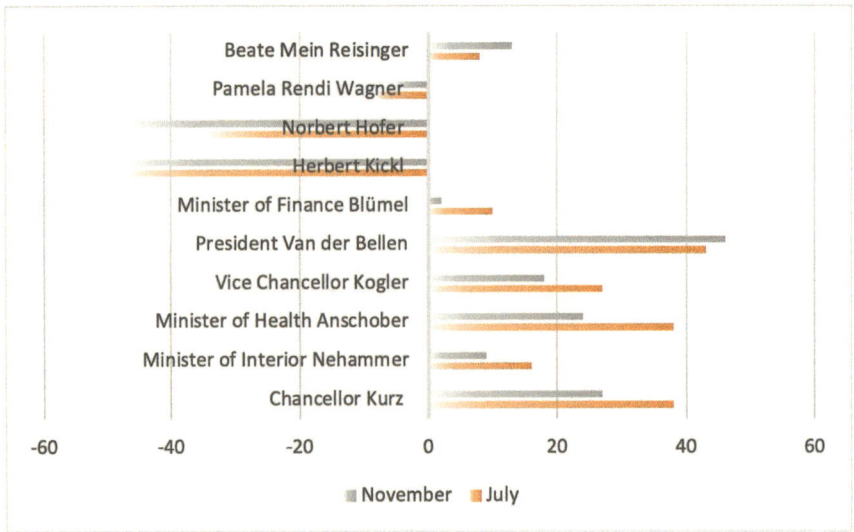

Figure 4: Confidence Rating Points July vs. November 2020. Source: Wolfgang Bachmayer, "APA/OGM Vertrauensindex BundespolitikerInnen Juli 2020," OGM Research and Communication, 2020, accessed April 24, 2021, https://www.ogm.at/2020/07/13/apa-ogm-vertrauens index-bundespolitikerinnen-juli-2020/.

By the beginning of October, Minister Anschober announced that the number of new corona cases was getting too high and negatively impacting the economy.

Therefore, he proposed that additional regional measures should be implemented to decrease the numbers.[56] However, regional solutions as foreseen by the traffic light system did not come. Instead, speculations of a new lockdown ran rampant with viable solutions, including either a "lockdown lite" beginning on November 2 or a two to three week hard lockdown starting on November 16. Members of the government gave contradictory messages about the probability of a new lockdown: Economic Minister Schrambock (new ÖVP) told the press that the lockdown scenarios were likely given the increasing numbers. At the same time, Minister Anschober said he could not imagine another lockdown,[57] further confusing the public.

With 2,551 new cases per day by October 23, Minister Anschober told people to stay at home. Two days later, Chancellor Kurz and Vice-Chancellor Kogler also pleaded with the population to take the pandemic seriously, signifying that public trust and cooperation with governmental guidelines were low. With over 4,000 daily cases just a few days later, the government announced plans for new measures and called upon the social partners and the *Länder* to help communicate the decision. The involvement of the other actors helped the coalition divide the responsibility of sending the country back into a lockdown, thereby dispersing the blame.

On November 14, Austria made headlines as the country with the most new COVID-19 cases (10,000 per day) worldwide.[58] This led the government to move from its "lockdown lite," implemented just a week prior, into a second hard lockdown beginning November 14 (Table 3), wherein everything would close, and an all-day curfew would be put in place. The opposition's critic was particularly harsh: FPÖ Party head Herbert Kickl stated, "Kurz, Kogler, Anschober, and Nehammer are trying to carry the Austrian Republic to its grave,"[59] and SPÖ party head Pamela Rendi-Wagner said, "this new lockdown is no more than a

---

56 Austrian Press Agency, "Corona-Zahlen 'Stabil, Aber Auf Deutlich Zu Hohem Niveau,'" Wiener Zeitung, 2020, accessed April 26, 2021, https://www.wienerzeitung.at/nachrichten/politik/oesterreich/2077313-Anschober-Wir-muessen-runter-mit-diesen-Zahlen.html.
57 Wiener Zeitung 2020.
58 Austrian Press Agency, "Österreich Mit Höchster Neuinfektionsrate Weltweit," Die Presse, accessed May 2, 2021, 2020, https://www.diepresse.com/5897665/osterreich-mit-hochster-neu infektionsrate-weltweit.
59 Freiheitlicher Parlamentsklub, "FPÖ – Kickl Zu Lockdown: Regierung Hat Nichts Dazugelernt," Austrian Press Agency, 2020, accessed April 30, 2021, https://www.ots.at/presseaus sendung/OTS_20201114_OTS0031/fpoe-kickl-zu-lockdown-regierung-hat-nichts-dazugelernt.

confirmation of guilt of the complete loss of control."[60] As far as the *Länder* were concerned, the six[61] led by the new ÖVP stood behind the government's lockdown, while the three[62] SPÖ-led *Länder* showered the government with criticisms for its indecisiveness.

In-between the second Lockdown on November 14 and a third lockdown that would come on December 26, the government announced plans for mass testing. There were several issues with this plan. The first was the lack of support from health experts, who spoke out against the mass testing plan, stating that single mass tests not only gave people a false sense of hope but only provided a snapshot of the population's state.[63] A better solution would be to increase testing in general.[64] Then, IT issues within the Ministry of Health led to delays, especially in Vienna.[65] These problems persisted, forcing the *Länder* to rely on their own software to document the tests. Finally, the mass testing uptake amongst the population was low. Only around 22% of the population participated[66] signifying, once again, a lack of willingness to comply with governmental guidelines.

On December 27, Austria received its first vaccine shipment but did not announce the vaccination start date until January 12. The government held the distributed vaccines back, except for photo opportunities, for more than two weeks. SPÖ party whip Jörg Leichtfried criticized this harshly, stating, "the difference between Austrian and Israel regarding vaccinations is that in Israel 1 million people were vaccinated and in Austria, there were 1 million pictures taken of the Chancellor at a vaccination site in Vienna."[67] After massive criticism, Anschober promised that 30,000 people would be vaccinated within the second week of January. This resulted in disapproval from the *Länder*, who were responsible

---

60 Daniela Kittner, "Rendi-Wagner: 'Der Weg in Den Dritten Lockdown Ist Programmiert,'" Kurier, 2020, accessed April 28, 2021, https://kurier.at/politik/ausland/rendi-wagner-der-weg-in-den-dritten-lockdown-ist-programmiert/401097894.

61 Vorarlberg, Tirol, Salzburg, Upper Austria, Lower Austria, and Styria.

62 Carinthia, Burgenland, and Vienna.

63 András Szigetvari, and Karin Pollack, "Taskforce Im Gesundheitsministerium Gegen Massentestung Wie in Der Slowakei," der Standard, 2020, accessed April 29, 2021, https://www.derstandard.de/story/2000121950069/taskforce-im-gesundheitsministerium-gegen-massentestung-wie-in-der-slowakei.

64 Luís Carlos Lopes-Júnior et al., "Effectiveness of Mass Testing for Control of COVID-19: A Systematic Review Protocol," *BMJ Open* 10, no. 8 (August 1, 2020): e040413, accessed May 3, 2021, https://doi.org/10.1136/bmjopen-2020-040413.

65 Josef Gebhard, "Corona-Massentests: Cyber-Attacke Und Datenpanne Legte Website Lahm," accessed April 29, 2021, Kurier, 2020, https://kurier.at/chronik/wien/corona-massentests-cyber-attacke-legte-anmelde-website-lahm/401116881.

66 Austrian Press Agency 2020c.

67 ORF, "Zeit Im Bild 5.1.21" (Austria: ORF, 2021).

for deciding whom they would vaccinate, but had no power over the distribution of the vaccines themselves. Without vaccines, which had not been distributed at the time of the announcement, the *Länder* could not vaccinate.

This delayed vaccination start as well as the problems surrounding the distribution of the vaccines presumably attributed to the decrease in citizens' trust in the government, as well as their distrust in the vaccines (Figure 5). To counteract the increasing skepticism, the government announced the commencement of the initiative "Austria Vaccinates," an information campaign to increase the transparency around the Austrian vaccination plan.[68] Despite the national government's efforts to turn around the slow vaccination start, opposition parties criticized the government as being "chaotic" and moving at a "snail's pace," accusing them of letting thousands of vaccinations lie around for weeks.[69] Criticism surrounding vaccination took another turn when it was uncovered that local politicians were getting their vaccines before the elderly.[70]

To make matters worse, the government announced an extension of the third lockdown until at least January 24 (Table 3). This was extended again until at least February 7, with the government stating that the incidence rate needed to, ideally, decrease to 50.[71] Citizens were becoming increasingly upset by the government's contradictory messages. The opposition's criticism ranged from the government being completely incompetent (NEOS) to the fact that lockdowns were superfluous (FPÖ).[72] Even Economic Chamber President Harald Mahrer (new ÖVP) demanded that the government re-open businesses.

---

68 Austrian Red Cross, "Österreich Impft," oesterreich-impft.at, 2021, accessed July 18, 2021, https://www.oesterreich-impft.at/.

69 ORF, "Zeit Im Bild 13.1.21" (Austria: ORF, 2021).

70 Gabriele Scherndl, Oona Kroisleitner, and Thomas Neuhold, "Kaum Konsequenzen Für Impfvordrängler," der Standard, 2021, accessed July 20, 2021, https://www.derstandard.at/consent/tcf/story/2000123472048/kaum-konsequenzen-fuer-impf-vordraengler.

71 Kleine Zeitung, "Inzidenz-Zahl 50 Unerreichbar Neuinfektionen in Österreich Erneut Bei Über 1500," Kleine Zeitung, 2021, https://www.kleinezeitung.at/oesterreich/5932709/Inzidenz Zahl-50-unerreichbar_Neuinfektionen-in-Oesterreich-erneut.

72 ORF, "Zeit in Bild Österreich 4.01.2021" (Austria, 2021).

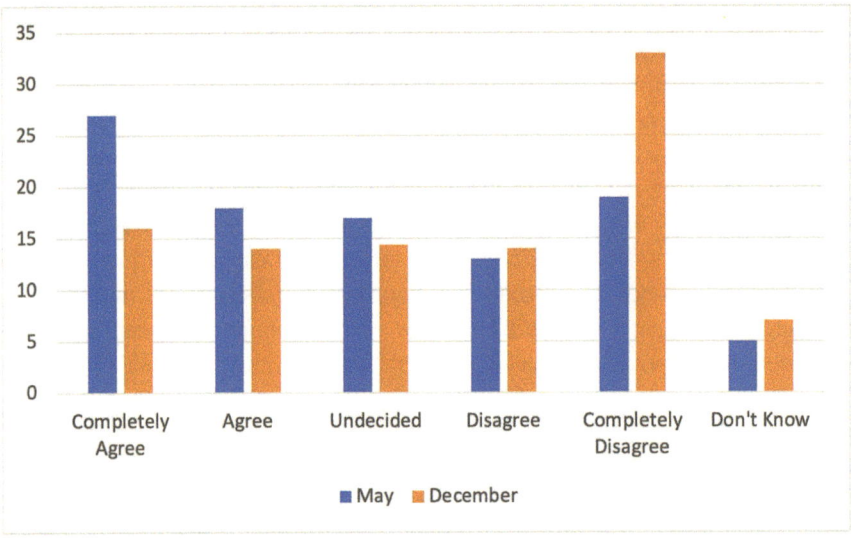

Figure 5: Vaccination willingness in Austria in May 2020 vs. December 2020. Source: attitudes towards coronavirus vaccination in May and December 2021 (data: ACPP, each N = approx. 1500, weighted). Jakob-Moritz Eberl, Julia Partheymüller, and Katharina T. Paul, "Impfbereitschaft in Österreich Stabil – Doch Nicht Jeder Impfstoff Gleich Beliebt" (Vienna, 2021), https://viecer.univie.ac.at/corona-blog/corona-blog-beitraege/blog104/.

Table 3: Lockdowns in Austria.

Lockdowns	Announced	Implemented	Extended	Extended	Ended
First lockdown	March 13	March 16			April 14
Lockdown Lite	October 30	November 3			Transferred into second lockdown
Second lockdown		November 17			December 6
Third lockdown	December 18	December 26	January 24	February 7	February 7 and then May 19*
Easter Lockdown	March 22	April 1	April 18		May 2[73]

* February 7 marked small openings (stores, services) while May 19 marked the opening of restaurants, sports clubs, and cultural attractions.

73 Burgenland ended its lockdown two weeks prior, on April 18.

By the beginning of February, the pressure to relax measures became too great. Although the seven-day incidence for 100,000 people was at 108 (not 50), the government relaxed measures allowing shops and services to open. On February 27, the government, in combination with the *Länder*, the social partners, and the opposition, announced additional opening steps, including outdoor seating in restaurants by March 27. Several days later, the national government also made the executive decision to place *Länder* and districts under quarantine if their incidence rate increased. At the same time, the national government issued a recommended travel warning for the province of Tyrol due to an outbreak of the South African COVID-19 strain. Governor Platter accepted the national government's decision to decrease the mobility of the Tyroleans but did not accept isolating the province, stating "the data does not call for such measures."[74] This demonstrated the national government's powerlessness against the will of the *Länder*, a concept well known as federalism.

At this point in the pandemic, the confidence index showed a continuation of the November decline, with practically all politicians' scores decreasing. The sustained loss of confidence could be attributed to increased dissatisfaction with the crisis management of those responsible coupled with the ongoing corruption proceedings surrounding high-ranking members of the ÖVP (see Figure 6). What this second wave demonstrated was how well the government dispersed blame. The more the government had to impose strict lockdowns, the more important it was for them to pull in other actors (*Länder*, Social Partners, and even the opposition) into the decision-making process. This helped divide the blame, thereby likely preventing the confidence ratings of the governmental officials from diminishing completely. While Chancellor Kurz and Minister Blümel saw further decreases in their confidence ratings (-7 and -5 respectively), their blame avoidance strategies both in terms of the pandemic management as well as with the corruption charges they were both facing seemed to have prevented more drastic losses. As we will see in the next section, what helped the government, especially Chancellor Kurz, to disperse the blame even more was the tactic of blaming the EU for a failed vaccination strategy.

In addition to the blame game, this second wave appeared to be a turning point with regards to *Länder* allegiances to the national government. Firstly, the *Länder* were no longer as compliant with national government regulations. The Länder, both ÖVP and SPÖ-led, increasingly chose to disregard national government requests (Luger in Linz and Platter in Tyrol). In addition, the SPÖ-led *Länder* more often than not found themselves on the side of the opposition

---

74 ORF, "Platter Erteilt Isolation Tirols Absage," orf.at, 2021, https://orf.at/stories/3200190/.

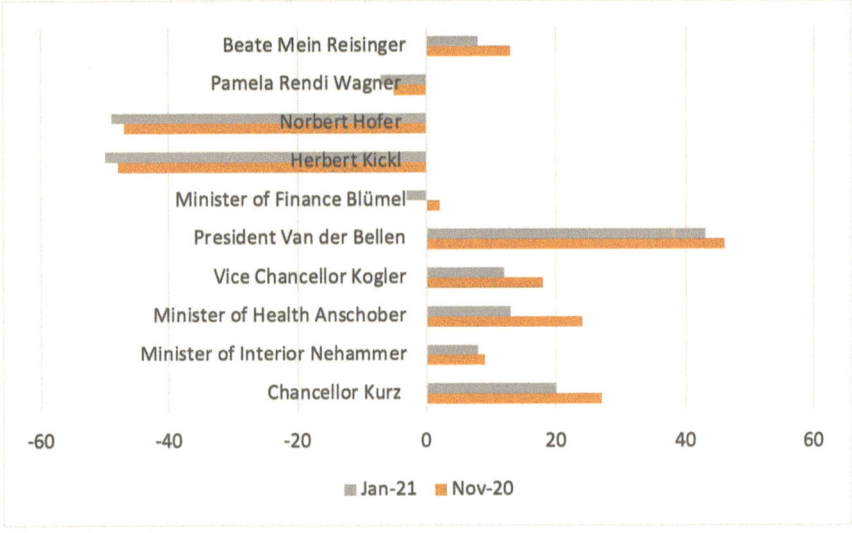

Figure 6: Confidence Ratings November 2020 vs. January 2021. Source: Wolfgang Bachmeyer, "Kommentar OGM/APA-Vertrauensindex Bundespolitiker Jänner 2021," OGM Research and Communication, 2021, accessed April 24, 2021, https://www.ogm.at/2021/01/15/ogm-apa-ver trauensindex-bundespolitiker-jaenner-2021/.

criticizing governmental measures for being chaotic and delayed, while the ÖVP-led *Länder* commonly supported governmental decisions, especially when they came directly from Chancellor Kurz.

Third Wave (March – May 2021)

The third wave reaffirmed the Austrian government's struggle with COVID-19. Events during this period showed further decreasing trust scores, renewed attempts to blame failed policies, and a nation on the brink of democratic backsliding. The first part of this section will surround the corona measures, including the vaccine distribution issues, the "Eastern lockdown," and the country's relaxation measures. The second half of the section will move into the corruption scandals plaguing new ÖVP government members.

On March 24, the government announced that the Eastern provinces of Vienna, Burgenland, and Lower Austria needed to increase their measures and close all stores and services due to the drastically increasing numbers, specifically ICU numbers (Table 3). Burgenland and Lower Austria initially disagreed but then put their *Länder* on a six-day "Easter Lockdown" from April 1 to April 7. On

March 29, Governor Ludwig (SPÖ, Vienna) announced that he would extend Vienna's lockdown until April 11; Burgenland (SPÖ) and Lower Austria (ÖVP) wanted to wait. By March 31, all three *Länder* extended their lockdowns for an additional week (Table 3). While calls for a national solution became increasingly loud, with Health Minister Anschober pleading for a single solution, the government stuck to their regional plan.

The disagreements that ensued with these three Eastern provinces highlights the delicate situation in which the *Länder* found themselves. Without the national government taking responsibility for lockdowns, it was up to the governors of these three *Länder* to make the unfavorable decision. The governors were put in a lose-lose situation as lockdowns, at this point, were increasingly unfavorable, and exploding case rates and increased hospitalizations were also to be avoided. The unanswered question that remains is whether the national government would have made the same decision, to decentralize COVID measure decisions, if the majority of ICU patients were located in ÖVP *Länder*. The guess is that this would have likely led to a quicker national lockdown to appease ÖVP governors.

Table 4: ICU beds per *Land* per million inhabitants.[75]

Länder	Governor Party	ICU
Vienna	SPÖ	122
Burgenland	SPÖ	71
Lower Austria	ÖVP	69
Upper Austria	ÖVP	49
Styria	ÖVP	49
Salzburg	ÖVP	39
Carinthia	SPÖ	23
Tyrol	ÖVP	44
Vorarlberg	ÖVP	15

Also, in April, when vaccination willingness was at an all-time high among citizens (Figure 7), it had become clear that the vaccination process was not progressing as quickly as Chancellor Kurz had announced it would due to vaccine distribution issues. To push the blame from himself, Kurz stated that the EU had created a vaccine Bazar where Austria and other countries were put at a dis-

---

75 Source: ORF, "Zeit Im Bild 6. April 2021" (Austria: ORF, 2021).

advantage.[76] This accusation led to the immediate dismissal of Clemens Auer (new ÖVP), head of the vaccine coordination for Austria.

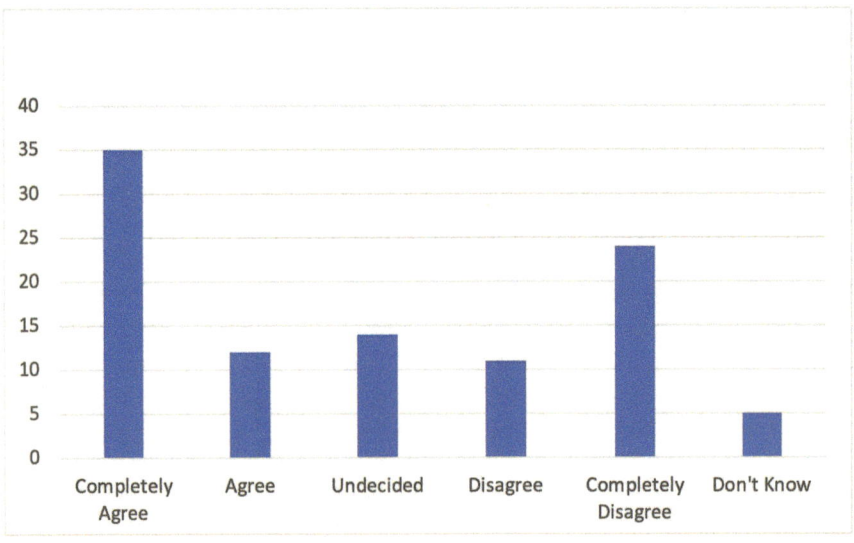

Figure 7: Vaccination willingness in Austria as of March 2021. Source: Eberl, Partheymüller, and Paul, "Impfbereitschaft in Österreich Stabil – Doch Nicht Jeder Impfstoff Gleich Beliebt." Attitudes towards coronavirus vaccination in March 2021 (data: ACPP, each N = approx. 1500, weighted).

As a likely distraction from the vaccine debacle, Chancellor Kurz announced (May 3) that the openings of all stores nationwide would come in May if the numbers decreased. He also promised that all people that wanted to be vaccinated would receive this opportunity within the next 100 days.[77] This garnered the Chancellor much criticism especially from governor Doskozil of Burgenland, who stated that "he (Kurz) show[ed] no leadership, and he [was] not making politically sound decisions." As of April 4, Austria had a vaccination rate of 20.19

---

76 Johanna Hager and Ingrid Steiner-Gashi, "Kurz: 'EU-Lieferungen Erfolgen Nicht Nach Bevölkerungsschlüssel,'" Kurier, 2021, accessed July 2, 2021, https://kurier.at/politik/inland/live-bundeskanzler-ueber-impfstofflieferungen-aus-der-eu/401216244.

77 David Krutzler, Gabriele Scherndl, and Klaus Taschwer, "Können in Den Nächsten 100 Tagen Alle Impfwilligen Geimpft Werden?," der Standard, 2021, accessed July 8, 2021, https://www.derstandard.at/story/2000125620311/koennen-in-den-naechsten-100-tagen-alle-impfwilligen-geimpft-werden.

doses per 100 people,[78] counted as a single dose. By June 3 (two months later), this number was 60.49, a far cry from Kurz's promise.

The "Eastern lockdown" was extended for a second time on April 12 for Vienna and Lower Austria while Burgenland was still deciding. The two *Länder* designated on May 2 as the end of the lockdown and made a compromise regarding schools; these would open again on April 25. SPÖ head Rendi-Wagner once again pleaded for an Austria-wide solution regarding lockdowns, stating that the number of cases as well as the number of patients in ICUs needed to decrease across the board. On April 13, Burgenland decided to stick with April 18 as the end date for its lockdown.

Also, on April 13 Health Minister Anschober stepped down, citing mental health problems as his primary reason for leaving. In addition, he stated that "by the 3rd wave, we (the Greens specifically within the Ministry of Health) noticed that the conflicts of interest increased with great strength, and I felt very left alone."[79] Not surprisingly, Anschober did not thank Chancellor Kurz or the new ÖVP in his resignation speech, signifying a very turbulent relationship with the coalition partner.

Again, to appease the public and distract from the negative press surrounding coalition difficulties and vaccination distribution problems, Chancellor Kurz announced first on April 16 and then on April 23 with a definite date that the uniform relaxation of measures for all *Länder* and all branches would begin on May 19. Heath experts and the Green coalition members were more reserved, signaling that this might be too soon.[80] For the first time since summer 2020, this opening would also include the opening of restaurants indoors and outdoors, hotels, and sport and cultural institutions. A "Green pass" (a negative test, vaccination, or any person cured of COVID-19 in the last six months) would be required to profit from the openings. The government announced that if the numbers increased in the future, then the *Länder* would need to set their own measures.

---

78 Our World In Data, "COVID-19 Vaccine Doses Administered per 100 People, Apr 4, 2021," Creative Commons, 2021, accessed April 4, 2021, https://ourworldindata.org/grapher/covid-vaccination-doses-per-capita?time=2021-04-04&country=AUT~HRV~BGR~CZE~DNK~CYP~FRA~European+Union~
FIN~DEU~GRC~ISL~HUN~IRL~ITA~LUX~LVA~MLT~LTU~PRT~ROU~ESP~CHE~GBR.
79 Petra Stuiber, "Anschobers Rücktritt: Die Konsequenz Eines Alleingelassenen," der Standard, 2021, accessed July 18, 2021, https://www.derstandard.at/story/2000125785113/konsequenz-eines-alleingelassenen.
80 Irene Brickner, "Die Öffnung Kommt Zu Früh," der Standard, 2021, https://www.derstandard.de/story/2000126204382/die-oeffnung-kommt-zu-frueh.

While the news was good, tensions between the coalition partners (specifically Chancellor Kurz and the new Minister of Health Mückstein) intensified as there were communication inconsistencies. For example, Chancellor Kurz announced, without having discussed with the Health Minister, that further relaxations would ensue, such as reducing the distance rules or curfew. Mückstein commented that the Chancellor is "operating with vague promises more likely to cause uncertainty among the population."[81] Chancellor Kurz's need to announce further relaxation measures was not surprising given the fact that his ratings were plummeting (Figure 8). This was likely the result of Finance Minister Blümel being questioned, once again, from the Ibiza committee regarding chat conversations between Blümel, Kurz and former ÖBAG head Thomas Schmid.

The trust index ratings of April (Figure 8) showed that those primarily responsible for managing the COVID-19 pandemic were falling from grace due to increasing frustrations, failure to order vaccines, and the corruption scandals surrounding the new ÖVP.[82] Chancellor Kurz, who had been in first place for years (behind President Van der Bellen), lost 11 trust points since January and fell to fourth place.

This third wave demonstrated the government's ability to stay in power at all costs despite the botched vaccine strategy, the miscalculations regarding vaccination rates, corruption accusations, and heavy critic from opposition parties, *Länder*, and the social partners. A likely reason for this was the Chancellor's strategy of appealing to the public, deflecting criticism from himself and those closest to him, urging people to forget the past, and taking himself and those closest to him out of the spotlight when situations became too heated. In short, the Chancellor has mastered the political game of credit and blame: showing up when there were opportunities to claim credit (openings, vaccination milestones, upstaging the EU) and blaming people when things went poorly (Health Minister Anschober for the unconstitutional corona laws, the *Länder*

---

81 Austrian Press Agency, "Mückstein Findet Kurz-Vorstoß Zu Lockerungen 'Entbehrlich' – Köstinger Über Kritik 'Verwundert,'" der Standard, 2021, accessed July 18, 2021, https://www.derstandard.at/story/2000126856306/mueckstein-haelt-kurz-vorstoss-zu-lockerungen-fuer-en tbehrlich.

82 The Ibiza Committee hearing formed as a result of the Ibiza scandal in 2019. Finance Minister Blümel has not only been accused of hindering the highest courts from doing their job by failing to deliver evidence (Ibiza scandal) in a timely matter, he is also under investigation regarding the Casino Affair. Chancellor Kurz is under investigation in the Ibiza Committee for making false statements under oath. Both refuse to step down. Thomas Schimd (new ÖVP), head of the ÖBAG (Austria holding PLC, a national wealth fund), was accused of corruption and the trading of political offices.

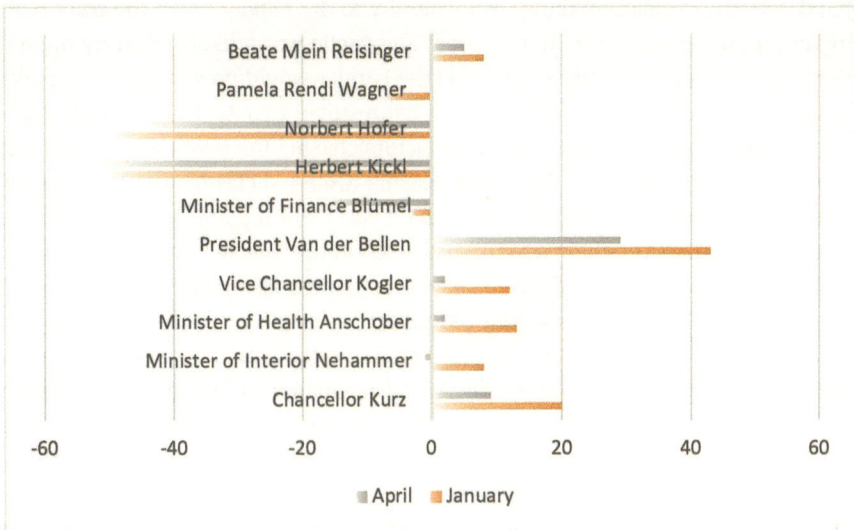

Figure 8: Confidence Rating Score January vs. April 2021. Source: Wolfgang Bachmayer, "OGM/APA-Vertrauensindex Bundespolitiker April 2021," OGM Research and Communication, 2021, accessed May 20, 2021, https://www.ogm.at/2021/04/09/ogm-apa-vertrauensindex-bundespolitiker-april-2021/.

for regional outbreaks, the EU for missing vaccines), thereby surviving (for now) increasing calls for new elections.

Tensions between the national government and the *Länder* remained, specifically with the SPÖ-led *Länder*.

Conclusion

Strong leadership and communication coupled with high levels of public support are essential to successfully guide a country through a pandemic such as COVID-19. In Austria, we saw the impact of resolute and united leadership making effective decisions without hesitation at the beginning of the first wave. This led to high levels of public support resulting in increased compliance with rules and regulations and a steady decrease in the case numbers resulting in a short lockdown and a quicker than usual return to normality, all of which allowed the government, especially Chancellor Kurz, to claim credit for having been successful.

Unfortunately, it is difficult for a government to uphold these high standards during a crisis. By the second wave, we saw the national government's attempt to hand over the decision-making responsibility to the *Länder* when the stark reality hit that the country was unprepared. This tactic was a likely effort by the national government to disperse blame as the Länder would now be forced to make unfavorable decisions, i.e. lockdowns. What resulted was Austrian officials arguing amongst themselves and with other actors chasing the pandemic rather than leading the fight against it. Due to increasing discrepancies resulting in general confusion (a patchwork instead of a unified vaccination plan, the end of the corona traffic light, overwhelmed authorities, contradicting statements by experts, rising infection rates, and delayed reactions), it was assumed that the public's satisfaction with politicians would plummet.

Surprisingly, however, this did not happen to the extent expected, although practically all politicians' values decreased compared to July 2020. The reason for this is likely the fact that the infection numbers exploded in the late fall, and terrifying images from intensive care units circulated, forcing citizens to accept the necessity of a further hard lockdown and support leadership.

However, what ultimately did pull down the confidence values were the corruption charges and blame mitigation strategies that shadowed the government throughout the third wave. Everything that went wrong was blamed on someone: not enough vaccines ordered, Clemens Auer (head of international affairs in the health ministry) was forced to step down; too few vaccines distributed, the European Union got blamed; corruption charges, the Economic and Corruption Prosecutor's Office got blamed for being politically biased and incompetent. Every blunder was craftily linked to a person or institution so that the government, particularly the new ÖVP members, would not be held politically responsible. On the other side, every positive occurrence (relaxation measures, increased state aid for businesses, rising vaccination rates) was announced by members of the new ÖVP, if not by Chancellor Kurz himself. Every opportunity to claim credit was taken, every opportunity the opposition, specifically the SPÖ, had to capitalize on the ÖVPs mistakes was overshadowed by internal conflicts, and every time the Green coalition partner could have voted against the ÖVP they decided being in power was more important than being true to their ideology. All are likely reasons as to why the government remained in power.

Part 2: **Regionalism: the Cases of Spain and Italy**

Juan-M. Trillo-Santamaría, Roberto Vila-Lage, and Valeria Paül

5 Are Internal Borders Gaining Momentum?

A Territorial Reading of Spain's Covid-19 Crisis Management

Introduction

Since the outbreak of the Covid-19 crisis in February/March 2020, the use of the term "border" has become widespread in the debate concerning measures to contain the pandemic when referring to the limits of Spain's autonomous communities (ACs). Primarily, the media, but also most of Spain's political classes, have standardized the use of this term, which until now had been restricted to the country's international borders. Yet, despite this, there has been virtually no academic discussion of this rapid resignification of the word "border" in Spain. Having said that, interestingly, prior to the pandemic, a line of research conducted from the perspective afforded by border studies had begun to draw attention to the growing territorial tensions between the ACs.[1] It is against this backdrop, therefore, that this chapter seeks to analyze how the Covid-19 crisis in Spain has been managed from a territorial perspective.

---

1 Xavier Oliveras and Juan-M. Trillo-Santamaría, "Fronteras en el contexto español: ¿barreras o puentes para la cooperación sanitaria?," *Documents d'Anàlisi Geogràfica* 60, no. 1 (2014): 135–59, DOI: 10.5565/rev/dag.64; Joan Tort and Ramón Galindo, dirs., *L'articulació geogràfica i jurídica dels municipis fronterers: radiografia de la cooperació en els límits autonòmics entre Catalunya, Aragó i la Comunitat Valenciana* (Barcelona: EAPC, 2018); Juan-M. Trillo-Santamaría and Valerià Paül, "¿Cooperación territorial alrededor de las fronteras interautonómicas?", in *España: Geografías para un estado posmoderno*, ed. Joaquín Farinós, Juan F. Ojeda, and Juan-M. Trillo-Santamaría (Madrid/Barcelona: AGE/Geocrítica, 2019), 269–85; Roberto Vila-Lage, Valerià Paül, and Juan-M. Trillo-Santamaría, "Fronteras autonómicas y áreas protegidas: Un análisis de tres reservas de la biosfera en la interfaz entre Galicia, Asturias y León," *Boletín de la Asociación de Geógrafos Españoles* 86 (2020): 1–47, DOI: 10.21138/bage.2966.

Juan-M. Trillo-Santamaría, Assistant Professor, Departamento de Xeografía, Universidade de Santiago de Compostela.
Roberto Vila-Lage, PhD Candidate, Departamento de Xeografía, Universidade de Santiago de Compostela. R. Vila-Lage holds a predoctoral research grant by the Spanish Ministry of Universities with reference FPU18/04624.
Valeria Paül, Associate Professor, Departamento de Xeografía, Universidade de Santiago de Compostela.

https://doi.org/10.1515/9783110745085-006

The chapter is organized as follows. First, we introduce the theoretical debate concerning the meaning of the term "internal border" in the broader framework of the European Union (EU) before examining the Spanish case in greater depth. Second, we describe the characteristics of Spain's local and regional map and the country's different tiers of government. Third, we break Spain's process of Covid-19 crisis management down into six phases (between January 2020 and June 2021) and describe their main characteristics and events. Finally, the last section discusses the findings presented in relation to the specific concepts identified and deployed in the second and third sections.

What are Internal Borders?

The pandemic caused by Covid-19 has been a direct affront to the borderless Europe of the Schengen Area. The internal borders of the EU which, in accordance with Article 26 of the Treaty on the Functioning of the European Union, should have disappeared to ensure the free movement of goods, persons, services, and capital, have been re-erected.[2] As a result, the internal borders of the EU today have, some would claim, come to emulate the EU's external borders,[3] where the latter are conceived as the upholders of "Fortress Europe."[4,5]

EU member-state solidarity is clearly threatened by the pursuit of individualist interests as countries seek to defend themselves from the effects of the virus by implementing somewhat selfish, egotistical policies. Indeed, some authors have even referred to the states in these times of pandemic as being "critically ill",[6] given their failure to collaborate and to adopt policies based on the principle of solidarity. However, reports commissioned by the European Parliament

---

2 Frederique Berrod, "The Schengen Crisis and the EU's Internal and External Borders: A Step Backwards for Security-Oriented Migration Policy?," *Borders in Globalization Review* 1, no. 2 (2020): 53–63, DOI: 10.18357/bigr12202019602; Jorrit Rijpma, "COVID-19, another blow to Schengen?," *Maastricht Journal of European and Comparative Law* 27, no. 5 (2020): 545–48, DOI: 10.1177/1023263X20954568.
3 Iker Barbero, "A Ubiquitous Border for Migrants in Transit and Their Rights: Analysis and Consequences of the Reintroduction of Internal Borders in France," *European Journal of Migration and Law* 22, no. 3 (2020): 366–85, DOI: 10.1163/15718166–12340080.
4 Mette Eilstrup-Sangiovanni, "Re-bordering Europe? Collective action barriers to 'Fortress Europe'", *Journal of European Public Policy* (2021): 447–67, DOI: 10.1080/13501763.2021.1881585.
5 See Chapter 10 of the present volume.
6 Eva Nossem, *UniGR-CBS Working Paper Vol. 8. The pandemic of nationalism and the nationalism of pandemics* (UniGR, 2020: 11), DOI: 10.25353/ubtr-xxxx-1073-4da7.

claimed that, while containment measures might not have been deployed in a coordinated fashion, the Schengen Area was not under threat.[7]

What seems undeniable, however, is that the nation-states of both Europe and other parts of the world responded to the crisis by adopting policies that reinforced their borders and, hence, the control they exercised over their respective territories.[8] Such has been the shift that the idea of a world without borders seems increasingly unattainable as we appear to head towards a "new global border regime."[9] This strengthening of state borders in response to the pandemic cannot be understood, however, without recognizing a prior trend in this very direction in recent years, notable in Europe because of the refugee crisis, among other causes. In the words of E. Opiłowska: "[T]he refugee crisis, Brexit, the revival of nationalist movements across Europe, and especially the outbreak of the Covid-19 pandemic and the resulting re-bordering measures have demonstrated that borders have remained strong and are still governed centrally by nation states."[10]

E. Medeiros et al.[11] have coined the expression "covidfencing" to refer to the systematic closure of borders attributable to Covid-19. Their study analyzes the impact this is having on the European cross-border regions,[12] which have seen neighbors that previously left their doors open to each other begin to erect fences or other types of barriers. The problems and inconveniences that the closure of state borders have had for border people constitute the basis of various studies that describe a range of disruptions[13] that include: accessibility, mobility, work,

7 Sergio Carrera and Ngo Chun-Luk, *In the Name of Covid-19: Schengen Internal Border Controls and Travel Restrictions in the EU* (Brussels: Policy Department for Citizens' Rights and Constitutional Affairs European Parliament, 2020), https://www.europarl.europa.eu/thinktank/en/document.html?reference=IPOL_STU(2020)659506.

8 Anna Casaglia et al., "Interventions on European Nationalist Populism and Bordering in Time of Emergencies," *Political Geography* 82 (2020): 1–9, DOI: 10.1016/j.polgeo.2020.102238.

9 Steven M. Radil, Jaume Castan Pinos, and Thomas Ptak, "Borders Resurgent: Towards a Post-Covid-19 Global Border Regime?," *Space and Polity* 25, no. 1 (2021): 132–40, DOI: 10.1080/13562576.2020.1773254.

10 Elżbieta Opiłowska, "The Covid-19 crisis: the end of a borderless Europe?," *European Societies* 23, no. 1 (2021): 590, DOI: 10.1080/14616696.2020.1833065.

11 Eduardo Medeiros et al., "Covidfencing Effects on Cross-Border Deterritorialism: The Case of Europe," *European Planning Studies* 29, no. 5 (2021), DOI: 10.1080/09654313.2020.1818185.

12 Birte Wassenberg and Bernard Reitel, *Critical Dictionary on Borders, Cross-Border Cooperation and European Integration* (Brussels: Peter Lang, 2020).

13 COTER, *Report. Public Consultations on the Future of Cross-Border Cooperation* (Brussels: Committee of the Regions, 2021), accessed June 15, 2021, https://portal.cor.europa.eu/egtc/about/Documents/4525_COTER_Report_on_the_Consultations-Future_of_CBC.pdf; Francisco Lara-Valencia et al., *COVID-19 and Cross-Border Mobility* (Tempe: Transborder Policy Lab, Arizona State Uni-

public services, and economic, social, and cultural activities, among others. These studies concur in granting a significant role to structures of cross-border cooperation if these barrier effects are to be overcome.

This research dedicated to the study of the impact of border closures on European border areas focuses on a specific type of border: the so-called "internal border," that is, a border equivalent to an international border between two EU member-states.[14] As discussed above in relation to the Schengen Area and "Fortress Europe," "external borders," therefore, are those shared with non-member-states, that is, those that mark the outer limits of the EU. However, this exclusive use of internal/external borders is, to our mind, overly restrictive, reducing as it does the scale of analysis to just one: that of the state. We consider it especially pertinent to broaden the focus and to reflect on the impact of Covid-19 on other territorial borders, such as those that exist within states. Thus, here, we defend the use of the concept of "internal border" to refer to administrative limits within a nation-state, and operating at a range of different scales, including federated states, regions, provinces, municipalities, etc.

It should be stressed that very little research related to the pandemic has taken an intra-state perspective. Some studies have, however, focused their attention on federal states, including, for example, the United States and Australia. In the former case, W. Lyu and G. Wehby[15] examine rates of coronavirus disease in the border counties of the adjacent states of Illinois and Iowa associated with different state policies concerning stay-at-home orders. In the second case, K. Moloney and S. Moloney[16] analyze how responses to various recent pandemics have contributed to shaping Australian identity and union. Clearly, this study refers to both "external borders," on the one hand, and to "domestic inter-

---

versity, 2021), DOI: 10.13140/RG.2.2.29353.72807; Medeiros et al., "Covidfencing Effects on Cross-Border Deterritorialism," MOT (Mission Opérationnelle Transfrontalière), *La crise du covid-19 aux frontières: retours d'expérience du réseau de la MOT* (Paris : MOT, 2020), accessed June 15, 2021, http://www.espaces-transfrontaliers.org/fileadmin/user_upload/documents/Documents_MOT/Articles_MOT/MOT_Covid-19_aux_frontieres_retours_experiences-06-2020.pdf.

14 Joni Virkkunen, "Disease control and border lockdown at the EU's internal borders during the COVID-19 pandemic: the case of Finland," *Baltic Region* 12, no. 4 (2020): 83–102, accessed June 15, 2021, https://www.ssoar.info/ssoar/handle/document/72226.

15 Wei Lyu and George L. Wehby, "Comparison of Estimated Rates of Coronavirus Disease 2019 (COVID-19) in Border Counties in Iowa Without a Stay-at-Home Order and Border Counties in Illinois With a Stay-at-Home Order," *JAMA Network Open* , no. 5 (2020), DOI: 10.1001/jamanetworkopen.2020.11102.

16 Kim Moloney and Susan Moloney, "Australian Quarantine Policy: From Centralization to Coordination with Mid-Pandemic COVID-19 Shifts," *Public Administration Review* 80, no. 4 (2020): 671–82, DOI: 10.1111/puar.13224.

nal borders" or "subnational borders" on the other, when examining the boundaries between states that implement different policies. Furthermore, the analysis includes other scales of study, including the subregional.

All of the research described up to this juncture does not, in fact, represent any great novelty in the broad multidisciplinary field of border studies,[17] which has paid more attention to the analysis of external (that is, international) borders at the expense of internal borders (that is, the internal borders of nation-states). In particular, studies of territorial and cross-border cooperation continue to focus almost exclusively on international borders. For example, there have been interesting contributions about the border barriers and obstacles that continue to exist within the EU. For example, a report published by the European Commission[18] points to the need to review existing practices and this has led to a proposal for a possible European cross-border mechanism to overcome legal and administrative obstacles in the field of cross-border cooperation.

If we focus exclusively on Spanish academic research, the same conclusion can be drawn.[19] Only a very small number of studies to date address the border effect in relation to the country's internal boundaries, that is, by seeking to employ a theoretical and methodological perspective that analyzes its internal borders by analogy with its external borders. This is the case, for example, of X. Oliveras and J.-M. Trillo-Santamaría,[20] a pioneer study of cooperation between ACs in the field of healthcare. In its wake, a number of studies have examined specific territorial areas or sectors, including the border areas between Catalonia, Aragon, and the Valencian Community[21] and the areas between Galicia, Asturias, and Castile and Leon.[22] These studies tend to focus specifically on the deficiencies and shortcomings in the cooperation between the ACs.[23] In what is

---

17 Anne-Laure Amilhat-Szary and Grégory Hamez, *Frontières* (Malakoff: Armand Colin, 2020); James W. Scott, ed., *A Research Agenda for Border Studies* (Cheltenham: Edward Elgar, 2020).
18 European Commission, *Easing Legal and Administrative Obstacles in EU Border Regions* (Luxembourg: EU, 2017), accessed June 15, 2021, https://ec.europa.eu/regional_policy/en/in formation/publications/studies/2017/easing-legal-and-administrative-obstacles-in-eu-border-re gions.
19 Lorenzo López-Trigal, "Investigación geográfica sobre las fronteras de la Península Ibérica," *Polígonos: Revista de Geografía* 29 (2017): 327–46, DOI: 10.18002/pol.v0i29.5213.
20 Oliveras and Trillo-Santamaría, "Fronteras en el contexto español."
21 Tort and Galindo, dirs., *L'articulació geogràfica i jurídica dels municipis fronterers.*
22 Trillo-Santamaría and Paül, "¿Cooperación territorial alrededor de las fronteras interautonómicas?"; Vila-Lage, Paül, and Trillo-Santamaría, "Fronteras autonómicas y áreas protegidas."
23 Joan Romero, "El gobierno del territorio en España. Organización territorial del Estado y políticas públicas con impacto territorial," in *Actas del XXV Congreso de la Asociación de Geógrafos*

often considered a quasi-federal state,[24] there would appear to be a need to promote a greater degree of federal culture in Spain and, as such, stronger horizontal intergovernmental relations.

In short, this chapter seeks to address a research gap that has been detected both internationally and within Spain: namely, that while a wide theoretical and practical literature has been compiled on the bridging (cooperation) and barrier (absence of cooperation) effects of external borders of the state, very little research has been conducted on the internal borders of the state. However, this particular research question has gained considerable momentum in recent times. Indeed, the management of the Covid-19 pandemic offers a highly pertinent case study for reflecting on territorial management in the Spanish framework of the so-called "State of Autonomies."

The Spanish Local and Regional Map and Tiers of Government

As discussed above, J. Gómez Mendoza et al. and E. Aja and J. Romero,[25] among others, concur that Spain today might be defined as a quasi-federal country, despite prevailing difficulties in classifying the Spanish political and territorial model as such. The country's main territorial units, the ACs, are devolved entities made up of two types (see Figure 1):

1. ACs that are defined as "nationalities" and which consider themselves as possessing a national character. In these entities, nationalist parties with varying degrees of strength often form part of the ACs Governments (Figure 3). These nationalisms tend to collide with Spanish nationalism, a sentiment that is especially common in the Spanish parties that have held office over the last four decades, above all those that lean to the right.[25, 26]

Españoles, ed. Fernando Allende et al. (Madrid: AGE/UAM, 2017), 2379–93, DOI: 10.15366/ntc.2017.

24 Josefina Gómez Mendoza, Rubén C. Lois, and Oriol Nel·lo, eds., *Repensar el estado. Crisis económica, conflictos territoriales e identidades políticas en España* (Santiago de Compostela: USC, 2013); Eliseo Aja, *Estado autonómico y reforma federal* (Madrid: Alianza, 2014); Romero, "El gobierno del territorio en España."

25 Xosé-Manoel Núñez Seixas, *Suspiros de España: el nacionalismo español (1808–2018)* (Madrid: Crítica, 2018).

26 Spanish nationalism is hardly regarded as such. In this sense, it is a typical case of "banal nationalism"; Michael Billig, *Banal Nationalism* (London: Sage, 1995).

2. ACs characterized by their regional character, yet which regard themselves as forming an integral part of the Spanish nation. Regionalist parties exist in some of these ACs, but only a few currently hold office (Figure 3).

This distinction between nationalities and regions is provided for under Article 2 of the 1978 Spanish Constitution, which grants these entities autonomy with executive and legislative powers. However, the judiciary remains highly centralized, including the superior courts of justice of the ACs, with the judges being appointed by Madrid. Indeed, various international institutions, including GRECO,[27] claim that the main political parties exercise undue political control over the judiciary. Whatever the case, from Article 3 onwards, the Constitution refers to all of these entities as ACs, implying that any previous distinction between the two types becomes blurred. Currently, the concept of AC is widely used, having been coined, it is claimed, to avoid the conflictual use of "nationality" – inherently related to national identity – referring to territories within the Spanish State rather than to Spain as a whole.

According to J. García Álvarez,[28] the Spanish "State of Autonomies" – developed under the framework of the Constitution and consisting, since the early 1980s, of 17 ACs (Figure 1) – responded to two major demands. On the one hand, it aimed to address the nationalist aspirations of the Basque Country and Catalonia, which in the late 1970s urged Spain to officially recognize their identity concerns. In this sense, the notion of "nationality" was the outcome of this process, and, indeed, the first Statutes of Autonomy were passed for the benefit of the three *de facto* constitutional nationalities (2nd transitional provision of the Constitution): the Basque Country (1979), Catalonia (1979), and Galicia (1981). On the other hand, the "State of Autonomies" aimed to de-centralize Spain in accordance with the prevailing trend in Western Europe. This implied generalizing the model of ACs to the whole of the country – with the exception of Ceuta and Melilla, designated as Autonomous Cities in the 1990s. Indeed, some of these ACs eventually attained nationality status (most notably Andalusia, following a controversial referendum held in 1981 in this respect) (Figure 1). However, some of the ACs emerged in the late 1970s-early 1980s without being rooted in previously recognizable regions in historical and geographical terms,

---

27 GRECO, *Prevención de la corrupción respecto de miembros de Parlamentos nacionales, jueces y fiscales. Cuarta ronda de evaluación* (Strasbourg: Council of Europe, 2019), accessed June 15, 2021, https://rm.coe.int/cuarta-ronda-de-evaluacion-prevencion-de-la-corrupcion-respecto-de-mie/168098c68e.
28 Jacobo García Álvarez, *Provincias, regiones y comunidades autónomas. La formación del mapa político de España* (Madrid: Senado, 2002).

such as the union of (Old) Castile and Leon in one common AC, the creation of single ACs for Madrid, Cantabria and La Rioja, etc.

Today, it would appear almost impossible to modify the map that was drawn up in the 1980s, as the current quest for secession of Leon from (Old) Castile makes evident.[29] There is also a broad-based homogenizing perception – a sense that all the ACs are the same, especially as far as the second type of ACs are concerned. The lack of specific recognition of the singular national character of Catalonia, for example, diluted in the 17 ACs, is one of the reasons underlying the rise of the pro-independence movement that has gained momentum during the second decade of this century. A pivotal event was the Constitutional Court ruling in 2010 that substantial sections of the 2006 reform of the Statute of Autonomy of Catalonia were unconstitutional. This included the subtle definition in its preamble of Catalonia as a "nation."

Constitutionally speaking, the ACs are the aggregation of contiguous provinces aimed at providing self-government, based on claims of common identity (or a sole province itself becoming an AC). This is ironic given that the provincial map of Spain, consisting of 49 provinces and established in 1833 (in 1927 a fiftieth province was added), is the map *par excellence* of the vision of Spain as a single, united territory and of the exercise of the homogenous territorial power of the Spanish State in a centralist fashion – see J. García Álvarez[30] and J. Burgueño[31] on the provincial division of Spain. Importantly, the 1833 map divided up historical territories such as Catalonia, Galicia, and the old Kingdom of Valencia into several provinces. Likewise, in the first half of the nineteenth century, the municipal map was drawn up for the whole of Spain, with a reduction in the number of municipalities being made in the mid-twentieth century.[32] As of 2020, there are 8,131 municipalities in Spain.

Some ACs have created their own territorial subdivisions for the purposes of delivering their devolved policies, for instance, health management regions which are quite commonly at odds with the provincial map (for instance, Galicia;

---

29 Valerià Paül et al., "¿Hacia una comunidad autónoma leonesa? Una interpretación urgente del *Lexit* de inicios de 2020 desde la perspectiva de la Nueva Geografía Regional," *Scripta Nova* 25 (2021): 3, DOI: 10.1344/sn2021.25.32289.

30 García Álvarez, *Provincias, regiones y comunidades autónomas*.

31 Jesús Burgueño, *La invención de las provincias* (Madrid: Catarata, 2011).

32 Jesús Burgueño and Montse Guerrero, "El mapa municipal de España. Una caracterización geográfica," *Boletín de la AGE* 64 (2014): 11–36, DOI: 10.21138/bage.1687.

and see J. Burgueño[33] for a discussion on the health management regions in Catalonia – Figure 6). In addition to this, there are supra-municipal territories recognized by the respective ACs which do not necessarily take into account the provincial map and which introduce new tiers of government. In this respect, cases in point are the following: the counties (*comarcas*) existing in Catalonia, Aragon, and El Bierzo in Castile and Leon;[34] the islands in the two archipelagic ACs, each with its own island councils; and some institutionalized metropolitan areas (e. g. Barcelona and Vigo).

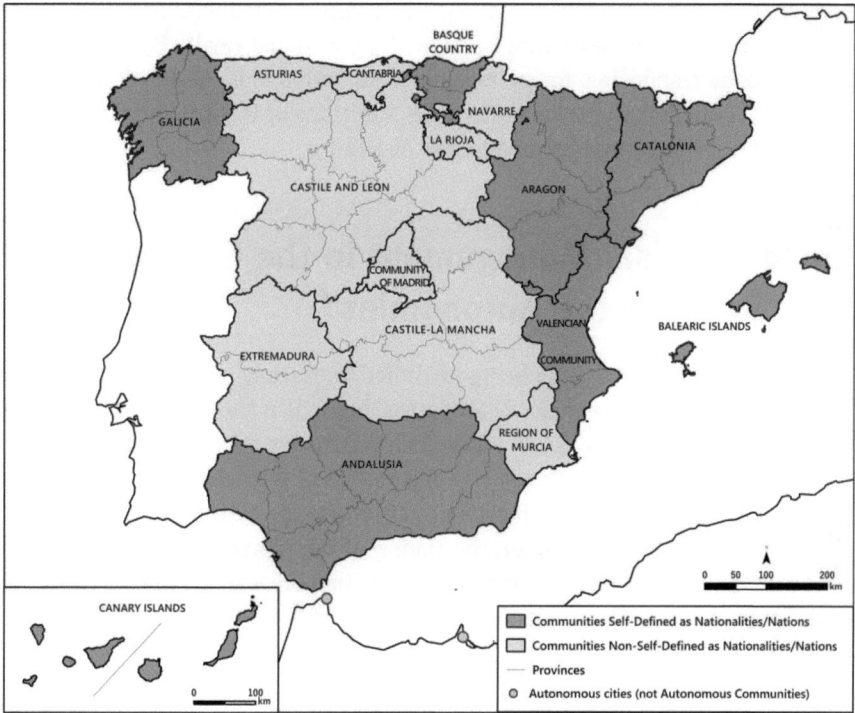

Figure 1: The "State of Autonomies": the 17 ACs. Source: authors' own.

33 Jesús Burgueño, "El territori de Catalunya s'organitza en... regions sanitàries?," in *Nova Geografia de la Catalunya post-covid*, ed. Jesús Burgueño (Barcelona: Societat Catalana de Geografia, 2021), 51–65.
34 Joan Carles Membrado Tena, "Entes territoriales de escala comarcal en la Administración local española," *Documents d'anàlisi geogràfica*, 62, no. 2 (2016): 347–71, DOI: 10.5565/rev/dag.300.

As for the political dimension of territorial decentralization, it should be stressed that since the early 2000s, all the ACs have attained similar political competences, including management of the public health system. Before 2001, however, two distinct classes of AC could be identified: those that exercised their own competences in the field of healthcare (broadly speaking, the "nationalities") and those that did not (essentially those characterized by their "regional character," as discussed above). In 2001, all the ACs became responsible for their own healthcare, thus ushering in a highly decentralized system of healthcare management.[35] Yet, the Spanish Government continued to ensure the effective coordination of health matters (Act 14/1986), with the creation, among other instruments, of the Inter-territorial Council of the National Health System (Act 16/2003), a body responsible for overseeing coordination and cooperation between the AC Governments (represented by their Ministries of Health) and the Spanish Government (represented by its Minister of Health).

Covid-19 Crisis Management in the Context of the "Spain of the Autonomies"

From the first case of Covid-19 being identified to the time of writing (June 2021), Spain was immersed in a major health crisis, but it also had to face a major conflict in its territorial governance. Figure 2 shows the six main phases that can be identified in this pandemic from the perspective of our territorial analysis. Although the detailed study of the health data emerging from Covid-19 crisis is not the objective of this chapter, the timing of the phases identified is shown here with the corresponding death count. Our aim here is to provide an overview of the impact of the pandemic in Spain in each of these six stages.

Phase I: Detection of First Cases of Infection

The first phase ran from the outbreak of the Covid-19 crisis in Spain, which can be traced to January 31, 2020, when the first case was detected on La Gomera (Canary Islands), to March 14, 2020, with the declaration of a nationwide State of Alarm. In general, these days were characterized by a general ignorance of and a sense of skepticism about the virus.

---

35 Aja, *Estado autonómico y reforma federal*; Oliveras and Trillo-Santamaría, "Fronteras en el contexto español."

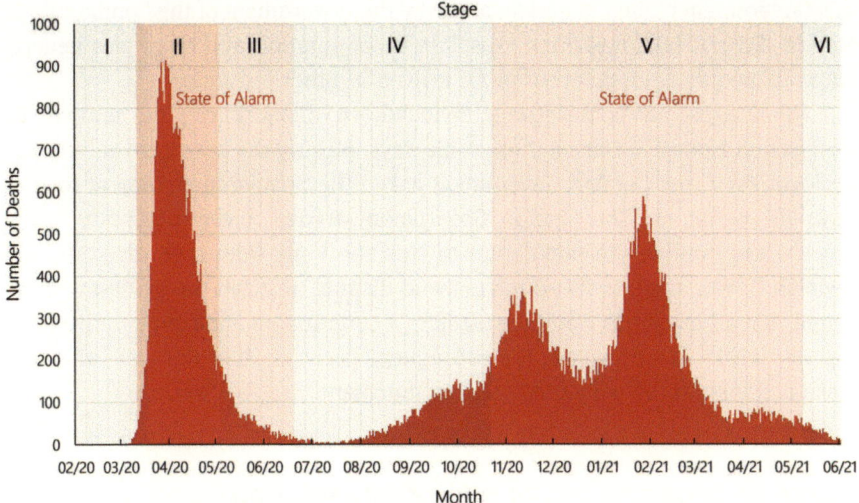

Figure 2: Number of daily deaths from Covid-19 in Spain and the main stages identified in the pandemic from a territorial perspective (February 2020-June 2021). Source: based on data from Spain's National Epidemiology Centre.

Initially, the crisis was managed within the existing legal framework, that is, a model in which all health management policy decisions lay with the ACs. During February, a month in which the number of cases detected was still low, the ACs were taking a "wait and see" approach. In March, the first steps were taken to prevent the virus from spreading. Thus, between March 6 and 13, 2020, all the ACs introduced regulations to this end.[36]

This first phase was not free of tension and ushered in a whole series of disagreements and conflicts between the Spanish Government and the ACs Governments, as well as between the different ACs Governments. A good example of these discrepancies of opinion concerned the need to apply stricter measures, such as perimeter lockdowns. For example, the Government of the Community of Madrid – the AC that accounted for almost half the cases of infection and which was considered a major zone of the transmission of Covid-19 – began to apply restrictive measures (including, working from home, closure of schools and other educational centers, and limiting numbers in typical places of gathering); however, no restrictions were placed on citizen mobility. Many of the other

---

36 Earlier, on February 14, 2020, the Balearic Islands created an infectious disease management commission. For more information on AC regulations and Covid-19: https://www.boe.es/bib lioteca_juridica/codigos/codigo.php?id=396&modo=2&nota=0 (accessed June 15, 2021).

ACs Governments failed to understand why the Government of the Community of Madrid did not take measures to isolate its population and there was general alarm as people from this central AC arrived in other territories.

The disagreements concerning the lockdown of Madrid cannot, however, be analyzed in isolation. During those same days, lacking the powers to enforce the decision itself, the Catalan Government asked the Spanish Government to shut down its perimeter. The Catalan Government argued it was necessary to act quickly and confine the population to stop the virus from spreading. Yet, the Spanish Government, in its efforts to avoid dispute, rejected the request and declared that all measures would be taken in a coordinated and collaborative fashion with all 17 ACs. However, the subsequent declaration of the State of Alarm was testimony to the inaccuracy of this statement.

Phase II: Recentralization and Strict Isolation

The State of Alarm is an emergency mechanism provided for under the Spanish Constitution via which the Spanish Government can adopt extraordinary powers in the face of major catastrophes, health crises or the paralysis of essential services. On March 14, 2020, the first nationwide State of Alarm of the crisis was declared.[37] During this period, the Spanish Government assumed the mantle of the highest "competent authority," while the Ministers of Defence, Interior, Transportation, Mobility, and Urban Agenda and Health were named "delegated competent authorities' in their respective areas of responsibility. Initially, the State of Alarm was supposed to have a duration of 15 calendar days, any extension requiring the approval of the Spanish Parliament. However, it was in fact to be extended on six occasions, being lifted eventually on June 21, 2020.

We can identify two major phases in the State of Alarm declared in mid-March. The first, which corresponds to phase II of our analysis, ran from its declaration until May 4, when a de-escalation was initiated. This stage was characterized by the confinement of people to their homes and restrictions on any type of non-essential activity.

Despite the critical nature of the healthcare situation, the political tension and territorial conflicts did not cease. For example, the presidents of Catalonia and the Basque Country called on the Spanish Government to respect the powers

---

37 This was actually the second State of Alarm to be declared under the 1978 Constitution, as the mechanism had been invoked for a month (between December 15, 2010 and January 15, 2011), when an air traffic controller strike had led to a blockade of Spanish airspace.

of the ACs in combatting Covid-19. However, competences in the field of health and security (recall these two ACs operate their own police forces) now corresponded to what was identified as the "sole command" of the competent authority. Unsurprisingly, the Catalan and Basque Governments compared the situation to the application of Article 155.[38] But most of the ACs Governments positioned themselves alongside the Spanish Government. Some of the ACs Governments, including those governed by the PSOE (Spanish Socialist Workers' Party, center-left) as well as by the PP (People's Party, center-right), came out in support of the recentralization of decision-making (Figure 3).

Despite this initial show of support, as the days passed, confrontation increased. The pandemic began to overwhelm the healthcare system and the exchange of accusations became constant. The relationship between the Government of the Community of Madrid, one of the ACs most seriously affected by Covid-19, and the Spanish Government was especially tense. The AC's president, Isabel Díaz Ayuso, went so far as to claim that the Spanish Government was impeding the arrival of medical supplies and that the loss of autonomy was significantly undermining her ability to respond to the crisis. Thus, the opposition of other ACs Governments to the State of Alarm – ACs Governments that had initially supported the measure – was now added to that of Catalonia and the Basque Country. This was especially the case in those ACs where Spain's main opposition party, the People's Party, was in power (Figure 3). Thus, the Governments of Galicia, Murcia, and Andalusia all issued critical statements about the management of the crisis, calling for greater coordination and collaboration between the ACs Governments and the Spanish Government.

In its turn, the Spanish Government also demanded greater collaboration and coordination in areas such as education and in relation to sensitive issues such as the death count. Paradoxically, it sought to justify the adoption of unilateral measures by resorting to the urgency of the situation, without consulting the ACs. Yet despite everything, the first three extensions of the State of Alarm were approved without excessive problems (Figure 5).

One aspect of this phase that should be highlighted were the weekly meetings (held by videoconference) of the Meeting of Presidents. This political body, not specifically provided for under the Constitution, was created in 2004 by Zapatero's Government (PSOE), and includes the President of Spain and the Pres-

---

38 An Article of the Spanish Constitution by which the Spanish Government can suspend the autonomy of an AC if it "does not comply with the obligations that the Constitution or other laws impose upon it, or acts in a way that seriously undermines the general interests of Spain," It was applied between October 27, 2017 and June 2, 2018 in Catalonia in response to the so-called process of independence.

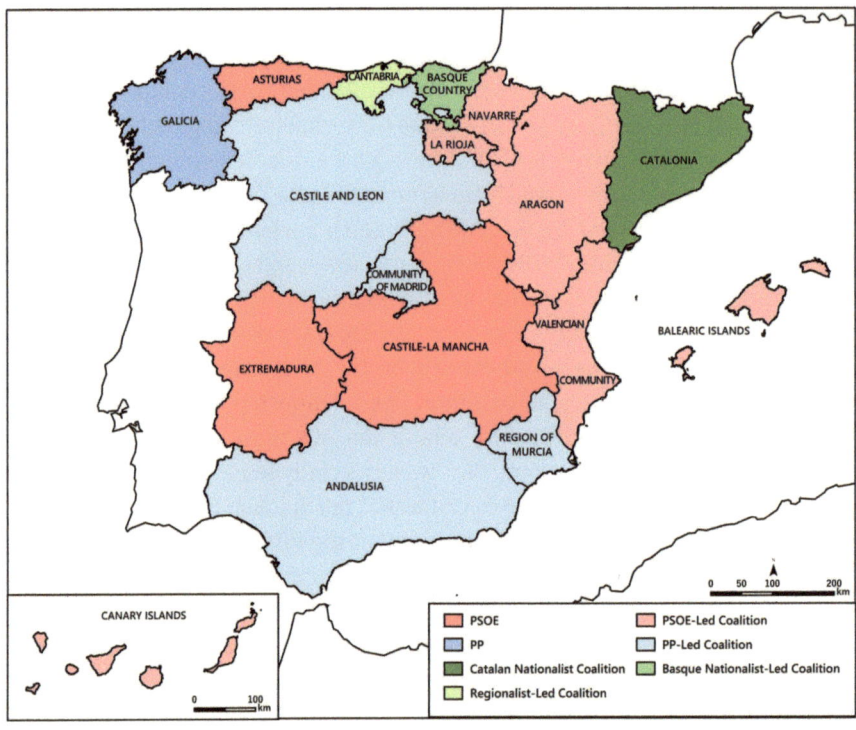

Figure 3: Political parties governing in the 17 ACs as of June 2021. Source: authors' own.

idents of the 17 ACs and the Cities of Ceuta and Melilla. The aim was to form a body for dialogue, cooperation, and coordination between the Spanish Government and the ACs Governments. It should be noted that, since its creation, only six Meetings had been held up to 2020, the last one in 2017. In the period of the first State of Alarm (phases II and III of our analysis), 14 were held, all of them virtual.

Phase III: Provincial De-escalation

This third phase ran from the beginning of the de-escalation process (May 4, 2020) until the end of the first state of alarm (June 21). During this period, although the situation remained grave, the number of infections fell and the previously introduced restrictive measures could be relaxed. Against this backdrop, the Presidents of the Basque Country and Catalonia were no longer the only ones who sought to have the State of Alarm lifted. The ACs Presidents in the People's

Party were also in favor of lifting the emergency measure. However, the Spanish Government opted to extend the State of Alarm and initiate a process of de-escalation in which, theoretically, the ACs would have a bigger role to play.

The watchwords that characterized this phase were "co-governance" and transition to a 'new normal." The first sought to draw a line under what had occurred in the previous months of "sole command." However, by opting to make the territorial unit of reference the province, the Spanish Government granted the ACs Governments merely a supporting role[39] (Figure 4). The Spanish Government established that each province should start from a so-called "zero or preliminary phase" and, if it met the requirements, it could progressively advance through the other three phases in which the number of permitted activities increased. In the event of a deterioration in the indicators, the provinces could also be sent back to an earlier phase. Once the three phases had been successfully overcome, the so-called "new normal" was reached.

Despite the Spanish Government's declarations of "co-governance," in practice, the role that the ACs Governments played was secondary. The latter were able to make their own proposals known, but the ultimate decision regarding a transition into a new phase lay with the Spanish Minister of Health. Only the culmination of the last phase and entry into the "new normal" were the exclusive decision of the ACs Governments. This de-escalation plan was not to the liking of many ACs, especially those not governed by the PSOE. These ACs Governments expressed their displeasure with the situation, which they considered to show a complete lack of transparency, communication, and coordination. During the weeks of de-escalation, the Spanish Government was accused of not applying common criteria for moving from one phase to another and its way of acting was even described as dictatorial.

Voting on the last three extensions of the State of Alarm differed significantly from the first three votes. Support in the Spanish Parliament gradually fell and the main opposition party, the People's Party, withdrew its support, which meant the votes of the different peripheral nationalist (PNV, ERC, CC, etc.) and regionalist (UPN, Teruel E., PRC, etc.) parties were indispensable in ensuring the PSOE-UP coalition government was able to get the necessary support for the extensions (Figure 5).

---

39 In the case of the Canary and Balearic Islands, the island was considered the territorial unit of reference. Ceuta and Melilla were also considered individually. The ACs Governments, however, were able to propose other territorial units which they felt should be subject to differential treatment (for example, health regions).

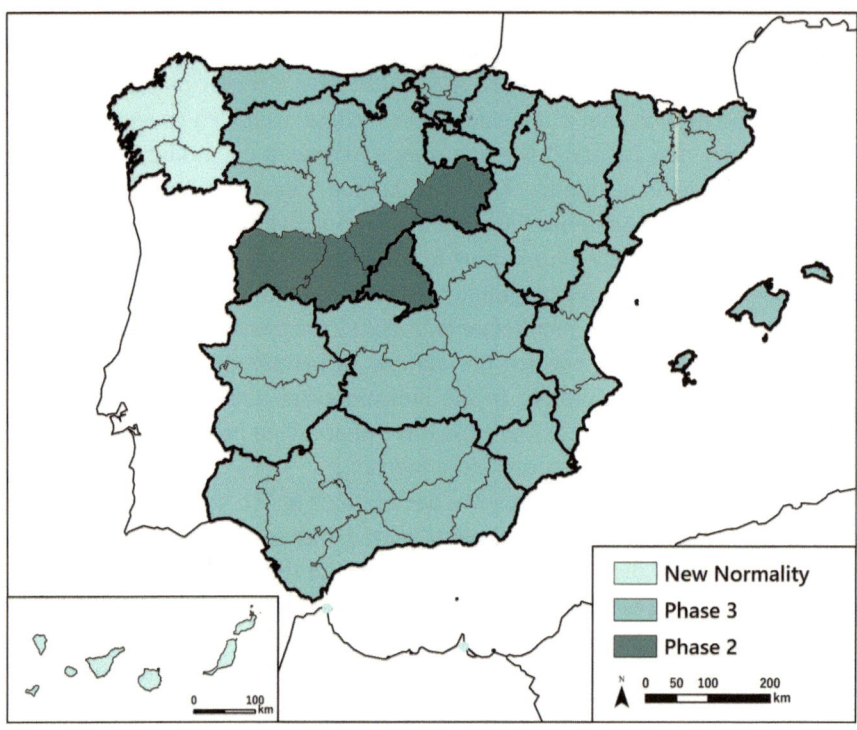

Figure 4: Situation of the provincial de-escalation as of June 17, 2020. Source: authors' own.

Phase IV: "New Normal"

The fourth phase coincided with the period between the first and second States of Alarm, that is, between June 21 and October 25, 2020. In this period, the "new normal" was officially established. The ACs Governments, in keeping with their wishes of the previous months, were in charge of managing the waning crisis. However, it was during this phase that the role of Spain's Inter-territorial Council of the National Health System gained in importance. The country's external borders were once again opened up and there were no longer any restrictions on internal mobility.

Outbreaks of the virus required the occasional isolation of municipalities or regions. But now the different political spheres seemed to enter a brief period of truce, reducing the territorial conflicts of the previous months. However, in August the infection rate rose and the tension between the ACs Governments and the Spanish Government rose with it. Some of the former took a stance diametri-

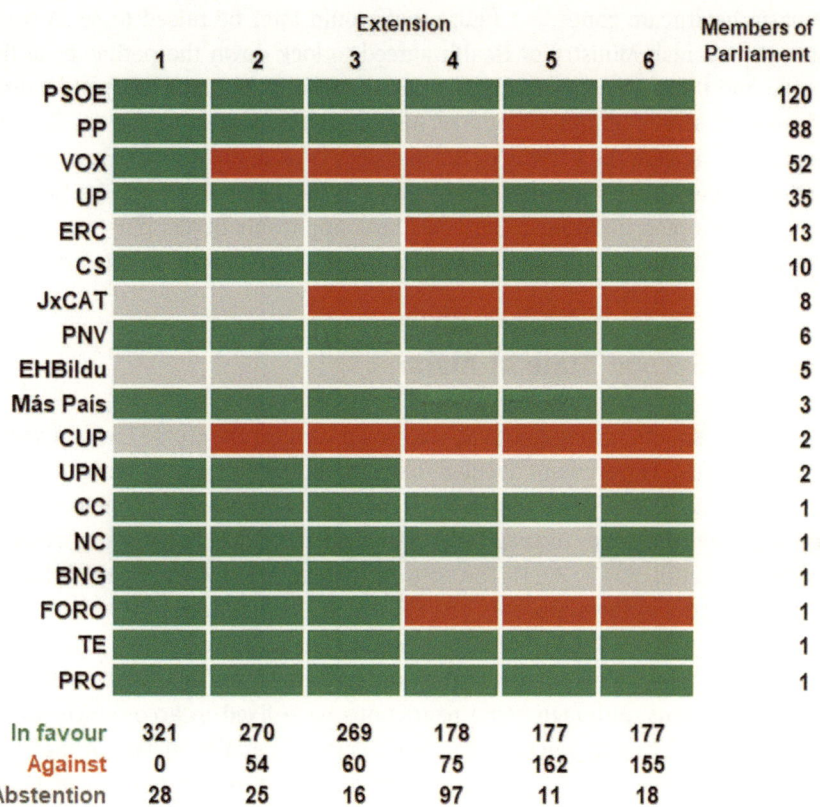

	Extension						Members of Parliament
	1	2	3	4	5	6	
PSOE							120
PP							88
VOX							52
UP							35
ERC							13
CS							10
JxCAT							8
PNV							6
EHBildu							5
Más País							3
CUP							2
UPN							2
CC							1
NC							1
BNG							1
FORO							1
TE							1
PRC							1
In favour	321	270	269	178	177	177	
Against	0	54	60	75	162	155	
Abstention	28	25	16	97	11	18	

Partido Socialista Obrero Español (PSOE), Partido Popular (PP), Unidas Podemos (UP), Esquerra Republicana de Catalunya (ERC), Ciudadanos (CS), Junts per Catalunya (JxCAT), Euzko Alderdi Jeltzalea-Partido Nacionalista Vasco (PNV), Euskal Herria Bildu (EHBildu), Candidatura d'Unitat Popular (CUP), Unión del Pueblo Navarro (UPN), Coalición Canaria (CC), Nueva Canarias (NC), Bloque Nacionalista Galego (BNG), Foro Asturias (FORO) Teruel Existe (TE), Partido Regionalista de Cantabria (PRC).

Figure 5: Spanish Parliament voting on extensions to the first State of Alarm. Source: authors' own.

cally opposed to the one they had taken in the previous phase and asked the latter for a common strategy to combat the pandemic.

As in the earlier phase, the case that best reflects the growing tension occurred in the Community of Madrid. Following a meeting between the Presidents of the Spanish Government and the Community of Madrid, the positions of the two appeared to be much closer. However, a few days later, with a rise in the infection rate, the Government of the Community of Madrid restricted mobility in

37 basic healthcare zones,[40] a figure that would later be raised to 45. A week later, the Spanish Ministry of Health agreed to lock down the perimeter of the capital and those of a further eight municipalities in the Community of Madrid. However, Madrid's Supreme Court of Justice, at the request of the AC Government, ruled against the validity of the decision, considering these measures a violation of the citizens' fundamental rights. In the light of events, the Spanish Government opted to decree a State of Alarm applicable in just nine municipalities of the Community of Madrid and thus restricted mobility in this area.

Phase V: Second State of Alarm

The general situation throughout Spain took a turn for the worse (second wave) and the Spanish Government decided to decree a new nationwide State of Alarm on October 25, 2020. A day later the XXIII Meeting of Presidents was held. On this occasion, the emergency measure was prolonged just once, albeit for a period of six months (until May 9, 2021). The vote on the extension in the Spanish Parliament failed to win the support of the PP, which abstained.

Compared to the State of Alarm decreed in March 2020, the differences were significant. The ACs Governments were now considered as "delegated competent authorities"; thus, although some restrictions were fixed in accordance with a previously established general scale, they enjoyed certain powers of management. For example, the ACs Governments could choose the number of hours of night-time curfew to impose and whether or not to implement perimeter closures (Table 1).

Table 2 provides an example of the variety of restrictions in place as of February 2021. The power of the ACs Governments to close the perimeter of other territorial areas within the AC was one of the most notable of these measures. We examine three of these ACs in greater depth. First, the case of Catalonia which, as discussed above, presents an internal division into health regions which, broadly speaking, coincide with the map of *vegueries* or regions made up of several *comarcas* or counties and which have been repeatedly proposed as a replacement for Catalonia's four *Spanish* provinces[41] (Figure 6). The AC's management of the pandemic was focused on these nine health regions (or *vegueries*) given that they, unlike the "artificial" provinces, have within their territory one or more of Catalonia's major hospitals and present more homogenous geographical char-

---

40 Areas in which a specific health center provides healthcare.
41 Burgueño, "El territori de Catalunya s'organitza en… regions sanitàries?"

Table 1: Main characteristics of the State of Alarm of October 25, 2020.

Competent authority	Spanish Government
Delegated competent authority	President of the AC or Autonomous City
Limitation of the freedom of movement of people	Limited to between 23:00 and 06:00 The ACs Governments being able to extend or shorten the beginning or the end of this curfew by one hour
Perimeter closures	The entry and exit of people from the territory of each AC is restricted*, ** The ACs Governments being able to limit the entry and exit of people from territorial areas at a lower tier than that of the AC, that is, depending on their internal territorial divisions. *Following the pertinent communication to the Spanish Ministry of Health, each AC Government is able to modify, adapt or suspend this measure **This does not affect the border regime with other states
Limitation of the permanence of groups of people in public and private spaces	Maximum of six people, unless from the same household bubble The ACs Governments being able to reduce this number
Limitation of the permanence of people in places of worship	The ACs Governments regulate the number of people allowed to gather

Source: authors' own.

acteristics. In this regard, there exists a fairly broad consensus that the 2010 Constitutional Court ruling concerning the unconstitutional nature of the reform of the Statute of Autonomy of Catalonia marked the beginning of the independence process of the last decade.[42] Ironically, this ruling closed the door to any possible reform of the provincial map in Catalonia, which is *de facto* considered constitutionally frozen, and the *vegueries* or health regions have had to continue as mere internal divisions employed by the Catalan Government in relation to certain specific matters, such as healthcare.

The second case corresponds to that of Galicia, whose health regions, unlike those of Catalonia, overlap more closely with its provinces (Figure 6). The main

---

42 Paül and Trillo-Santamaría, "The Persistent Catalan-Spanish Turmoil."

exception are its two western provinces, which are both divided into three regions with an interprovincial region emerging around the Galician capital (Santiago de Compostela). This health map is more coherent with Galicia's urban system, in particular with the areas of influence of the five main cities of western Galicia. However, the tendency to be governed by the provincial divisions often gave rise to contradictions between the decisions taken and implemented based on the provincial map and the reality of healthcare needs in the Santiago de Compostela region in particular.

Finally, in the case of Madrid, decisions concerning the management of the pandemic were taken at the level of the basic healthcare zones. Indeed, the regional government recognized a total of 286 zones, centered at the neighborhood level or lower. However, opting to make decisions at this scale gave rise to numerous criticisms, not least because epidemiological indicators were not available at this level (which means taking decisions about perimeter closures is far from easy) and because the policing of zones at this scale is especially challenging.

Table 2: Restrictions by AC in February 2021

AC	Perimeter closure	Other territorial units locked down	Night-time curfew	Social gatherings
Andalusia	Yes	Provinces and municipalities with high incidence	22:00 – 06:00	Maximum of four people except for funerals
Aragon	Yes	Provinces and four municipalities	22:00 – 06:00	Maximum of four people
Canary Islands	Yes*	Two islands	22:00 – 06:00	Depending on the island, varies from two, four or six people
Cantabria	Yes	Four municipalities	22:00 – 06:00	In general, maximum of six people. In four specific municipalities, a maximum of four people
Castile and Leon	Yes	Provinces	22:00 – 06:00	Maximum of four people
Castile-La Mancha	Yes	None	22:00 – 07:00	Maximum of six people
Catalonia	Yes	All municipalities	22:00 – 06:00	Maximum of six people and two cohabitation bubbles

Table 2: Restrictions by AC in February 2021 *(Continued)*

AC	Perimeter closure	Other territorial units locked down	Night-time curfew	Social gatherings
Community of Madrid	No	Basic health zones and municipalities	22:00–06:00	Only cohabitants
Navarre	Yes	None	23:00–06:00	Maximum of six people
Valencian Community	Yes	Municipalities over 50,000 inhabitants on weekends and public holidays	22:00–06:00	Maximum of two people in public spaces. Only cohabitants in spaces for private use
Extremadura	No	22 municipalities	22:00–06:00	Maximum of six people
Galicia	Yes	All municipalities	22:00–06:00	Only cohabitants
Balearic Islands	No	Two islands	22:00–06:00	In three islands, only cohabitants. In the other islands, a maximum of six people
La Rioja	Yes	All municipalities	22:00–06:00	Only cohabitants
Basque Country	Yes	All municipalities	22:00–06:00	Maximum of four people
Asturias	Yes	17 municipalities	22:00–06:00	Maximum of four people. Only household cohabitants
Region of Murcia	Yes	23 municipalities and one consortium	22:00–06:00	Maximum of two people in public spaces

*The entry restriction does not apply to travelers who have taken a PCR test
Source: authors' own.

During this period, two particularly critical moments were experienced as regards the ongoing healthcare crisis: the second wave reached its peak (October/November 2020) and the third wave emerged (January-March 2021). However, in terms of the political and territorial conflict, the tensions recorded were constant. Some ACs Presidents accused the Spanish Government of not providing them with sufficient tools to deal with the pandemic. This dispute even reached the Courts. We mention two of these legal cases. First, the case of Castile and Leon, where the AC Government decided to fix a later curfew than that established under the parameters of the State of Alarm. The second case corresponds to that of Galicia, whose AC Parliament passed a law-making vaccination mandatory (Galician Act 8/2021). Both measures were challenged by the Spanish Government before the Courts.

Even in those moments when the infection rate fell, disputes between the ACs Governments and the Spanish Government concerning the measures to be applied were constant. Thus, in the days before Christmas and Easter – when special measures were agreed to by the Inter-territorial Council of the National Health System – tensions ran high. Similarly, in April, faced by the potential shortage of vaccines, some ACs Governments studied the possibility of purchasing supplies of vaccine unilaterally. The EU was obliged to remind them that this was the competence of the state.

Phase VI: Confusion

On May 9, 2021, more than six uninterrupted months of the State of Alarm were finally brought to an end. By this date, Spain's most elderly citizens had been vaccinated and the situation, from a healthcare perspective, had improved notably. However, the lifting of the emergency measure ushered in another turbulent episode in the relations between the ACs Governments and the Spanish Government.

Some ACs Governments claimed not to have the necessary tools to combat the pandemic and urged the Spanish Government to provide some type of solution (for example, the Basque Government demanded the continuation of the State of Alarm, since it ensured more restrictive measures could be taken). Restrictions affecting fundamental rights, such as the freedom of movement, could no longer be applied directly and had to be ratified by the Courts. ACs Governments seeking to apply restrictions of this kind (night-time curfews or perimeter closures, for example) had to go to the superior court of justice sitting in each AC and, if denied, could appeal to the Supreme Court – the Spanish Government approved Royal Decree-Act 8/2021 to make these measures lawful. The Galician President, Alberto Núñez Feijóo, referred to this situation as the "judicialization of the pandemic" resulting from the inaction of the Spanish Government; the judiciary itself was also critical of this way of regulating the measures, in a typical display of the political posturing of the judiciary.

Disagreements and conflict followed hard on each other over the course of the following weeks. One of the main disputes concerned the vaccination protocol for the second dose of the Oxford/AstraZeneca vaccine. The Spanish Government proposed that it be replaced by Pfizer, while some ACs Governments, including Madrid and Galicia, recommended injecting Oxford/AstraZeneca and, if not, insisted upon obtaining a signed consent from the person to be vaccinated

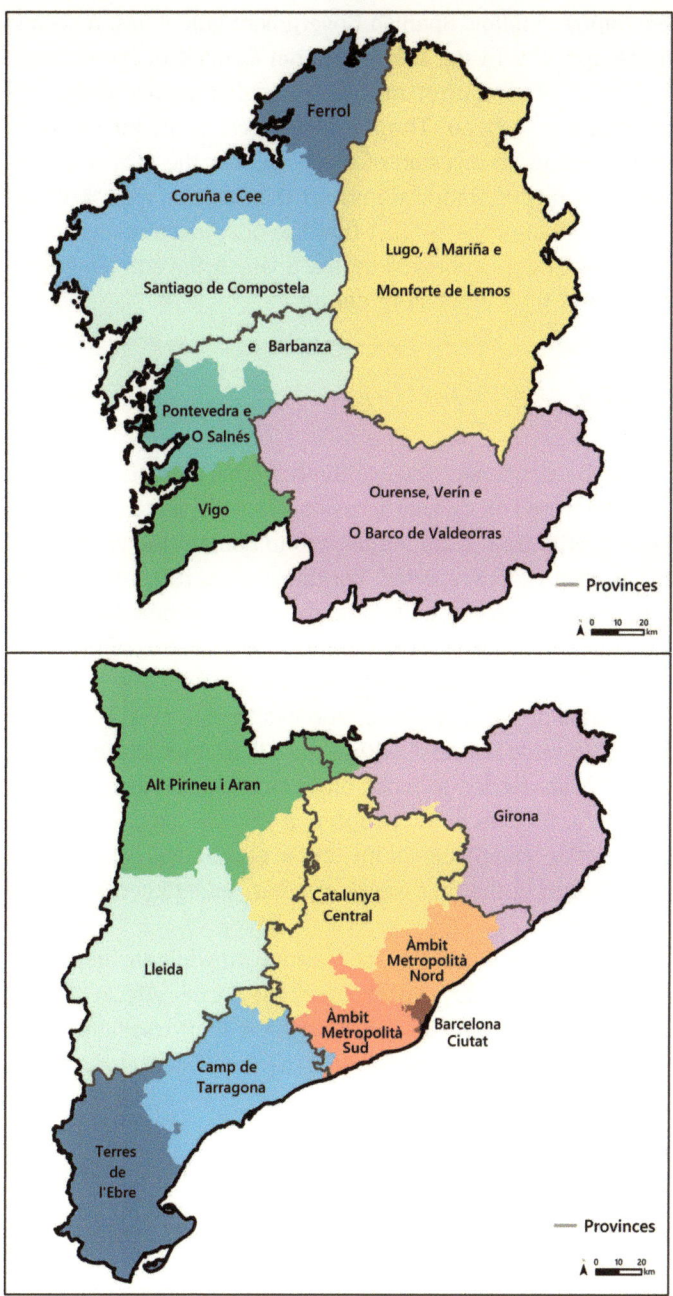

Figure 6: Health regions of Galicia and Catalonia during the pandemic. Source: authors' own.

indicating they were happy to follow Spanish Government guidelines. A second dispute concerned the approval in the Inter-territorial Council of the National Health System of a series of measures, including restrictions on restaurants and bars and on nightlife in general. The Basque Government, for example, claimed that this amounted to an invasion of the powers of the ACs, while the Government of the Community of Madrid described the measure as a "political imposition." Such is the extent of the conflict that the ACs Governments threatened not to apply the regulations approved by the Spanish Government, while the latter reminded them of their mandatory nature.

Final Reflections

From the beginning of the pandemic, Spain's international borders with both Portugal and France were closed on various occasions, in what was a widespread response of the states to withdraw in on themselves to contain the virus.[43] Evidence of this trend has been widely reported. For this reason, rather than reiterating this finding, the chapter has chosen to analyze a parallel process and one that has received less attention from within academia: the bolstering of the Spanish State's internal borders that consequently occurred at various territorial scales – for example, that of the ACs, provinces and health regions. It is our contention that the use of "internal borders" within the EU to refer to the borders between member-states[44] has tended to mask other "internal borders," that is, the ones specifically discussed herein. By adopting a broader agenda and time framework, this contribution complements an initial geopolitical study of the Spain–Catalonia conflict during the first weeks of crisis, undertaken by two of the authors of this chapter.[45]

This chapter has enabled us to draw, at least, two worthwhile theoretical inferences. On the one hand, it provides evidence that the barrier effects of international borders in relation to the Covid-19 crisis[46] have their correlation in a state's internal borders. Our analysis of the Spanish case has detected six phases

---

43 Berrod, "The Schengen Crisis and the EU's Internal and External Borders"; Rijpma, "COVID-19, another blow to Schengen?"

44 Barbero, "A Ubiquitous Border for Migrants in Transit and Their Rights"; Virkkunen, "Disease control and border lockdown at the EU's internal borders."

45 Paül and Trillo-Santamaría, "The Persistent Catalan-Spanish Turmoil."

46 COTER, *Report. Public Consultations on the Future of Cross-Border Cooperation*; Lara-Valencia et al., *COVID-19 and Cross-Border Mobility*; Medeiros et al., "Covidfencing Effects on Cross-Border Deterritorialism"; MOT, *La crise du covid-19 aux frontières.*

characterized by different perimeter closures at different scales. All of them have had a major impact on their respective populations, including a curtailment of mobility and disruptions to their daily lives. This process has taken place, in particular, although not limited to, the border areas of all of the internal borders that have been erected.

On the other hand, we have shown that the main internal borders at stake are those erected between the 17 ACs. These borders have been resignified with the management of the conflict described here, adding pressure to Spain's dysfunctional territorial model, which strives to be federal in definition but fails to fulfil the requisite conditions[47]). Indeed, in the course of the six phases described, we have witnessed constant tensions between the Spanish Government and the ACs Governments, regardless of the specific measures that have been implemented. During the first State of Alarm, the ACs Governments criticized the centralizing policies adopted, considering them an encroachment on their devolved powers (phase III). Yet, when the Spanish Government switched strategies and initiated greater decentralization (phases IV, V, and VI), some ACs Governments denounced the lack of coordination and the general chaos. Clearly, when the political colors of the governments at loggerheads did not coincide, the tensions were much greater. However, the situation cannot simply be reduced to a matter of conflicts between parties that lean more to the left or to the right. Indeed, in the Spanish case, different conflicting national sensitivities – or regional, depending on the case – clearly emerge.[48] In Spain, several nations, with varying degrees of official recognition and varying degrees of adherence among the population, coexist, and these may or may not coincide with one or more of the 17 ACs. The different nationalist movements – or regionalist in some cases – in question erect "external borders" for their respective "national [or regional] territories."[49] Note that, in this game of scales, what are "external borders" for the nations/regions are "internal borders" for the Spanish State.

In their turn, nationalist – and regionalist – movements create their own internal territorial divisions which they defend zealously. For this reason, Spanish State nationalism will always prefer the provincial scale as its map *par excellence*,[50] in its efforts to subtly undermine the role of the ACs, as occurred in

47 Josefina Gómez Mendoza and C. Lois Gonzalez, eds., *Repensar el estado*; Aja, *Estado autonómico y reforma federal*; Romero, "El gobierno del territorio en España."
48 Paül and Trillo-Santamaría, "The Persistent Catalan-Spanish Turmoil"; Núñez Seixas, *Suspiros de España: el nacionalismo español*.
49 Joan Nogué, *Els nacionalismes i el territori* (Barcelona: El Llamp, 1991).
50 García Álvarez, *Provincias, regiones y comunidades autónoma*; Burgueño, "El territori de Catalunya s'organitza en... regions sanitàries?"

phase III of the crisis. Moreover, some ACs with openly nationalist Governments, as is the case of Catalonia, reject this territorial division in favor of another: the *vegueria* and the *comarca* or county, both of which respond to their territorial self-representation.[51] Thus, what we find is a face-off between internal borders at various scales based on conflicting maps of the same territory.

However, in the case of Madrid its healthcare map does not respond to a specific nationalist imaginary. Yet, it is worth stressing that the scale represented by its 286 basic healthcare zones areas has been used by the Government of the Community of Madrid (the PP in coalition with *Ciudadanos*) as a weapon against the Spanish Government (a coalition led by the PSOE). Thus, in the face of constant demands from the Spanish Government during phase V to "shut Madrid down," the Government of the Community of Madrid responded that it would shut down only those neighborhoods it deemed necessary, but not the entire city or region. Recall that, in phase IV, the Spanish Government, following the annulment by the Supreme Court of a previous ministerial decision, declared a specific State of Alarm in order to be able to close the perimeter of the capital and a further eight municipalities. In short, the tensions between the Government of the Community of Madrid and the Spanish Government acquired a clearly political nature, with the former taking on the role of the opposition and acting with particular firmness and obduracy. Indeed, it would not be going too far to claim that this confrontation reached levels of tension greater than those recorded between the Catalan Government (ruled by Catalan nationalist parties) and the Spanish Government.[52] Such was the tension that a strong nationalist – in this case, Spanish nationalism – discourse emerged: the Government of the Community of Madrid defended its *Spanishness* as the capital of the State and as the ultimate embodiment of Spanish identity. This political tension between parties ended up being transferred to the judiciary, which, as mentioned previously and as reported by GRECO,[53] is unduly influenced by the political parties. In practice, this means that the courts may end up ruling in favor of the Spanish Government or the ACs Governments based on purely political criteria.

The criticisms that emanate from the ACs Governments (above and beyond those that are purely political in nature) are based on the evident failure of the mechanisms of horizontal cooperation, consubstantial to all federal state systems. For example, although between March 15 and June 14, 2020, more Meetings of the Presidents were held than ever (14), they did not function as a mech-

---

51 Membrado-Tena, "Entes territoriales de escala comarcal"; Burgueño, "El territori de Catalunya s'organitza en... regions sanitàries?"
52 Paül and Trillo-Santamaría, "The Persistent Catalan-Spanish Turmoil."
53 GRECO, *Prevención de la corrupción.*

anism for debate and the reaching of agreements, but rather for the transmission of the decisions taken by the Spanish Government to the ACs Governments. As for the Inter-territorial Conference of the National Health System, the deficiencies – and tensions – identified in its governance confirm the weaknesses described elsewhere – see J. Ruiz González[54] and E. Aja[55] – regarding these so-called "sectoral conferences" (multilateral bodies with the representation of the Spanish Government and the ACs Governments): the disproportionate importance of the former in their operation and an excessive dependence on the Spanish Minister on duty, among others.

In short, what emerges from the territorial analysis conducted here of Spain's Covid-19 crisis management is, on the one hand, the virtual absence of any effective mechanisms of coordination, collaboration, and cooperation. This can be attributed to the limitations of the "State of Autonomies," which, since at least the first decade of the present century, has been characterized by the erection of a blockade that has prevented any movement towards the expected horizon of a more federal state. On the contrary, Spain seems to have moved in the opposite direction, in large part, as described above, due to the persistence of a centralized and politicized judiciary. On the other hand, Spain provides an extraordinarily rich case study from a geopolitical perspective, which includes that of its internal borders. As we have seen, various coexisting nationalisms and regionalisms have erected conflicting and overlapping borders at different scales. At the time of writing, Covid-19 is still very much present in our lives and just what the next phases might hold remains unknown. However, in Spain, the crisis can never be simply a circumstantial matter of health management, but, in common with any issue that affects this country, it inevitably acquires a territorial reading.

---

54 José Ruiz-González, "La cooperación intergubernamental en el Estado Autonómico: situación y perspectivas," *REAF* 15 (2012): 287–328, accessed June 15, 2021, https://raco.cat/index.php/REAF/article/view/252678.
55 Aja, *Estado autonómico y reforma federal.*

Michel Martínez Pérez

6 Covid-19, Territorial Structure, and Nationalisms

The Case of Spain and its Internal Borders

When the first COVID-19 cases were revealed in Spain, in February 2020, Pedro Sánchez had been in power as President of the Spanish government for less than a month. A couple of weeks later, on March 14, 2020, the head of the first coalition government in Spanish democratic history (with *Unidas Podemos* [Together we can] led by Pablo Iglesias), the Spanish President had to renounce part of the territorial singularity of his country and the *a priori* federalist ideology of his floundering government. Indeed, while Spain has, since its 1978 Constitution, been one of the most decentralized countries in Europe and the world, and while the leaders of the coalition government steadfastly supported the federal state, Pedro Sánchez made the decision to stand alone at the helm of the crisis unit. The adoption of the State of Emergency (*Estado de alarma*) that day established a single command protocol (*mando único*)[1] for the Spanish central government.

Faced with the COVID-19 surge, and in line with the war metaphors used by many leaders, the head of the Spanish executive together with the ministers of the Interior, Transports, Defence, and Health were the only ones to decide. As the most vulnerable citizens began dying by the hundreds every day,[2] this wartime mode made a sole decision-making authority seem like the only way forward. The governments of the Autonomous Communities, including their presidents and ministers of health, were excluded from any decision-making and were informed of the measures to be applied at regular interterritorial conferences or multilateral summits. Some would later say that despite the ruling parties being firm believers in the autonomy of the communities and in subsidiarity, Spain be-

---

1 Gobierno de España, Consejo de Ministros, "Coronavirus COVID-19 El Gobierno decreta el estado de alarma para hacer frente a la expansión de coronavirus COVID-19," March 14, 2020, accessed July 9, 2021, https://www.lamoncloa.gob.es/consejodeministros/resumenes/Paginas/2020/14032020_alarma.aspx.
2 Redaction, "Nuevo récord de fallecidos de coronavirus en un día en España," *El País*, March 28, 2020, accessed July 9, 2021, https://elpais.com/sociedad/2020-03-28/nuevo-record-de-fallecidos-de-coronavirus-en-un-dia-en-espana-832-en-las-ultimas-24-horas.html.

Michel Martínez Pérez, Associate Professor, Toulouse Capitole University, FRAMESPA UMR 5132 / CRIMIC EA 2561.

https://doi.org/10.1515/9783110745085-007

haved like a centralized country (such as France) at a time when it could have demonstrated its alignment with a semi-federal state model, one that would be closer in theory to the German federal state. Ironically, the health sector is undoubtedly the one area in which the Spanish regional state, comprised of 17 Autonomous Communities and two autonomous cities, was closest to the federal model and in which the semi-federal structure of Spain could have been made concrete through the pandemic response.

Beyond addressing the question of the territorial organization of the Spanish state as a regional state, halfway between a federal state and a centralized one, this chapter will present a brief historical overview before turning to the question of the management of the pandemic in Spain and the different types of internal borders used in the various stages of lockdown and gradual processes of opening up. We will see the political significance of the use or the contestation of a given "demarcation," which testifies to a territorial structure and a local and national network that is still under discussion.

Spain: The Response of a Decentralized, Regional State in Response to Nationalist Challenges

Spain is not formally a federal state in the strictest sense. "The State of Autonomies" or "the Autonomous State" (*Estado de las autonomías* or *Estado autonómico*), as it is named in Spanish, reflects the fact that Spain is a regional state: the central state delegates a certain number of powers to the communities. In fact, the Spanish regional model, established in 1978 in the midst of the democratic transition, allowed for a relegation of the high centralism of the Franco regime (1939–1975) to the past and a return to the territorial model established by the Second Spanish Republic (1931–1939). Under the former Republican regime, autonomy was granted to politically, linguistically, and culturally distinctive regions in which most of the population did not identify as being Spanish (mainly Catalonia and the Basque Country[3]). The republican territorial model was therefore initially asymmetrical and clearly designed for the two most differentiated territories from a "national" point of view. However, little by little, other regions

---

3 Under the Second Republic, the parties of Catalan or Basque allegiance were hegemonic in these two territories due, among other things, to a regional nationalism that emerged in the last third of the nineteenth century from the ashes of a Spanish Empire incapable of preventing the consolidation of alternative nationalisms in these two regions.

maneuvered into position to obtain a Statute of autonomy (Galicia, Aragon, Valencia, Andalusia, Castile) which never saw the light of day due to the military *coup d'état* in July 1936 against the Popular Front government and thus against the Republic, whose secular character particularly irritated the pillars of the monarchist and military establishment. Very quickly, these two camps diverged on the question of the political autonomy of the regions: would autonomy be the best way to put an end to separatism (among republicans) or would it fuel secessionism (on the monarchist right)? Would the extension of autonomy to all territories effectively accelerate a separatist process that would shatter Spain, or would it be the best way to drown the autonomy of the two main "cultural nations" in a generalized wave of autonomy being granted to territories that requested it? This debate still rages today, with no resolution in sight.

In 1936 (the year of the putsch) as in 1978 (which witnessed the adoption of the Constitution at the height of the democratic transition) or after 18 months of the COVID-19 pandemic (2021), the territorial question remained unanswered for one main reason: the absence of consensus on the political and territorial definition of Spain.[4] Beyond the issue of regime (monarchy or republic?), which is settled for now by the (monarchist) Constitution, Spain is still torn between Jacobin, centralist (despite the state of autonomy), and peripheral or nationalist ideologies (which espouse a maximalist interpretation of the new regional state as repairing the excesses of Francoism).[5] Thus, in order to assert itself as an indivisible State, must Spain assimilate all its peripheries into a centralized, linguistically, and culturally Castilian model or could it truly integrate the different cultural nations that composed it on an equal footing, and in so-doing lead to the construction of a plurinational State? Unfortunately, there is no single or simple answer to this question. Different ideological families still clash on this subject. The Constitution of 1978 enshrines the political autonomy of the communities and the existence of "cultural nations" (*nacionalidades*), thus implicitly recognizing a plural State in which citizens, especially in Catalonia and the Basque Country, can legitimately feel a sense of belonging to a nationality which is not necessarily Spanish. The ambiguity that was necessary for

---

4 José Álvarez Junco, *Mater Dolorosa. La idea de España en el siglo XIX* (Madrid: Taurus, 2001); Xosé-Manoel Núñez Seixas, *Suspiros de España. El nacionalismo español (1808–2018)* (Barcelona: Crítica, 2018).

5 Javier Moreno Luzón, *Construir España: nacionalismo español y procesos de nacionalización* (Madrid: Centro de Estudios Políticos y Constitucionales, 2008); Ismael Saz and Ferran Archilés, *Estudios sobre nacionalismo y nación en la España contemporánea* (Zaragoza: Prensas Universitarias de Zaragoza, 2011).

securing consensus during the writing of the Constitution[6] today leaves room for interpretations favoring the Jacobins (and thus the indivisibility of a centralized Spanish nation) and the autonomists (and therefore State respect for regional autonomy) in equal measure.[7]

Broadly speaking, the territorial question has not ceased to trouble Spain since the decline of its colonial Empire and the "existential" crisis of 1898, a year marked by the loss of its last colonies (Cuba, Puerto Rico, and the Philippines). The regions least assimilated to Castilian Spain (Catalonia and the Basque Country) are also those which went through an intensive period of industrialization in the second half of the nineteenth century. Just like Cuba, Catalonia, and the Basque Country consider themselves to be "prisoners" of a dilapidated, archaic, decadent, and ineffective state. The experience of the past century and a half has nevertheless underscored an understanding that nationalisms feed on each other and that political developments follow a pendulum-like movement.[8] In other words, when Spain imposes a Hispano-Castilian vision and a Castilian standardization on the peripheries (on the Basque and Catalan peripheries in particular), it gives rise to the emergence or intensification of regionalism, na-

---

6 Francisco González Navarro, *España, nación de naciones. El moderno federalismo* (Pamplona: Eunsa derecho, 1993); José Luis de la Granja, Justo Beramendi, and Pere Anguera, *La España de los nacionalismos y las autonomías* (Madrid: Síntesis, 2001).

7 Preliminary title, article 2: "The Constitution is founded on the indissoluble unity of the Spanish nation, common and indivisible homeland of all Spaniards. It recognizes and guarantees the right to autonomy of the nationalities and regions which compose it and the solidarity among them." Concerning the use of the term "Jacobin" in the political context of contemporary Spain, it is often used as a synonym for "centralist," with post-Revolution France held up as perfect model of a centralized state. This centralism was adopted in Spain for many decades without knowing any of the successes of the French case. See the column by Lluís Roura in *El País*, professor of history at the Autonomous University of Barcelona in 1998, in which he expresses surprise at the usage of this term: Lluís Roura, "Antijacobinos irredentos," *El País*, May 5, 1998, accessed August 23, 2021, https://elpais.com/diario/1998/05/05/catalunya/894330441_850215. html. For a more complete study: Jean-Baptiste Busaall, *Le spectre du jacobinisme. L'expérience constitutionnelle française et le premier libéralisme espagnol* (Madrid: Casa de Velázquez, 2012).

8 After the First Federal Republic (1874), Spain experienced a period of Restoration (1876–1931) which tolerated a first military dictatorship that was close to Mussolini-style fascism, being hyper-nationalist and therefore very anti-Catalanist (1923–1930). There followed the Second Spanish Republic, a regional state in which the autonomy of the regions was used by military putschists to topple the regime (1936). Francoism, a period marked by cultural and linguistic genocide in non-Castilian regions, was replaced by the current Constitution (1978) which attempted to blend the central state and the autonomy of the communities; Xosé-Manoel Núñez Seixas, *Los nacionalismos en la España contemporánea (siglos XIX y XX)* (Barcelona: Hipòtesi, 2001).

tionalism or even demands for independence.[9] Moreover, this "pancastillan" vision of Spain has often been imposed by authoritarian regimes or dictatorships (notably that of Franco). It is therefore the image of Spain as a unified whole that is excoriated in the territories where local identity is gaining ground and fostering a perspective that is instead positive, modern, democratic, republican, and linked to local nationalisms. By contrast, when Spain assumed its plural character (during the Second Republic and the Parliamentary Monarchy of 1978), peripheral nationalisms became involved in democratic political movements that were integrated into the political functioning of the whole State. These parties were thus legitimized and their voices were channeled: they were a part and parcel of the system and of political debate and their ideology was not persecuted even though their political ambitions (the creation of an independent Basque Country and Catalonia) were not compatible with the fundamental rule of the state.

Even today, the political conflicts that stem from the clash of different nationalisms permeate all the debates and seem to spill over onto the whole of Spanish politics. It was therefore to be expected that the management of the COVID crisis in Spain would have "national" and "territorial" interpretations.

Managing the Pandemic in Spain

The central government helmed by Pedro Sánchez, in coalition with *Unidas Podemos* (UP) was, at least on paper, a "plurinationalism friendly" executive. This self-described "most progressive government in history"[10] drew on the presence of UP to lend a left-leaning sheen to the majority-holding social democrats of the PSOE. In terms of territorial issues, Podemos has since its beginnings espoused a "confederal" vision of Spain, manifested most notably through regional alli-

---

9 At the beginning of the twenty-first century, one could observe that the greatest victories of the nationalist and independence parties of the peripheral territories (Galicia, Aragon, Valencia, Balearic Islands, Canaries, Navarre, in addition to Catalonia and the Basque Country) were achieved during periods of central government when the Popular Party, and its uninhibited Spanish nationalism, was in power (in 2003 and 2017 in particular). On the contrary, in 2008, the nationalist parties collapsed in favor of the plural Spain discourse of José Luis Rodríguez Zapatero and the PSOE, which played a strategic role at that key moment in blocking the PP, whose exclusionary nationalism repulsed the peripheries.

10 En Comú Podem, Asens, "Está en nuestras manos que en 2020 tengamos el gobierno más progresista de la historia de la democracia española," December 30, 2019, accessed July 12, 2021, https://encomupodem.cat/es/asens-esta-en-nuestras-manos-que-en-2020-tengamos-el-gobierno-mas-progresista-de-la-historia-de-la-democracia-espanola/.

ances with local parties,[11] and has long defended the need to organize an independence referendum in Catalonia.[12] The PSOE is opposed to this outcome for the Catalan crisis but considers Spain to be a federal state (a vision which is much clearer in the peripheral federations than in the federations of central and southern Spain, where the Jacobin and anti-nationalist tendencies of the periphery are just as strong).[13] The "national" strategy is therefore not shared by the two parties of the government coalition, and their rivalry is more evident in the difference between the "federal" (PSOE) and "confederal" (UP) approaches. However, Pedro Sánchez did not hesitate for a moment during the electoral campaign (2019) to (re-)use the current Spanish flag (constitutional but monarchist) so that it would not be "surrendered" to the right and to the growing extreme right.[14] For Sánchez, it was a question of elucidating a discourse that was "national" in scope and of asserting the "national" character of the PSOE, even if it meant casting aside the most federal and multinational vision of Spain in the wake of the independence crisis in Catalonia which seemed to catalyze anti-independence discourse across the rest of Spain.[15] It was indeed crucial for the Socialists to be seen as a transversal party which

11 Iolanda Mármol, "Las alianzas de Podemos retan a Iglesias y le piden independizarse," *El Periódico de Catalunya*, April 17, 2016, accessed July 12, 2021, https://www.elperiodico.com/es/politica/20160417/las-alianzas-de-podemos-retan-a-iglesias-y-le-piden-independizarse-5058711. Unlike the PSOE, a single political party uniting regional federations throughout Spain, Podemos has forged alliances with parties "to the left of the PSOE," with a territorial or even regionalist/ nationalist slant, in order to forge a political force out of those who have become alienated from the PSOE (except when blocking the Popular Party). This structure and its local alliances give Podemos a "confederal" nature, a term used by the party during meetings and political actions organized in the periphery; https://podemos.info/caminando-juntas-reunion-espacio-con federal/, accessed August 23, 2021.
12 Ana Marco, "Podemos recupera su defensa del referéndum pactado en Cataluña," *El País*, October 13, 2019, accessed July 12, 2021, https://elpais.com/politica/2019/10/13/actualidad/1570960689_497344.html.
13 The structure of the PSOE (political party) is federal: one federation of the PSOE per region. Thus, in the Balearic Islands, for example, the PSOE is formally called the Socialist Party of the Balearic Islands (PSIB) and qualifies itself as "territorial federation of the PSOE in the Balearic Islands" (PSIB-PSOE). The same pattern is reproduced in the other 16 regions of Spain. However, the Catalan federation (PSC) is the only one to act as an autonomous party within the federation. From 1977 to 1982, the PSC deputies in the Spanish parliament even constituted a parliamentary group distinct from that of the PSOE.
14 Juan Ruiz Sierra, "Sánchez recurre a una enorme bandera de España y se presenta como un "patriota"," *El Periódico de Catalunya*, June 21, 2015, accessed July 12, 2021, https://www.elperiodico.com/es/politica/20150621/sanchez-recurre-bandera-espana-presenta-patriota-4292622.
15 "El PSOE y el federalismo," *El Periódico de Catalunya*, April 12, 2020, accessed July 9, 2021, https://www.elperiodico.com/es/opinion/20191030/editorial-el-psoe-y-el-federalismo-7708011.

could win the Spanish legislative elections by achieving excellent results in all regions of Spain, including the Basque Country and Catalonia.[16] The federalism of the PSOE could thus be described as that of a federal state in which independence tendencies would be nonexistent (Mexico, Germany, Brazil, Austria, Argentina, United States). According to the socialists, the application of this federalism to Spain would produce the perfect cohesive structure for the State because it would make it possible both to satisfy the demands of peripheral nationalists (Basque and Catalan in particular) and to administer the rest of the territories, as accomplished in the federal states cited above, without any hidden nationalist motives.

However, in order to face the first COVID 19 surge, Pedro Sánchez insisted on implementing a "single command" protocol and piloting health measures at the level of the central state by effectively canceling the mechanisms of regional action. Criticized by both peripheral nationalists[17] and the right-wing opposition (who suddenly became pro-autonomy, perhaps none more so than the president of Madrid, Isabel Díaz Ayuso[18]), the recentralization spearheaded by Sánchez was justified by the unprecedented and exceptional nature of the health crisis and by a need for clarity at a moment when governments around the world seemed to be stumbling around in the dark. The government feared that without this concentration of decision-making power, regional dissonance or contradictory measures implemented across territories might prove politically fatal because human lives were at stake. It is in this context of general panic that must also be understood the decisions of heads of state and of government to unilaterally close the land borders of the European continent, even if it meant

---

16 This is not the case with the Popular Party, for example, which has become marginal in Catalonia and the Basque Country due to an increasingly exclusionary Spanish (Hispano-Castilian) nationalist discourse. In 2020, the PP retained only six deputies (out of 75) in the Basque parliament. In 2021, in the Catalan parliament, the PP kept only three (out of 135). In the legislative elections of 2019, the PP obtained only two seats out of the 48 Catalan representatives in Madrid while in the Basque Country it only obtained one (out of 18 seats).

17 "Las comunidades del PP y los nacionalistas elevan el tono contra el mando único de Sánchez," *La Voz de Galicia*, April 12, 2020, accessed July 9, 2021, https://www.lavozdegalicia.es/noticia/sociedad/2020/04/12/pp-nacionalistas-endurecen-tono-contra-mando-unico-sanchez/0003158671236403115084.html.

18 Javier Portillo, "Madrileñismo, el arma identitaria de Isabel Díaz Ayuso," *Huffington Post*, October 10, 2020, accessed July 12, 2021, https://www.huffingtonpost.es/entry/madrilenismo-el-arma-identitaria-de-isabel-diaz-ayuso_es_5f89aa6cc5b6dc2d17f64abb.

abandoning the free movement of European citizens sanctioned by the EU and the Schengen Agreement.[19]

Focusing back on the recentralization of the Sánchez-Iglesias government, this arrangement was doubly paradoxical for another reason: as mentioned above, public health in Spain is the domain in which Spain was already partly functioning as a federal state.[20] Indeed, like education, public health in all its aspects is one of the sovereign powers to have been delegated ("transferred," as is said in Spain) to what would later become Autonomous Communities: Catalonia and the Basque Country in 1979, and Galicia and Andalusia in 1980. The same happened in the other communities: first in the Valencian Country, then in the Canary Islands, and finally in all the others. In 2001, the autonomous cities of Africa (Ceuta and Melilla) joined all the other autonomous regions that had already been transferred the authority and funding needed to manage matters of public health. While greatly diminished, the Ministry of Health is nonetheless not a hollow shell. It plays a role in intergovernmental coordination and regularly organizes multilateral "summits" to that end. Public health administration is thus undoubtedly the most federal structure that Spain has put in place, one that is ideologically compatible with the federalism of the PSOE.[21] However, Pedro Sánchez did not feel compelled to reinforce this crisis-shaken federalism and instead preferred to "recentralize" health (and manage the crisis in the French style) rather than approach it in the German style at a time when federal and centralized systems were being closely judged in a spirit of competition between states as to who managed the pandemic best. Such a strategic move raises one major question: is centralism the true orientation of the PSOE, or was the pandemic simply too risky for experimentation? While no definitive answer can be given here, it is clear that this issue continues to imbue Spanish territorial and political debate.

---

19 "Epidémie de coronavirus: confinement, fermeture des frontières, état d'urgence... Quelles sont les principales mesures prises par les pays européens?," *France Télévisions Info*, March 18, 2020, accessed July 12, 2021, https://www.francetvinfo.fr/sante/maladie/coronavirus/epi demie-de-coronavirus-confinement-fermeture-des-frontieres-etat-d-urgence-quelles-sont-les-principales-mesures-prises-par-european-countries_3872959.html.

20 José María Pérez Medina, "Dinámica de las conferencias sectoriales. Entre la intergubernamentalidad y la cooperación administrativa," *Revista d'Estudis Autonòmics i Federals*, 31 (2020): 48, accessed October 18, 2021, DOI : https://doi.org/10.2436/20.8080.01.44; Serafín Pazos-Vidal, "Federalismo sanitario en tiempos de coronavirus," *Agenda pública*, April 14, 2020, accessed October 18, 2021, https://agendapublica.es/federalismo-sanitario-en-tiempos-de-coronavirus/.

21 Ana Carbajosa and Marc Bassets, "La pandemia examina el federalismo alemán y el centralismo francés," *El País*, April 17, 2020, accessed July 12, 2021, https://elpais.com/internacional/2020-04-17/la-pandemia-examina-el-federalismo-aleman-y-el-centralismo-frances.html.

Indeed, like Spain and its ambiguous territorial structure, the PSOE swung from one position to the other: even if the party is a federal one and is, in theory, federalist, it is obvious that centralist Jacobin reflexes can emerge at any time, especially in moments of crisis. Well aware that his decision to adopt a *"mando único"* was being contended, Pedro Sánchez sought to make up for his "recentralized" approach by holding recurring meetings with the Conference of Presidents of the Autonomous Communities. This body had been created under the leadership of another socialist president, José Luis Rodríguez Zapatero, who had made "plural" Spain one of his main political slogans in order to win back over the Catalans and Basques who had joined the smaller parties during the markedly nationalist presidency of José Maria Aznar (2000–2004) but was then largely forgotten during the presidency of Mariano Rajoy.[22] The use of this formal gathering, designed to project onto the public stage the image of Spain as a diverse country, coming together for a common purpose, embodied the federalist will and spirit of presidents Zapatero and Sánchez. Conversely, the fact that Mariano Rajoy summoned this meeting only twice during his two terms (2011–2018) illustrates the political culture of the Popular Party which seems to distinguish between central (and sole?) power and that of the regional level, where the political autonomy of the communities would only allow for the administrative management of powers delegated by the central government.[23]

However, even though Pedro Sánchez convoked the Conference of Presidents more frequently (including 17 times since the start of the pandemic, mostly over videocall), another centralist tendency was observable in the intergovernmental network of Spain during the health crisis. The decisions of the central government were in fact territorialized by the provinces, the equivalent of the French *départements*, and thus by the administrative entities that existed prior to the Autonomous Communities. This political choice was far from insignificant and represented a cause for much concern and irritation for several regional governments.[24]

---

22 José Marcos, "La crisis del coronavirus reactiva los engranajes del Estado autonómico," *El País*, August 1, 2020, accessed July 12, 2021, https://elpais.com/espana/2020-08-01/la-crisis-del-coronavirus-reactiva-los-engranajes-del-estado-autonomico.html.
23 Luis Á. Gálvez Muñoz, "La conferencia de presidentes autonómicos o la historia interminable de la cooperación horizontal en el estado autonómico," in *"El futuro territorial del Estado español. ¿Centralización, autonomía, federalismo, confederación o secesión?"*, ed. Joan Oliver Araujo (Valencia: Tirant lo Blanch, 2014), 351–58.
24 Ferran Bono, "Siete autonomías se oponen al desconfinamiento por provincias y el Gobierno se abre a revisarlo," *El País*, April 29, 2020, accessed July 12, 2021, https://elpais.com/espana/2020-04-29/la-generalitat-valenciana-pedira-a-sanchez-realizar-la-desescalada-por-areas-sanitarias-y-no-por-provincias.html.

Internal Borders and Entities in the Management of the Pandemic: a Problematic Issue

Initially, the national policies and the decisions of Pedro Sánchez and his Minister of Health (the Catalan and very federalist Salvador Illa) were relayed across Spain via the 50 provinces. The incidence rate and therefore the different alert levels (that could lead to a lockdown) or the lifting of lockdown restrictions were calculated province by province, which generated waves of discontent in border areas where "interprovincial" traffic is very frequent for professional, personal, and socio-cultural reasons. This return to the province, and thus to the geographical demarcations created in 1833 and modeled after the French *départements* in order to break up the historical entities of former peninsular kingdoms, brought back to life a form of centralism imposed at the local scale that was very difficult to accept in many autonomic communities. It should be noted that the establishment of the Autonomous Communities by the Spanish Constitution of 1978 did not lead to the abolition of the Spanish provinces, which undoubtedly served as way for the central government to maintain a measure of territorial control to counterbalance the new regional powers. Indeed, the new Autonomous Communities were often formed through the merger of several federated provinces (the four Catalan provinces, for example).[25] In this sense, the *Carta Magna* of 1978 thus made up for the disappearance of historic territories caused precisely by the establishment of the provinces in 1833. In addition, seven provinces decided, for various reasons, to become autonomous communities themselves (Madrid, Murcia, La Rioja, Balearic Islands, Navarra, Asturias, and Cantabria). In these specific cases, the question of the recourse to provincial organization during the pandemic was not necessarily seen as a politicized issue but was instead viewed as an obstacle to mobility imposed by the central state. This situation was particularly hard to accept in Madrid, where workers commute on a daily basis from neighboring provinces, in the regions of Castile–La Mancha or Castile and León.

According to autonomists/nationalists, however, the province-based implementation of the various health measures evidenced that the federalist spirit of the PSOE was only an illusion and that in a crisis the centralizing nature of any

---

25 Article 143: In the exercise of the right to self-government recognized in Article 2 of the Constitution, bordering provinces with common historic, cultural, and economic characteristics, island territories and provinces with historic regional status may accede to self-government and form Autonomous Communities in accord with the provisions contained in this Title and in the respective Statutes: https://www.congreso.es/constitucion/ficheros/c78/cons_ingl.pdf.

Spanish government would prevail. This centralization would be compounded by another instinctive response: to consider Spain as being divided into provinces (linked only to Madrid), thus circumventing the communities, the truly autonomous entities. In the communities of central Spain, which were closely integrated into the State by virtue of being Castilian and/or Castilian-speaking, the strategy of resorting to the province seemed natural and did not shock anyone, except when it came to the aforementioned limitations imposed on residents' mobility. Neither was there any turmoil in the Basque Country, as the three provinces of Euskadi corresponded exactly to the three historical provinces of Biscay, Gipuzkoa, and Araba, which had associated with the Crown of Castile since the eleventh century. In Catalonia, however, the province-centered response was incomprehensible and considered unacceptable. Autonomous Catalonia had hastened since the early 1980s to develop (or rather, recover from the republican *Generalitat* of 1936) its own administrative division, with its 41 *comarques* (communities of municipalities) federated into seven *vegueries* since 2010[26] – a situation that highlighted the artificial and arbitrary character of the provinces imposed by the centralized State in 1833 and instituted as the sole local entities (beyond the municipalities) permitted during the Franco era. In Catalonia, local leaders (who are almost always Catalanists) have such an aversion to the concept of the Spanish province that, when it is necessary to refer to them – the province, for instance, is always the electoral district for the Catalan and Spanish legislative elections –, they prefer to use the term *demarcació*.[27]

Beyond Catalonia, the territorialization of pandemic management efforts via the provinces sparked controversy in several neighboring territories in which economic activity is largely cross-border. When the lifting of lockdown measures was decreed province by province after the strict and generalized lockdown of March and April 2020, many "cross-border" Spanish citizens were impacted. Derogations were of course possible for compelling reasons (e. g. work, medical appointments, examinations, etc.), but these excluded the purchase of food or basic necessities. For municipalities belonging to one province while being economically oriented towards a town in another neighboring province (which is a

---

26 Parlament de Catalunya, Llei 30/2010, del 3 d'agost, de vegueries, accessed July 12, 2021, https://www.parlament.cat/document/cataleg/48036.pdf.
27 This is the case in the media (public as well as private). In the example below, the term "demarcacions" is used to refer to the results of Spanish legislative elections in which the electoral district is the province. Even in this case where the use of the term "province" would be appropriate, it is that of "demarcació" which is preferred.

relatively common occurrence[28]), this return to the province was difficult to accept. The province as an administrative entity often proved unsuitable, and it was exactly the arbitrary nature of these internal borders that provoked an outcry, especially – but not only – in Catalonia.

During the second wave of the pandemic (from late summer to autumn of 2020), the legal framework of the state of emergency was made available to the autonomous communities in a spirit of "co-governance" on the part of the Sánchez-Iglesias government.[29] After the first spike in cases and the recentralized response discussed above, the central government sought to share decision-making responsibilities – as well as the risks that came with them. Indeed, this reorientation was interpreted by some as an effort to counter the criticisms coming from the opposition (from the PP and the nationalist parties), while others would say that it was a subtle way of sharing responsibility for controversial decisions, mistakes, and other failures.[30] Beyond this new controversy, the outbreak of the second wave pushed Catalonia to immediately set up local (municipal) or cantonal (to use the equivalent of the Catalan *comarca*) lockdowns. Better adapted to demographic and economic realities, the borders of the *comarques*[31] came under much less fire in Catalonia, even though they often presented a greater obstacle to mobility.[32] It is worth noting that for practical reasons, the Catalan *comarques* respect the borders of the four Catalan provinces, and thus none of them straddles two or more provinces (the *comarques* were created in 1936, by which point the provinces were already over 100 years old and well embedded in the popular imagination).

---

28 Lucía Palacios, "Trabajadores de ida y vuelta," *El Comercio*, October 6, 2019, accessed July 12, 2021, https://www.elcomercio.es/economia/trabajo/movilidad-laboral-2018-20191006155854-ntrc. html.

29 Gobierno de España, "Sánchez afirma que la unidad y la cogobernanza permitirán doblegar la segunda ola del COVID-19," Congreso de los Diputados, Madrid, miércoles 9 de septiembre de 2020, accessed July 12, 2021, https://www.lamoncloa.gob.es/presidente/actividades/Paginas/2020/090920-sanchezcongreso.aspx.

30 Gregoria Caro, "Sánchez descarga en las comunidades la responsabilidad de solicitar el estado de alarma por territorios," *ABC*, August 25, 2020, accessed October 19, 2021, https://www.abc.es/espana/abci-sanchez-descarga-comunidades-posibilidad-solicitar-estado-alarma-territorios-202008251412_noticia.html.

31 In Catalan, the plural of "comarca" is "comarques."

32 There are 41 *comarques* versus four provinces: the area of the *comarques* is therefore much smaller. Also, relatives are likely to depend on different *comarques* (and therefore encounter different restrictions).

Surprisingly, Aragon – which also counts 33 well-developed *comarcas*[33] – as is the case in Catalonia, and was thus well situated to respond to demographic and economic realities on the ground while also respecting the borders between the three provinces – chose not to impose lockdowns based on *comarcas*. Less sensitive than Catalonia in regard to the very existence of the provinces, the Aragonese government embraced the administrative division of the province in managing the local perimeter of lockdowns. Mobility between Aragonese provinces was thus prohibited for several months (except in cases of compelling reasons); similarly, it was impossible to travel to the capitals of these provinces, which had long been locked down. In this sense, lockdowns were implemented in an overlapping and multi-layered way: a municipal lockdown for the three provincial capitals (the cities of Huesca, Zaragoza, and Teruel); a lockdown by the provinces (the three homonymous provinces); and a regional lockdown. The reality of this situation meant that movement was only authorized between towns and villages within the same Aragonese province, provided it did not require passing through the provincial capital. All of these lockdowns were referred to as "perimeter-based," insofar as a municipal, provincial or community border designated the outer limits of the area placed under lockdown.

In other territories such as the Valencian Community (or Valencian Country) or Castile and León, it was the healthcare zones (demarcated within autonomous communities for the management of public health) which were taken into account for the different response levels, up to "perimeter-based" lockdown. This choice was intriguing, pragmatic and, above all, politically transversal. Indeed, the Valencian Country, ruled by a plural and autonomist left-wing party, is a very populated and relatively small territory (and therefore very densely populated) while Castile and León, ruled by a center-right party, is the largest region of Spain and one of the least populated (and in fact a demographic desert in places). As different as these two examples may be, healthcare zones turned out to be, in both cases, the most relevant territorial division for responding to the pandemic.[34] The Community of Madrid, an eminently urban and densely populated region, has also chosen to manage the different alert thresholds by healthcare zones. However, this scale in a metropolitan area like Madrid has shown limita-

---

33 In Spanish, the plural of "comarca" is "comarcas."
34 Diari Oficial de la Generalitat Valenciana, Num. 8936/25.10.2020 : 40467, accessed July 12, 2021, https://dogv.gva.es/datos/2020/10/25/pdf/2020_8862.pdf; Junta de Castilla y León, "Tasa de Enfermos por zonas básicas de salud," accessed October 19, 2021, https://analisis.datosa biertos.jcyl.es/explore/dataset/tasa-enfermos-acumulados-por-areas-de-salud/custom/?dis junctive.zbs_geo.

tions (there were exemptions allowing professional mobility) and has proved to be not very effective in controlling the evolution of the pandemic.[35]

Conclusion

During the first wave of the COVID 19 pandemic, the Spanish government (PSOE-UP) of Pedro Sánchez and Pablo Iglesias, although committed to the autonomy of the communities and to the (con)federal spirit, displayed a "centralized" response when faced with widespread panic. This progressive government effectively renounced the semi-federal nature of Spain and behaved like a centralized state. Later, during the initial lifting of restrictions (May-June 2020) and then during the second wave (September 2020), the recourse to the territorial entity known as the "province" (one that is very politically charged in certain territories) drew further criticism of this "recentralization" and highlighted the blurred nature of these territorial demarcations in the national and local management of the crisis. During the second wave of the pandemic, the government also put in place a form of "co-governance" by leaving to the executive authorities of the autonomous communities the legal framework of the state of emergency and the possibility of deciding on the various restrictions they deemed appropriate to the evolution of the health crisis. The more regionalized management of this second wave received its own criticism from (some of) the regional leaders themselves and from a segment of popular opinion (the most Jacobin, or, in other words, pro-centralization, section). Indeed, for the former it was electorally challenging to potentially be held responsible for unpopular measures, while, for the latter, the lack of a single decision-maker (the central government) was further proof of the disintegration of the state.

However, "co-governance" enabled the regions to decide on perimeter-based lockdowns within the most relevant administrative divisions, as informed by the criteria of regional governments (districts, communes, communities of communes [*comarcas/comarques*], healthcare zones, provinces, and/or entire regions). If in the use of healthcare zones (in the Valencian Country and Castile and León) one can see a pragmatic and apolitical approach, the use of the provinces in Aragon or of the *comarcas* in Catalonia can seem to have (consciously or unconsciously) political overtones. Beyond these very political con-

---

35 Isabel Valdés, "Por qué las restricciones por zonas básicas de salud no son efectivas," *El País*, March 1, 2021, accessed October 19, 2021, https://elpais.com/espana/madrid/2021-03-01/por-que-las-restricciones-por-zonas-basicas-de-salud-no-son-efectivas.html.

troversies surrounding the selection of internal delimitations, the COVID-19 crisis also undeniably gave rise to situations that can only be described as absurd. When the borders between countries began to reopen, some internal boundaries remained closed, which resulted in a situation in which it was impossible to go directly from Barcelona to Madrid (except for compelling reasons) while it was theoretically possible to take the same trip via Paris, Rome, Lisbon, Brussels etc. The arrival of young French people looking to party in Madrid even as the inhabitants of the capital city could not leave their area or host family members from outside this territory thus led to heated debates. During the summer of 2021, the French and German governments recommended their fellow citizens not to travel to Spain for the holidays, while a higher percentage of the Spanish population was fully vaccinated than in these two countries.[36] As for COVID-19-related mortality, since the dark days of the first wave, Spain's numbers had generally been better than those of the United Kingdom or Italy, for example, and comparable to those of France.[37] Future research will give us the insights necessary to understand whether the territorial organization of States had an impact on the management of this pandemic.

---

36 Vincent Coste, "Covid-19: le point sur la vaccination en Europe, pays par pays," *Euronews*, October 14, 2021, accessed October 18, 2021, https://fr.euronews.com/2021/01/14/covid-19-le-point-sur-la-vaccination-en-europe-pays-par-pays.
37 Redaction, "Muertes por COVID-19 en el mundo: ¿Qué país cuenta con más fallecidos por habitante?," *Radiotelevisión española, RTVE*, June 4, 2021, accessed October 18, 2021, https://www.rtve.es/noticias/20210604/paises-muertos-coronavirus-poblacion/2012350.shtml.

Anna Malandrino and Giliberto Capano

7 Institutional Mayhem as Usual

Intergovernmental Relations between the Central Government and the Regions in Italy during the Early Stages of the COVID-19 Pandemic

List of abbreviations

3T = Test, trace, treat
DL = Decree-law
DPCM = Decree of the Prime Minister
DPR = Decree of the President of the Republic
IGR = Intergovernmental relation
L. Cost = Constitutional Law
LEA = Essential level of assistance

Introduction

The COVID-19 pandemic represented – and at the time of writing still represents – a challenge that goes beyond public health issues. Indeed, it has also exacerbated the challenges at the heart of the Italian institutional framework. This chapter focuses on the evolution of the Italian response to the COVID-19 pandemic, specifically on the intergovernmental relations (IGRs) that characterized the Italian multi-level governance system from the end of January 2020 until May 2021. This timeframe covers the first three pandemic waves and the subsequent decline of the epidemiological threat that followed each wave. In doing so, the chapter reconstructs the key dynamics that affected IGRs of different types (horizontal and vertical) in terms of their level of conflict, their capacity to share goals, their level of agreement on policies and practices, and the clarity of each level's role. It also outlines the expected effects of these dynamics on the Italian regionalist – or quasi-federalist – configuration.

Anna Malandrino, Postdoctoral scholar and adjunct professor, University of Bologna.
Giliberto Capano, Professor of Political Science and Public Policy, University of Bologna.
The original version of this chapter was revised. Unfortunately the affiliation of Anna Malandrino was not included. We apologize for the mistake.

https://doi.org/10.1515/9783110745085-008

Our analysis builds on a critical examination of the policy measures adopted at different governmental levels and of the stances taken by Italian subnational units, i.e., regions, and by the central government throughout the evolution of the epidemiological crisis. To grasp the nature of IGRs from the point of view of policymaking, we examine policy documents, institutional communication documents as available on the website Regioni.it, policy and politics literature, and public opinion data. We code these sources qualitatively based on an analytical framework that devotes its attention to the key dimensions of IGRs between the central government and the regions. Two questions guide our research. First, how did internal IGRs evolve during the pandemic? And second, was the pandemic able to change the typical institutional dynamic of Italian regionalism/quasi-federalism in non-crisis times?

To contextualize our analysis, the chapter first provides a brief account of the main features of Italian regionalism by presenting the institutional context in which IGRs developed during the pandemic (Section 2). It then outlines and defines the key dimensions that constitute the analytical framework, which we employ to understand the reality of IGRs during the pandemic (Section 3). As will be shown, intergovernmental dynamics were crucial for determining the public policy response to the virus (Section 4). Moreover, we believe that these dynamics might play a role in changing the political landscapes in which regions operate and generate greater difficulties for them to challenge the quasi-federal arrangement that currently characterizes the Italian governance context (Section 5).

Institutional Context: Italian Regionalism

The Italian political system builds on a regional constitutional arrangement that includes 20 regions and two autonomous provinces. Five of these regions hold a special status (*regioni a statuto speciale*) that grants them more autonomy than the remaining ones. In 2001, a constitutional reform[1] provided the other 15 regions with more concurrent legislative powers and the opportunity for single regions to negotiate with the central government to obtain specific policy competences. As a result, regions are now especially autonomous in terms of health policy, including the organization and management of healthcare delivery. In fact, Italy's healthcare is a policy area of "undisputed regional government re-

---

1 Constitutional Law no. 3/2001 of October 18, 2001, Amendments to Title V of Part Two of the Constitution, https://www.normattiva.it/uri-res/N2Ls?urn:nir:stato:legge.costituzionale:2001-10-18;3~art10.

sponsibility."[2] While the central government establishes the general planning criteria and guidelines for the healthcare system, provides funding for it, and designs and ensures essential levels of assistance (LEAs), regions have full responsibility and autonomy for organizing, managing, and delivering healthcare services throughout their territory.[3] This high degree of organizational decentralization results in the very different design of key activities from region to region, even in terms of public/private dynamics.[4]

Despite this regional autonomy, the central government is primarily responsible for dealing with emergencies that threaten public health. However, since the management of those emergencies falls within the broader concept of health protection, including both public health and collective prevention or medical care measures and actions, the regions and their healthcare policy competences play a role in it, as well. The Italian Constitution does offer some instruments in the case of an emergency, such as granting the central government the power to replace regional authorities in the face of serious threats to public safety, but does not provide a general regulation on emergency management. However, primary legislation regulates emergency management and calls on both the central government and the regions.[5]

Thus, overall, the way Italian regionalism is designed includes a high level of constitutional asymmetry,[6] which some scholars define as "semi-federalism."[7]

2 Joan Costa-Font and Gilberto Turati, "Regional healthcare decentralization in unitary states: equal spending, equal satisfaction?," *Regional Studies* 52 (2018): 977, accessed May 26, 2021, DOI: 10.1080/00343404.2017.1361527.

3 Gianluca Fiorentini, Matteo Lippi Bruni, and Cristina Ugolini, "Health Systems and Health Reforms in Europe: the Case of Italy," *Intereconomics* 43 (2008), accessed May 26, 2021, DOI: 10.1007/s10272–008–0253-z; Federico Toth, "Like Surfers Waiting for the Big Wave: Health Care Politics in Italy," *Journal of Health Politics Policy and Law* 40 (2015), accessed May 26, 2021, DOI: 10.1215/03616878–3161186.

4 Sabina Nuti, Tommaso Grillo Ruggieri, and Silvia Podetti, "Do university hospitals perform better than general hospitals? A comparative analysis among Italian regions," *BMJ Open* 6 (2016), accessed May 26, 2021, doi:10.1136/bmjopen-2016–011426.

5 Paolo Giangaspero, "La normativa 'speciale' sulla gestione della pandemia da covid-19 sotto il profilo dei rapporti tra competenze statali e regionali," in *Virus in fabula. Diritti e Istituzioni ai tempi del covid-19*, ed. Gian Paolo Dolso, Maria Dolores Ferrara, and Davide Rossi (Trieste: EUT Edizioni Università di Trieste, 2020), accessed September 4, 2021, https://www.openstarts.units.it/handle/10077/30887; about collective prevention, see also Lino Cinquini et al., "Un modello di performance management per mitigare il problema dell'ambiguità nell'organizzazione della prevenzione collettiva: il caso della Regione Friuli-Venezia Giulia," *Mecosan: management ed economia sanitaria* 117 (2021), accessed September 4, 2021, DOI: 10.3280/MESA2021–117005.

6 Francesco Palermo and Alice Valdesalici, "Irreversibly Different. A Country Study of Constitutional Asymmetry in Italy," in *Constitutional Asymmetry in Multinational Federalism – Managing*

Additionally, following the 2001 reform, IGRs have also become more complex and conflictual. First, the reformed constitution is ambiguous in its attribution of powers, which has provoked a persistent jurisdictional conflict between the central government and the regions.[8] Second, in recent years, some northern regions have begun to firmly[9] request the implementation of the constitutional provisions that grant the regions more policy competences from the central government.[10] These requests act as a significant indicator of the centrifugal nature of Italian regionalism, which becomes even clearer in health policy.[11] Constitutional asymmetry has the potential to favor institutional differentiation and this, in addition to the characteristics of the respective regional political systems, which are mostly presidential systems,[12] creates a powerful opportunity for regional issues to become "politicized,"[13] in addition to provoking constant conflictual interinstitutional relationships. Thus, these pre-existing characteristics

---

Multinationalism in Multi-Tiered Systems, ed. Patricia Popelier and Maja Sahadzic (Cham: Palgrave Macmillan, 2019), accessed May 26, 2021, DOI: 10.1007/978-3-030-11701-6.

7 Marco Brunazzo, "Italian Regionalism: A Semi-Federation is Taking Shape – Or is It?," in *Territorial Choice: The Politics of Boundaries and Borders,* ed. Harald Baldersheim and Lawrence E. Rose (London: Palgrave Macmillan, 2010), accessed May 26, 2021, DOI: 10.1057/9780230289826_10.

8 Andrea Lippi, "Evaluating the 'Quasi Federalist' Programme of Decentralisation in Italy since the 1990s: A Side-effect Approach," *Local Government Studies* 37 (2011), accessed May 26, 2021, DOI: 10.1080/03003930.2011.604543.

9 Brunetta Baldi and Filippo Tronconi, "Tra centro e periferia. Le elezioni regionali e il difficile approdo al federalismo fiscale," in *Politica in Italia. I fatti dell'anno e le interpretazioni. Edizione 2011,* ed. Elisabetta Gualmini and Eleonora Pasotti (Bologna: Il Mulino, 2011), accessed May 26, 2021, DOI: 10.978.8815/304339.

10 Brunetta Baldi, "Autonomismo o federalismo? Modelli di sviluppo per il regionalismo italiano," *Economia e Società Regionale* 37 (2019), accessed May 26, 2021, DOI: 10.3280/ES2019-003003; Davide Vampa and Arianna Giovannini, "Autonomia differenziata come processo dal basso: i referendum regionali in prospettiva comparata," *Economia e Società Regionale* 37 (2019), accessed May 26, 2021, DOI: 10.3280/ES2019-003007.

11 Joan Costa-Font and Scott L. Greer, "Health System Federalism and Decentralization: What Is It, Why Does It Happen, and What Does It Do?," in *Federalism and Decentralization in European Health and Social Care,* ed. Joan Costa-Font and Scott L. Greer (London: Palgrave Macmillan, 2013), accessed May 26, 2021, doi:10.1057/9781137291875_1; Joan Costa-Font and Gilberto Turati, "Regional healthcare decentralization."

12 Fabio Padovano and Roberto Ricciuti, "Political competition and economic performance: evidence from the Italian regions," *Public Choice* 138 (2009), accessed May 26, 2021, DOI: 10.1007/s11127-008-9358-y.

13 Franca Maino, "The Italian Health System: Cost Containment, Mismanagement, and Politicization," *Italian Politics* 24 (2008): 216, accessed May 26, 2021, http://www.jstor.org/stable/43486427.

of Italian regionalism and its centrifugal dynamics set the stage for a fragmented political environment and politicization on the eve of the pandemic.

Theoretical Background and Analytical Framework

IGRs embody "the processes and institutions through which governments within a political system interact. All countries, whether unitary or federal, have IGRs of some sort, provided that they have more than one level of government."[14] Italy is no exception. However, in the real world of politics, the distribution of power through constitutional arrangements matters less than the way IGRs actually work in practice. It is therefore not a coincidence that federal countries undergo a continuous process of change[15] in the face of specific contingencies.[16] This is also true of other countries that possess different configurations and which, despite their form (as more or less unitary), are also subject to constant readjustments in their IGRs.[17]

The COVID-19 pandemic and the declaration of a state of emergency reshuffled decision-making responsibilities and entrusted the central executive with more powers. At the same time, crisis management also involved the regions as key actors. Throughout the emergency, they adopted restrictions and numerous ordinances for the benefit of public health, and they regulated how crucial public services such as healthcare and education were provided. In this context, the COVID-19 pandemic and the response to it in Italy can be considered as a litmus test of how IGRs really operate. Indeed, worldwide, the type of political sys-

---

14 John Phillimore, "Understanding Intergovernmental Relations: Key Features and Trends," *Australian Journal of Public Administration* 72 (2013): 229, accessed May 26, 2021, DOI: 10.1111/ 1467-8500.12025.

15 Robert Agranoff and Beryl A. Radin, "Deil Wright's Overlapping Model of Intergovernmental Relations: The Basis for Contemporary Intergovernmental Relationships," *Publius: The Journal of Federalism* 45 (2015), accessed May 26, 2021, DOI: 10.1093/publius/pju036; Sabine Kropp and Nathalie Behnke, "Marble cake dreaming of layer cake: the merits and pitfalls of disentanglement in German federalism reform," *Regional & Federal Studies* 26 (2016), accessed May 26, 2021, DOI: 10.1080/13597566.2016.1236335.

16 Arthur Benz, "Gradual Constitutional Change and Federal Dynamics – German Federalism Reform in Historical Perspective," *Regional & Federal Studies* 26 (2016), accessed May 26, 2021, DOI: 10.1080/13597566.2016.1226813.

17 Arthur Benz and Jörg Broschek, eds., *Federal Dynamics: Continuity, Change, and the Varieties of Federalism* (Oxford: Oxford University Press, 2013), accessed May 26, 2021, DOI: 10.1093/acprof:oso/9780199652990.001.0001.

tem (unitary vs. federal or quasi-federal) itself was not the only variable that de-termined a country's ability to respond to this crisis.[18] Some unitary countries performed decently while others performed poorly. The same is true of federal countries.[19] Governmental capacities and policy design characteristics do, of course, matter. However, their impact cannot be assessed without understanding how internal intergovernmental dynamics develop in reality.

Therefore, to understand internal intergovernmental dynamics, we analyze five key dimensions:

- The type of relationship involved: relationships can be either vertical or hor-izontal (or a mix of both)[20] and can be defined as such by identifying the main actors that are involved in each IGR;
- The level of intergovernmental conflict: we define conflict as public criticism and accompanying actions between government levels[21] as well as a dynam-ic that requires attention during the processes of intergovernmental coordi-nation.[22] We assess the level of conflict by means of the frequency and strength of the identified criticism;
- The capacity to share goals: sharing goals is a structural foundation of col-laboration between different governmental levels.[23] We evaluate this capaci-ty by comparing whether the actions taken by the central government and the regions follow the same direction of action;
- Intergovernmental agreement on policy practices: this agreement is defined as an essential feature for effective policymaking, whose absence can lead to

---

18 Davide Vampa, "COVID-19 and Territorial Policy Dynamics in Western Europe: Comparing France, Spain, Italy, Germany, and the United Kingdom," *Publius* (2021), accessed September 5, 2021, DOI: 10.1093/publius/pjab017.

19 Tim Büthe et al., "Patterns of Policy Responses to the COVID-19 Pandemic in Federal vs. Uni-tary European Democracies" (paper prepared for presentation at the 2020 Annual Meeting of the American Political Science Association, September 10, 2020).

20 Beryl Radin, "The instruments of intergovernmental management," in *Handbook of public administration*, ed. Guy Peters and Jon Pierre (Los Angeles, London, New Delhi, Singapore: SAGE Publications 2003), 607–18, DOI: 10.4135/9781848608214.n49

21 André Lecours et al., "Explaining Intergovernmental Conflict in the COVID-19 Crisis: The United States, Canada, and Australia," *Publius* (2021): 1–24, accessed September 5, 2021, DOI: 10.1093/publius/pjab010.

22 Nicole Bolleyer, Wilfried Swenden, and Nicola McEwen, "A theoretical perspective on multi-level systems in Europe: Constitutional power and partisan conflict," *Comparative European Pol-itics* 12 (2014): 367–83, accessed September 5, 2021, DOI: 10.1057/cep.2014.18.

23 Allan Fels, Preface to *Collaborative Governance: A New Era of Public Policy in Australia?*, ed. Janine O'Flynn and John Wanna (Canberra: ANU Press, 2008), xi–xiv, accessed September 5, 2021, www.jstor.org/stable/j.ctt24h315.4.

contradictory and mutually destructive policies.[24] We assess the level of agreement through an analysis of the measures adopted or advocated at the examined government levels;
- The clarity of the roles of different government levels: this clarity refers to the level of definition of responsibilities at different levels of government, which is a structural foundation of collaborative IGRs whose absence can, however, particularly emerge and pose problems during crises.[25] We estimate this dimension by assessing the rules provided to solve this problem and the intergovernmental debates on the respective competences.

These dimensions provide us with a deep understanding of the characteristics of IGR dynamics in Italy over time. The response to the pandemic was a process that, like in the rest of the world, occurred through a number of waves and according to the pace at which the virus spread, rather than a response developed "in one shot." For this reason, this chapter analyzes IGR dynamics during a 16-month timeframe that includes three pandemic waves. This timeframe and our analysis of the key dimensions of IGRs allow us to assess the multifaceted dynamics of Italian IGRs during the COVID-19 pandemic over time and to test their capacity to change during the crisis. Moreover, these five dimensions represent different aspects of the government levels' capacity to coordinate, which is crucial for determining the success of policy responses to crises.[26] Furthermore, we assume that these five dimensions adapted depending on the specific phase of each pandemic wave during which they occurred. Two specific phases alternated through the three pandemic waves and characterized the policy dynamics: the building-up and scaling-down phases. The building-up stage refers to policies that represented the maximum response for containing the virus, i.e., when the levels of government adopted and enforced highly restrictive measures. In contrast, the scaling-down phase refers to the process through

---

24 Xun Wu et al., *The public policy primer: managing the policy process* (London/New York: Routledge, 2017).
25 Andrea Riccardo Migone, "Trust, but customize: federalism's impact on the Canadian COVID-19 response," *Policy and Society* 39 (2020): 382–402, accessed September 5, 2021, DOI: 10.1080/14494035.2020.1783788.
26 Brunetta Baldi and Stefania Profeti, "Le fatiche della collaborazione. Il rapporto stato-regioni in Italia ai tempi del COVID -19," *Rivista Italiana di Politiche Pubbliche* (2020): 278, accessed May 28, 2021, DOI: 10.1483/98731; Donald F. Kettl, "Contingent Coordination: Practical and Theoretical Puzzles for Homeland Security," *The American Review of Public Administration* 33 (2003), accessed May 28, 2021, DOI: 10.1177/0275074003254472; Tom Christensen et al., "Comparing Coordination Structures for Crisis Management in Six Countries," *Public Administration* 94 (2016), accessed May 28, 2021, DOI: 10.1111/padm.12186.

which the levels of government lifted restrictions. This distinction is analytically important. We can expect that the dimensions of IGR dynamics may have varied through the different phases and, specifically, that they may have experienced a lower level of consensus during the scaling-down phases due to the natural re-balancing of interests and priorities once the pandemic curve flattened and the virus was less perceived as a threat.

Public Policy and IGR Dynamics during the Pandemic

The organizational characteristics of the regional healthcare systems resulted in a great variety of policy responses to the epidemiological crisis.[27] Different regional healthcare delivery setups influenced the effectiveness of healthcare not only during the first wave,[28] which took all regions by surprise, but also in the following waves. Accordingly, national guidelines on health responses could not guarantee the uniformity of the policy outcome in different parts of the country. The different ways in which regions treated the disease (ranging from massive hospitalization to predominantly home-based approaches) impacted the course of the pandemic. However, some horizontal policy learning[29] occurred. Regions were able to draw lessons from others[30]: for instance, all regions learned from specific regions' early experiences (such as that of Veneto) that ordering not-heavily-affected patients to stay home was a more effective measure than the hospitalization of mild cases, and they reduced hospitalization at a later stage of the pandemic.[31] The Italian regions' differentiated organizational mod-

---

27 Mattia Casula, Andrea Terlizzi, and Federico Toth, "I servizi sanitari regionali alla prova del COVID-19," *Rivista Italiana di Politiche Pubbliche* (2020), accessed May 26, 2021, DOI: 10.1483/98732.

28 Giliberto Capano and Andrea Lippi, "Decentralization, Policy Capacities, and Varieties of First Health Response to the COVID-19 Outbreak. Evidence from Three Regions in Italy," *Journal of European Public Policy* (2021), forthcoming.

29 Colin J. Bennett and Michael Howlett, "The lessons of learning: Reconciling theories of policy learning and policy change," *Policy Sciences* 25 (1992), accessed May 28, 2021, DOI: 10.1007/BF00138786.

30 Richard Rose, "What is lesson-drawing," *Journal of Public Policy* 11 (1991), accessed May 28, 2021, DOI: 10.1017/S0143814X00004918.

31 Fabrizio Pecoraro, Daniela Luzi, and Fabrizio Clemente, "Analysis of the Different Approaches Adopted in the Italian Regions to Care for Patients Affected by COVID-19," *International Journal of Environmental Research and Public Health* 18 (2021), accessed May 28, 2021, DOI: 10.3390/ijerph18030848.

els also impacted vaccination policy. At first, different regions were able to choose the order in which they vaccinated social groups. For instance, Tuscany included lawyers among the people who could get vaccinated before others, considering them as operators of the justice system and therefore as essential workers.[32] Moreover, each region defined its own system for citizens to "book" a vaccination appointment or for invitations to vaccinate to be sent to citizens.[33] This fragmentation partly derived from the vague standards set at the central level that left regional authorities with a fair degree of discretion.[34] This later changed following the adoption of a new priority order at the national level.[35]

This diversity in terms of healthcare policy formulation and implementation went hand in hand with a lack of national monitoring and coordination of the regional strategies that sought to protect public health. National coordination was especially weak[36] in the face of regional politicization. The central government mostly led the pandemic response erratically across its various waves, and its initial lack of preparation[37] was only slowly addressed. It did not fully exploit the legislative and constitutional powers that enable its supremacy over the regions in exceptional cases, such as pandemics.[38] This initial choice was partly due to the weakness of the ruling coalition, characterized by the predominance of two main political forces, i.e. the Five Star Movement and the Democratic Party, with the former having been somewhat delegitimized by its

---

32 Bar Association of Florence, Letter to the President of the Tuscany Region, Prot. 4652, of April 2, 2021, accessed September 30, 2021, https://ordineavvocatilivorno.it/news/lettera-alla-regione-toscana-sulla-questione-vaccini.html.

33 See for instance Lombardy region, Deliberation no. 4353 of February 24, 2021, Approval of the regional vaccine plan for the prevention of SARS-COV 2 infections, accessed September 30, 2021, https://www.regione.lombardia.it/wps/portal/istituzionale/HP/istituzione/Giunta/sedute-delibere-giunta-regionale/DettaglioDelibere/delibera-4353-legislatura-11.

34 Ministry of Health, Decree of March 12, 2021, https://www.gazzettaufficiale.it/eli/id/2021/03/24/21A01802/sg.

35 Extraordinary Commissioner for the COVID-19 Emergency, Ordinance no. 6 of April 9, 2021, https://www.governo.it/sites/governo.it/files/CSCovid19_Ord_6_20210409.pdf.

36 Paola Mattei and Eloisa Del Pino, "Coordination and Health Policy Responses to the First Wave of COVID-19 in Italy and Spain," *Journal of Comparative Policy Analysis: Research and Practice* 23 (2021), accessed May 26, 2021, doi:10.1080/13876988.2021.1878886.

37 Giliberto Capano et al., "Mobilizing Policy (In)Capacity to Fight COVID-19: Understanding Variations in State Responses," *Policy and Society* 39 (2020), accessed May 26, 2021, DOI: 10.1080/14494035.2020.1787628.

38 Giliberto Capano, "Policy design and state capacity in the COVID-19 emergency in Italy: if you are not prepared for the (un)expected, you can be only what you already are," *Policy and Society* 39 (2020), DOI: 10.1080/14494035.2020.1783790; and Vampa, "COVID-19 and Territorial Policy Dynamics."

participation in the previous, heterogeneous ruling coalition (with *Lega Nord*) and its incapacity to meet the high expectations of policy reform that were associated with its ascendance to power as a challenger.[39] The choice not to shift power to the center undermined the central government's role and reinforced a general perception that regional presidents had more power than had actually been formally granted to them. The regions, for their part, often played the "blame game," thus contributing to delayed decision-making.[40] Regional presidents often acted as the representatives of local interests rather than as co-responsible actors of the national strategy. They also constructed joint positions, often expressed through the Conference of Regions and Autonomous Provinces (hereinafter referred to as "Conference of Regions"), an association of the Italian regions (and autonomous provinces) born in 1981 to promote regional lobbying activities vis-à-vis the national government.[41] This was also mirrored in the high levels of local consensus reached by some regional presidents in their own regions, such as those of Campania and Veneto, after the first wave (Figure 1).

However, IGR characteristics did not remain constant throughout the pandemic. In fact, they took different forms depending on whether they occurred as part of the building-up or scaling-down phases and whether they occurred during a specific pandemic wave.

The First Wave

Building-up

Amidst the policy response to the first wave, IGRs experienced several conflictual moments. Indeed, concurrently issued public health policies created a number of rules at the national and local levels that were sometimes contradictory, over crucial issues such as face mask usage, movement restrictions, and testing. These contradictory policies were a result of weak coordination within the vertical relationship of the governance levels.[42] The central government, on its part,

---

39 Nicolò Conti, Andrea Pedrazzani and Federico Russo, "Policy Polarisation in Italy: The Short and Conflictual Life of the 'Government of Change' (2018–2019)," *South European Society and Politics*, 25 (2020), accessed September 30, 2021, DOI: 10.1080/13608746.2020.1840110.

40 Capano, "Policy design and state capacity in the COVID-19 emergency in Italy."

41 Baldi and Profeti, "Le fatiche della collaborazione."

42 Anna Malandrino and Elena Demichelis, "Conflict in decision making and variation in public administration outcomes in Italy during the COVID-19 crisis," *European Policy Analysis* 6 (2020), accessed May 26, 2021, doi:10.1002/epa2.1093.

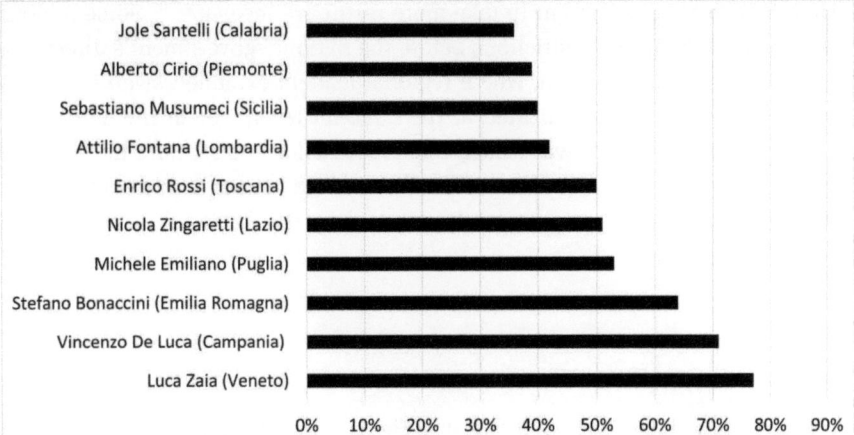

Figure 1: Public satisfaction with the actions of the presidents of Italian regions, as observed in July 2020. Authors' elaboration of available data released by Winpoll. Italian male and female population aged 18 and over, segmented by sex, age, provinces, in proportion to the universe of the population in the 11 most populous regions. Number of interviews: 3,500. Question posed: "Can you please tell me how satisfied you are with the performance of the president of your region?"

behaved erratically and often sought consensus. It thus pursued a kind of decision-making that disclosed a vocation for negotiation[43] and which resulted in time-consuming discussions on how to face the pandemic emergency. These discussions led to a slow response, as evident by the chronology of the decisions adopted. Italy registered its first COVID-19 cases when the Spallanzani Hospital in Rome admitted two Chinese tourists from Wuhan (China) on January 30, 2021,[44] a few days after they had arrived in Italy.[45] From that date, it took 39 days for the central government to issue the first national lockdown, which halted all non-essential business activities.[46] The awareness that there was a need to face a dangerous external threat gradually emerged among the regions and the central government. During this phase, some regional governments

---

43 Umberto Ronga, "Il Governo nell'emergenza (permanente). Sistema delle fonti e modello legislativo a partire dal caso Covid-19," *Nomos* (2020), accessed May 26, 2021, https://www.nomos-leattualitaneldiritto.it/wp-content/uploads/2020/05/Ronga-1-2020-coronavirus-D.pdf.
44 Paola Mattei and Eloisa Del Pino, "Coordination and Health Policy Responses."
45 Marta Giovanetti et al., "The first two cases of 2019-nCoV in Italy: Where they come from?," *Journal of Medical Virology* 92 (2020), accessed May 26, 2021, DOI: 10.1002/jmv.25699.
46 DPCM of March 11, 2020, https://www.gazzettaufficiale.it/eli/id/2020/03/11/20A01605/sg.

urged the central government to take more restrictive measures.[47] Some regions even imposed their own restrictions before the national government's directives, such as in the Veneto region, where regional leaders extended swab testing to categories beyond those indicated at the national level,[48] or in the Marche region, where an ordinance was issued that closed all schools before the national lockdown was declared[49] (indeed, the ordinance was immediately contested by the central government and promptly quashed by the Regional Administrative Court).[50]

Scaling-down

In the scaling-down phase, vertical IGRs continued to follow their usual conflict-ridden path while the horizontal relationships between regions started to improve. The final result for vertical IGRs was that regions were granted more autonomy to shape their scaling-down processes according to their specific local situations and socioeconomic trade-offs. However, these processes had to take place within the limits of the measures adopted at the national level and could only occur if the measures adopted were more restrictive than the national ones, as established by the national legislation adopted during the building-up phase.[51]

Over time, the presidents of the regions began to construct shared positions during their recurrent meetings, which culminated in the adoption of common guidelines for managing the reopening phase.[52] These guidelines provided mea-

---

47 Segreteria della Conferenza delle Regioni e delle Province autonome, "Coronavirus: richieste restrizioni più severe," *Regioni.it* 3803 (2020), accessed May 26, 2021, http://www.regioni.it/newsletter/n-3803/del-20-03-2020/coronavirus-richieste-restrizioni-piu-severe-20973/.

48 Paola Mattei and Eloisa Del Pino, "Coordination and Health Policy Responses."

49 Marche region, ordinance no. 1 of February 25, 2020, Measures to contain and manage the COVID-19 emergency, accessed September 30, 2021, https://www.regione.marche.it/ars/Aree-di-Attivit%C3%A0/Coronavirus/Normativa-regionale.

50 Regional Administrative Court for the Marche region, decision of February 27, 2021, http://www.issirfa.cnr.it/tar-marche-56-2020.html; see also Malandrino and Demichelis, "Conflict in decision making."

51 DL 19/2020 of March 25, 2020, art. 3, https://www.normattiva.it/uri-res/N2Ls?urn:nir:stato:decreto.legge:2020-03-25;19!vig=.

52 Conferenza delle Regioni e delle Province autonome, "Linee guida per la riapertura delle Attività Economiche, Produttive e Ricreative," Rome, June 9, 2020, 20/83/CR01/COV19, accessed May 26, 2021, http://www.regioni.it/home/aggiornate-linee-guida-per-riapertura-attivita-economiche-produttive-e-ricreative-2563/.

sures for the safe resumption of social and economic activities (such as those of restaurants, shops, swimming pools, museums, hairdressers, etc.) and covered aspects such as workplace sanitation, social distancing, and facial coverings. The presidents of the regions had sometimes opposed the national government's proposals that failed to adequately consider regional decisions and joint efforts, but these efforts were finally recognized and approved in the guidelines adopted at the central level, although with a few exceptions (for instance, discos and clubs were included in the regions' safe reopening guidelines but were still subjected to a suspension of their activities by national decree).[53] However, subsequently, there was also some degree of conflict on the horizontal level, i.e., between regions. This conflict mainly revolved around a split between regions in relation to the solutions proposed to prepare for the summer months. A minority of regions supported the introduction of health passports for tourists coming from other regions. However, the majority of regions opposed this proposal and agreed with the central government's argument that it was unconstitutional in nature.[54]

The Second Wave

Building-up

During the summer of 2020, many regions were unable to adapt local transportation services to the changed contingencies implied by the pandemic in preparation for the reopening of schools and to protect public health. Notwithstanding, through the joint effort of local authorities, regions, and the central government, a final agreement was reached which culminated in the adoption of public transportation guidelines.[55] On the other hand, many regions did not

---

53 Segreteria della Conferenza delle Regioni e delle Province autonome, "Linee guida per la riapertura delle attività economiche," *Regioni.it* 3844 (2020), accessed May 26, 2021, http://www. regioni.it/newsletter/n-3844/del-19-05-2020/linee-guida-per-la-riapertura-delle-attivita-econom iche-21233/; see also DL no. 33 of May 16, 2020, https://www.gazzettaufficiale.it/eli/id/2020/05/ 16/20G00051/sg.
54 Cf. DL 33/2020 of May 16, 2020, https://www.gazzettaufficiale.it/eli/id/2020/05/16/20G00051/ sg, as well as Segreteria della Conferenza delle Regioni e delle Province autonome, "Emergenza Covid-19 e spostamenti interregionali nell'agenda Governo-Regioni," *Regioni.it* 3852 (2020), accessed May 26, 2021, http://www.regioni.it/newsletter/n-3852/del-29-05-2020/emergenza-covid-19-e-spostamenti-interregionali-nellagenda-governo-regioni-21280/.
55 Segreteria della Conferenza delle Regioni e delle Province autonome, "Linee Guida trasporto locale: Toma, bene soluzioni condivise Governo-Regioni," *Regioni.it* 3901 (2020), accessed

manage to implement a consistent[56] 3T (test, trace and treat) strategy, due to in-efficiencies in the testing phase.[57] The central government itself was not fully prepared for a possible second wave, despite efforts by the Ministry of Health during the summer to get ready for this scenario.[58]

This general lack of preparedness was paired with regional resistance to the new restrictive measures that were adopted by the central government in October 2020 due to the resurgence of the pandemic. There were even regional demands asking the national government for the attribution of powers to adopt not only more but also less restrictive measures than those issued by the central govern-ment, as demanded by Sicily after the closure of gyms, restaurants, cinemas and theaters by the national government, which the region itself considered "unrea-sonable."[59] These demands sharply contrasted with the types of demands that characterized the first building-up phase. The central level responded to these demands for greater autonomy by adopting a radically new system of restrictions based on specific health indicators and risk levels, commonly known as the color-based or traffic-light system because of how the central government pre-sented it to the general public and its resemblance to the traffic regulation sys-tem based on three colors. This system replaced the previous system that only identified red zones as specific areas subject to more restrictive measures. The central government adopted this system at the beginning of November 2020.[60]

Overall during this phase, the central government's decision to react with the maximum response for tackling the virus was delayed because of tensions within IGRs. This delay was so severe that some causes of the second pandemic wave in Italy were identified as stemming from low coordination and political

---

May 26, 2021, http://www.regioni.it/newsletter/n-3901/del-07-09-2020/linee-guida-trasporto-lo cale-toma-bene-soluzioni-condivise-governo-regioni-21602/.

56 Giorgio Alleva and Alberto Zuliani, "Coronavirus: chiarezza sui dati," *Bancaria* (2020).

57 Fondazione Gimbe, "Coronavirus: tamponi, indietro tutta," press release, June 11, 2020, ac-cessed May 26, 2021, https://www.gimbe.org/pagine/341/it/comunicatistampa?pagina=12.

58 Ministry of Health and National Institute of Health, "Elementi di preparazione e risposta a COVID-19 nella stagione autunno-invernale," August 11, 2020, http://www.protezionecivile.gov. it/documents/20182/823803/Elementi+di+preparazione+e+risposta+a+COVID-19+nella+stagione +autunno-invernale/a0a052cd-b5d9-423f-ae68-45eb527b68cc; see also the document entitled "Prevenzione e risposta a COVID-19: evoluzione della strategia e pianificazione nella fase di transizione per il periodo autunno-invernale" (Rome: Ministero della Salute, Istituto Superiore di Sanità, 2020).

59 Segreteria della Conferenza delle Regioni e delle Province autonome, "Dpcm e pandemia: spiegazioni e proposte," *Regioni.it* 3937 (2020), accessed May 26, 2021, http://www.regioni.it/ newsletter/n-3937/del-27-10-2020/dpcm-e-pandemia-spiegazioni-e-proposte-21830/.

60 DPCM of November 3, 2020, https://www.gazzettaufficiale.it/eli/id/2020/11/04/20A06109/sg.

conflict between the central government, regions, and stakeholders, which led to "a relaxation of individual health behaviors, poor and conflicting communication to the general public, poor management of the public transport and the reopening of schools and companies after the summer."[61]

Scaling-down

The alert levels defined in the new system made the scaling-down process almost automatic since restrictions could be progressively lifted according to the values of a series of 21 indicators that gauged regional capacities in three areas. These areas can be summarized as follows: a) monitoring (process indicator); b) diagnosis and treatment (process indicator); c) virus transmission and healthcare system robustness/endurance (result indicator). These indicators became the basis for policy regimes of varied restrictiveness in different areas of the country from November 2020 on. There was some degree of consensus between the central government and the regions on the approval of these criteria,[62] which thus proved to provoke less conflict than previous policy processes. The outcome of this color-based system was by nature different depending on the evolving epidemiological and healthcare situation of each region, which was periodically "photographed" by means of ordinances issued by the Ministry of Health and addressed using (top-down) measures that had a variable degree of restrictiveness.

Some degree of vertical intergovernmental conflict did materialize around the reopening of schools after the Christmas holidays. According to national rules,[63] primary and middle schools were due to reopen on January 7, 2021 and high schools on January 11, 2021 with 50% in-class teaching. However, many regions were worried about the epidemiological situation and opposed these measures, opting to apply more restrictive ones. School re-openings were postponed variably until the end of January or even the beginning of February. The regions sought and obtained the opportunity to discuss the issue of

---

61 Francesco Chirico et al., "Coronavirus disease 2019: the second wave in Italy," *Journal of Health Research* (2021), doi:10.1108/JHR-10 – 2020 – 0514.
62 See the document entitled "Informativa urgente del Governo sui dati e sui criteri seguiti per la collocazione delle regioni italiane nelle aree rossa, arancione e gialla, previste dal DPCM 3 novembre 2020," speech of the Minister of Health at Camera dei Deputati (Parlamento Italiano), November 6, 2020, accessed May 28, 2021, https://www.salute.gov.it/portale/ministro/p4_3_1_1.jsp?lingua=italiano&id=70&label=parlamento&menu=ministro.
63 DL 1/2021 of January 5, 2021, https://www.gazzettaufficiale.it/eli/id/2021/01/05/21G00001/sg.

school reopening with the central government,[64] a symbol of collaborative efforts. In the meantime, by the end of January, the color-based system designated most Italian regions as having low levels of risk (i.e., they became "yellow"). As a result, they were less affected by restrictive measures.[65]

The inversion of support for more restrictive measures between the central government and the regions, with the former pursuing less restrictive measures and the latter opposing them and opting for more restrictive policies, reversed once more in February. At that time, the regions pushed to decrease the stringency of restrictions in the areas designated as yellow. In this regard, the president of the Conference of Regions and of the Emilia-Romagna region, Stefano Bonaccini, asked for the reopening in low-risk areas of cinemas, theaters, swimming pools, gyms, and restaurants in the evening.[66] However, this new trend confronted the new political contingencies and policy strategies triggered by the appointment of the new Prime Minister, Mario Draghi,[67] after the Conte government crisis. This was a political crisis triggered at the end of 2020 when the leader of the *Italia Viva* party (Matteo Renzi), which was at that time in the ruling coalition, started to threaten to withdraw its support for the government on grounds of its spending priorities for the Italian part of the EU recovery fund.[68]

---

64 Segreteria della Conferenza delle Regioni e delle Province autonome, "Emergenza Covid-19: didattica in presenza a scuola, urge confronto Governo-Regioni," *Regioni.it* 3984 (2021), accessed May 28, 2021, http://www.regioni.it/newsletter/n-3984/del-19-01-2021/emergenza-covid-19-didattica-in-presenza-a-scuola-urge-confronto-governo-regioni-22157/.
65 Ministry of Health, Ordinances of January 29, 2021, reg. no. 165, https://www.trovanorme.salute.gov.it/norme/dettaglioAtto?id=78698, and reg. no. 166, https://www.trovanorme.salute.gov.it/norme/dettaglioAtto?id=78699.
66 Segreteria della Conferenza delle Regioni e delle Province autonome, "Pandemia: nuove ordinanze territoriali e richieste di rimodulazione aperture," *Regioni.it* 4011 (2021), accessed May 28, 2021, http://www.regioni.it/newsletter/n-4011/del-23-02-2021/pandemia-nuove-ordinanze-territoriali-e-richieste-di-rimodulazione-aperture-22335/.
67 DPR of February 12, 2021, https://www.gazzettaufficiale.it/eli/id/2021/02/15/21A00995/sg.
68 Martin Bull, "The Italian government response to Covid-19 and the making of a prime minister," *Contemporary Italian Politics* 13 (2021), accessed September 30, 2021, DOI: 10.1080/23248823.2021.1914453.

The Third Wave

Building-up

The process of building up new restrictions in the face of the third wave of the pandemic was initially less conflictual than the previous two ones. This was due in large part to the settlement of the new central government, which was supported by a varied and "large" coalition in terms of political orientations. Indeed, the new government was endorsed by a large majority of the Italian Parliament, involving members of six different political parties (the Five Star Movement, the League, the Democratic Party, *Forza Italia*, *Italia Viva*, and Article One). These parties represented a wide array of political orientations, ranging from left-wing to right-wing ones, which was mirrored in the new composition of the Council of Ministers. The general agreement and consensus around the newly-appointed Prime Minister – a former president of the European Central Bank – was also due to his personal background and competences. Thus, his appointment by the President of the Italian Republic and his formation of a "technocratic government" – a type of government that is led by a non-political leader and whose formation is often resorted to in times of crisis in Italy[69] – were generally considered a necessity in a context of high political conflict that did not allow for the development of a "political" government.[70]

However, it was not long before the new Prime Minister faced difficulties due to regional discontent. The usual blame-game dynamic arose again between the Prime Minister and some presidents of regions. The Prime Minister reproached the regions for neglecting elderly people within the framework of the vaccination policy.[71] Meanwhile, some presidents of regions retorted that the vaccination plan had actually been adopted at the national level and therefore called on the central government to take responsibility. A similar blame-shifting dynamic

---

69 Luca Verzichelli and Maurizio Cotta, "Shades of Technocracy: The Variable Use of Non-partisan Ministers in Italy," in *Technocratic Ministers and Political Leadership in European Democracies*, ed. António Costa Pinto, Maurizio Cotta, and Pedro Tavares de Almeida (Cham: Palgrave Macmillan, 2018).

70 On the nature and function of technocratic governments in Italy including the Draghi cabinet, cf. also Nicola Lupo, "Un governo "tecnico-politico"? Sulle costanti nel modello dei governi "tecnici", alla luce della formazione del governo Draghi," *Federalismi.it* (2021), accessed May 28, 2021, https://www.federalismi.it/nv14/articolo-documento.cfm?Artid=45087.

71 Cf. the Prime Minister's speech to the Senate of the Republic, "Comunicazioni del Presidente del Consiglio dei ministri in vista del Consiglio europeo del 25 e del 26 marzo 2021," March 24, 2021, accessed October 1, 2021, https://www.senato.it/japp/bgt/showdoc/18/Resaula/1210019/index.html?part=doc_dc-ressten_rs-gentit_cdpdcdmivdced25e26m2021ec.

also occurred within horizontal relationships. In response to the criticism from the national level, some of the attacked regions blamed in turn other regions for their crisis management. However, the Prime Minister's political skill along with a more pronounced assumption of responsibility at the national level enabled a relatively fast building-up process and also granted Draghi a pivotal role in the design of the third scaling-down phase.

Scaling-down

The preparation of the highly anticipated third scaling-down phase, however, was not completely free from conflictual episodes, since the regions expressed their will to hasten the reopening phase with the adoption of less restrictive measures,[72] thus determining a further trend inversion in the relative stringency orientations of central and regional governments. However, in the face of the central government's progressive loosening of restrictions, the newly-elected president of the Conference of Regions, Massimiliano Fedriga, who replaced former president Stefano Bonaccini, applauded the so-called "re-opening decree."[73] Moreover, he welcomed it as a sign of progress[74] compared to the previous decree in April,[75] which had involved scaling-down measures for the gradual resumption of economic and social activities. It is worth noting that the third scaling-down phase also witnessed lower levels of conflict because of the lower number of COVID-19 cases following the launch and intensification of the vaccination campaign (cf. Figure 2) and because this campaign was expected to unroll more quickly in the upcoming months.

---

[72] Segreteria della Conferenza delle Regioni e delle Province autonome, "Piano riaperture in sicurezza con calo contagio," *Regioni.it* 4045 (2021), accessed May 28, 2021, http://www.regioni.it/newsletter/n-4045/del-12-04-2021/piano-riaperture-in-sicurezza-con-calo-contagio-22546/.

[73] DL 65/2021 of May 18, 2021, https://www.normattiva.it/uri-res/N2Ls?urn:nir:stato:decreto.legge:2021-05-18;65!vig=2021-05-24.

[74] Segreteria della Conferenza delle Regioni e delle Province autonome, "Decreto riaperture: Fedriga, 'E' stato fatto un passo avanti molto importante'," *Regioni.it* 4072 (2021), accessed May 26, 2021, http://www.regioni.it/newsletter/n-4072/del-18-05-2021/decreto-riaperture-fedriga-e-stato-fatto-un-passo-avanti-molto-importante-22707/.

[75] DL 52/2021 of April 22, 2021, https://www.normattiva.it/uri-res/N2Ls?urn:nir:stato:DECRETO-LEGGE:2021-04-22;52!vig=.

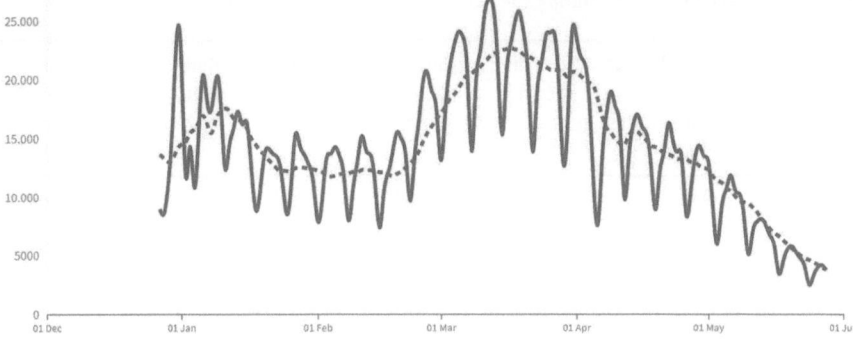

Figure 2: New daily COVID-19 cases over time since the launch of the vaccination campaign in Italy (from December 27, 2020 until the end of May 2021). Source: GEDI Visual, elaboration based on data released by the Italian Ministry of Health.

An Assessment of IGR Dimensions during the Pandemic

In regard to our first research question – how did internal IGRs evolve during the pandemic? – our analysis shows that there was a fluctuation in all five examined dimensions throughout the examined time period. Table 1 assesses the key dimensions of IGRs in light of the abovementioned review of the building-up and scaling-down phases that occurred during the three COVID-19 pandemic waves.

Overall, the evolution of IGRs fluctuated in terms of their level of conflict. Moreover, conflict intensity depended on the extent to which central and regional governments prioritized the same goals and policies. Whether the types of relationships were affected by coordination or conflict also changed throughout the pandemic. Vertical relationships were constantly relevant, while horizontal ones were occasionally relevant, in line with the nature of the constitutional sharing of responsibility in the healthcare sector. The average level of conflict was always fairly significant, except during the scaling-down phase following the third wave. This means that not even a pandemic was able to change the degree of intergovernmental conflict that has been a structural feature of the dynamics of the Italian quasi-federalist arrangement for a long time.[76]

---

76 Paola Mattei, "The Enterprise Formula, New Public Management And The Italian Health Care System: Remedy Or Contagion?," *Public Administration* 84 (2006), accessed May 28, 2021, DOI: 10.1111/j.1467–9299.2006.00624.x.

Table 1: Dimensions of IGRs during the COVID-19 pandemic at a glance.

	Building-up 1 March 2020 – May 2020	Scaling-down 1	Building-up 2 October – January 2020	Scaling-down 2	Building-up 3 March – April 2021	Scaling-down 3
Type of relationship	Vertical	Mixed	Mixed	Vertical	Mixed	Mixed
Level of conflict	Medium	Medium/high	Medium	Medium	Medium	Low
Capacity to share goals	High	Medium	Medium/Low	Medium	Medium	Medium/Low
Agreement on policy measures and practices	Low	Medium	Low	Low	Low	Low
Clarity of roles	Ambiguous	Partially ambiguous	Partially ambiguous	Clear	Partially ambiguous	Clear

Source: authors' elaboration.

The central and regional governments shared policy goals in the very first stage of the pandemic once they realized the extent of the epidemiological threat. These common policy goals translated into a substantially restrictive approach to public health measures given that all levels shared the perception that this external threat had to be tackled with stringent measures. However, the degree to which they shared policy goals began to oscillate once the central government and the regions were able to develop different views on the response to this epidemiological and socioeconomic crisis. Despite (or because of) the pandemic's continued severity, it represented still in 2021 an ambiguous problem that had a variety of policy responses even in the face of the greater availability of information.[77] Therefore, following the initial shock of the pandemic as a completely unexpected event, the capacity to share goals became deeply influenced by the

---

77 Martha S. Feldman, *Order without Design: Information Production and Policymaking* (Stanford, CA: Stanford University Press, 1989); Nicole Herweg, Nikolaos Zahariadis, and Reimut Zohlnhöfer, "The Multiple Streams Framework: Foundations, Refinements, and Empirical Applications," in *Theories of the Policy Process (4th edition)*, ed. Paul A. Sabatier and Christopher M. Weible (New York: Routledge, 2018), accessed May 26, 2021, DOI: 10.4324/9780429494284; James Q. Wilson, *Bureaucracy* (New York: Basic Books, 1989).

regions' different perspectives and interests, as shown by the many cases presented above in which regional problem framing and goal setting diverged from those of the central government. Additionally, these interests did not even remain stable over time, as shown by the frequent inversion of roles in advocating more restrictive or permissive measures compared to those proposed by the central government. These differing roles were also mirrored in the government levels' general inability to agree on policy measures and practices. The constant shift between preferences for more or less restrictive measures, embodied each time by central or regional government representatives, epitomized this disagreement. This lack of vertical coordination, which emerged during the first wave, did not improve during the second wave, as illustrated by the central government's lack of direction with regard to the implementation of the 3T strategy.[78]

Decree DL 19/2020 partially clarified the ambiguity of the respective roles, responsibilities, and competences of the central and regional governments. Article 3 of this decree specified that regions can adopt more restrictive measures for emergency management in consideration of specific health risk situations. This acknowledgment of regional competences was necessary because of the blurred constitutional arrangement of the responsibilities at the central and regional levels (cf. Section 2 of this chapter). However, the analysis shows that regions would have welcomed a less restraining approach from the national level on the extent to which they could enforce their own measures. This theme was later resumed when regions once again demanded the power to adopt less restrictive measures instead of just more restrictive ones. As of the second scaling-down phase, the competence-sharing mechanism seemed to work more smoothly, although there was some vacillation in the third building-up phase. Moreover, the presence of the new Prime Minister encouraged the clarification of institutional roles. He assumed a position that was more assertive than his predecessor's, who had possessed a style that was more like a broker between different interests.

Conclusions: Predicting Future Effects of IGRs during the Pandemic

To conclude, we found that the pandemic basically reproduced, and possibly magnified, pre-existing intergovernmental dynamics, which answers our second

---

78 Fondazione Gimbe, "Coronavirus: tamponi, indietro tutta."

research question as presented in the introduction. Our analysis raises some doubts about the effectiveness of institutional arrangements on health-related policy. However, at the time of writing, there are no efforts to provide long-term solutions to permanently solve the intergovernmental conflicts that this chapter identifies by using the pandemic as a litmus test. Our analysis reveals that the Italian IGR dynamics evolved during the pandemic in a predictable way based on the different government levels' default characteristics. This finding is particularly interesting because it contrasts with a different expectation, i.e., that these dynamics should be more cooperative given the exceptional magnitude of the challenge represented by the pandemic. This finding raises the question of whether and how crises can promote significant changes in inherited institutional dynamics in both federal and quasi-federal systems. In the Italian case, which embodies a quasi-federal arrangement, these dynamics not only seem to have remained the same but, in certain moments, some already-existing characteristics of IGRs were even exacerbated. Overall, Italian regionalism has shown all of its base-condition shortcomings even during the COVID-19 crisis. However, while it is evident that a reconsideration of the concurrent constitutional powers is needed, introducing significant changes will plausibly pose difficulties because, on the one hand, regions have been central to the management of the epidemiological crisis and, on the other hand, it can be expected that the northern regions will strongly oppose any attempt to decrease their current autonomy.

Moreover, in terms of political outcomes, the centrality of regions in the debate concerning the response to the pandemic might entail political reversals, especially in those regions that were perceived to have performed inadequately. Indeed, these reversals might become part of the feedback that public policy naturally triggers[79] and whose intensity is likely to be directly proportional to the perceived performance achievements (or failures) of the presidents of regions. The same reversal might not apply within the context of national elections. One main reason is that the large and diverse coalition government that managed the third wave might make it difficult to attribute clear responsibilities to different political parties and personalities.

While progress was made in terms of the certainty of roles at the national and regional levels, and there was certainly some degree of learning, regional differences in terms of healthcare infrastructures, their public health competence

---

79 Suzanne Mettler and Mallory Sorelle, "Policy Feedback Theory," in *Theories of the Policy Process (4th edition)*, ed. Paul A. Sabatier and Christopher M. Weible (New York: Routledge, 2018), accessed May 26, 2021, doi:10.4324/9780429494284.

sharing with the national government, and their incapacity to share policy goals and instruments might still eventually represent a challenge in the event of a future pandemic.

Part 3: **Devolution in a Post-Brexit (dis-)United Kingdom**

Fiona Simpkins

8 Scotland's SNP Government and the Management of the Covid-19 Pandemic

Devolved Power, Trust, and Support for Independence

Introduction

The divergent approaches adopted by Westminster and the devolved administrations regarding the management of the Covid-19 pandemic are neither surprising nor unusual given the wide-ranging powers that devolution conferred upon the devolved nations' new political legislatures when they were first created in 1999, in particular over public health services, education, policing, and justice matters. These are all major public services affected by the coronavirus pandemic and are the responsibility of the devolved administrations. Since its creation in 1999, the Scottish Parliament has in fact diverged from Westminster in significant ways over the management of public health services and, in doing so, has shown just how effective devolution could be in tailoring legislation more suited to the specific needs, characteristics, and infrastructures of each nation. This in turn has highlighted the more democratic processes involved by devolution as policy divergence is not only acceptable but necessary to better respond to local circumstances. As the democratically elected governments of the devolved nations have a duty to manage public services efficiently according to their own judgements and circumstances, it is natural that there should be a lack of uniformity across the UK.

Yet, the sudden outbreak of the current COVID-19 pandemic and the crisis that ensued revealed deep cracks between the United Kingdom's four constituent nations, throwing "into sharp relief the importance of productive working relationships between all levels of government."[1] While the resolution of the crisis was widely expected to supersede politics, emphasizing solidarity in times of cri-

---

1 Nicola McEwen et al., "Intergovernmental relations in the UK: time for a radical overhaul?," *Political Quarterly* 91–3 (2020): 632–40.

Fiona Simpkins, Associate Professor, Triangle UMR 5206 Université Lyon 2.

https://doi.org/10.1515/9783110745085-009

sis and the imperious need for the unity of the country,[2] it also demonstrated that "competent, democratically accountable local executive leadership, even without exercising legislative power, can itself play an important role in maintaining public trust in state decision making and fostering collective action."[3] This has been true of the devolved governments in Scotland and Wales as they commanded much higher levels of trust and public support than their UK counterpart under Prime Minister Boris Johnson, whose handling of the British response to the pandemic on the contrary undermined trust in UK institutions.

Despite an initially coordinated response to the challenges posed by the coronavirus crisis, the increasing differences in the four governments' management of the pandemic within their own territories have clearly illustrated the practical dimensions of devolution and the complexities of a multi-national state. The Scottish Parliament's extensive devolved powers have allowed the SNP government to shape a distinctive response to the coronavirus crisis and effective communication with the Scottish public. The pandemic has therefore provided the SNP government with the opportunity to build trust in its ability to manage a crisis and govern Scotland through extremely challenging times, perhaps developing its support base for independence at the same time. This chapter seeks to explore how the SNP government's management of the pandemic was perceived by the public in Scotland and to assess the subsequent impact of the coronavirus crisis on levels of support for independence there. It will first consider British inter-governmental decision-making processes over COVID-19 during the first year of the pandemic and examine in turn the structural and political drivers of policy divergence between Westminster and Holyrood. Perceptions of both the UK and the Scottish governments' handling of the pandemic will be analyzed to assess their impact on levels of support for independence in Scotland.

---

2 Over the first few months of the pandemic in the UK, a survey found that more adults on average thought that Britain would be united after it had recovered from the pandemic (46%) than thought it was united before the pandemic (24%): Office for National Statistics, "Unity and Division in Great Britain 24th April 2020 to 28th June 2020," *ONS Statistical Bulletin* (August 2020), accessed June 8, 2021, ons.gov.uk.

3 Ben Jackson, "A Crisis for Devolution?," *Political Quarterly* 91–3 (2020): 499–503.

Devolution as a Structural Driver of Divergence in Emergency Health Policy?

In the early years of devolution, the organization of the NHS was a key matter of debate and the first coalition government in Scotland moved quickly to achieve an integrated healthcare system with a flatter integrated structure than in England and Wales. It introduced a single tier of organization comprising 14 area health boards to assess needs, plan provision, allocate resources, and deliver services. The underlying approach to the 2004 NHS Reform (Scotland) Act was to bring together community-based services in a decentralized system and a rejection of a "command and control" management approach in favor of public participation. There remained some centralized aspects to the organization of public health services in Scotland and NHS National Service Scotland is still responsible for commissioning and performance management, national screening programs, specialist clinical services, and nationally managed clinical networks, but the overall approach was that of a more community-based system. Devolution also enabled Scotland to develop its own health priorities and avoid the delays entailed by the length of legislative procedures at Westminster. Scotland was therefore able to develop legislation that had no equivalent in England and Wales.[4]

The early years of the Scottish Parliament therefore introduced a divergent pattern for healthcare provision and services in Scotland and many of the emergency powers that were used during the pandemic to deal with the spread of infection were set out in the Public Health etc. (Scotland) Act 2008 which differed to varying degrees with the powers provided by the Public Health (Control of Disease) Act 1984 for England and Wales. The Public Health etc. (Scotland) Act 2008[5] includes provisions for quarantine orders, exclusion and restriction orders, quarantine and hospital detention orders, compensation for carers, provi-

---

4 This was the case for instance of the Adults with Incapacity (Scotland) Act, which provided for decisions to be made on behalf of adults who lacked legal capacity and was seen as an example of the new Parliament's commitment to serve the interests of vulnerable people, or the 2003 Mental Health (Care and Treatment) (Scotland) Act, which defined mental disorder as a mental illness and established new rights for users and carers as well as access to independent advocacy services. The policy divergence that proved most controversial, however, related to free care to the elderly introduced in Scotland in 2001 by former Labour First Minister, Henry McLeish, despite the policy having previously been strongly rejected for England and Wales by the Blair government.
5 "Public Health etc. (Scotland) Act 2008," last accessed June 8, 2021, https://covidlawlab.org/wp-content/uploads/2020/12/PH-Act-Scotland-2008.pdf.

sion of mortuaries, restrictions on the release and disposal of infected bodies, breach of orders and offenses as well as powers over international travel to name but a few. Part I of the Act furthermore details the public health responsibilities and duties of the Scottish Ministers, the Scottish Health Boards, and the local authorities. It provides for the duty of health boards and local authorities to co-operate and for the power of Scottish Ministers to intervene.

These provisions followed numerous experts' warnings that flu and virus pandemics had occurred with increasing frequency since the Asian flu of 1957 and that the threat of a pandemic should be the subject of contingency planning. These considerations combined with Scotland's increasingly divergent healthcare system to spur the Scottish Government to run its own simulation in 2018 to test the country's ability to deal with such a scenario. Exercise Iris was a table-top exercise held in March 2018 to assess NHS Scotland's response to a suspected outbreak of Middle Eastern Respiratory Syndrome (MERS-CoV). Like both previous UK-wide simulations (Winter Willow in 2007 and Exercise Cygnus in 2016), the simulation showed serious failings and recommended the need to test, track and isolate, stockpile equipment, shield the people who were most at risk in care homes, and the need for close coordination between the different levels of government. The different levels of the healthcare system in the UK remained uninformed of the findings and all three reports remained confidential until the Exercise Cygnus report was leaked in May 2020.[6] The Scottish Government only published its Exercise Iris report in June 2020, citing as its reason "the understandable interest in activity around preparedness or planning for infectious disease outbreaks."[7]

The common secrecy of the UK and Scottish governments over the failings of their simulations in emergency pandemic management perhaps mirrored their initial close coordination in the early phase of the crisis. Although the main body for inter-governmental coordination that was set up with the introduction of devolution in 1999, the Joint Ministerial Committee, was not mobilized, the First Ministers of the devolved legislatures were instead invited to attend the meetings of the Civil Contingencies Committee (i.e. COBRA, the Cabinet Office Meetings Room) as well as the meetings of the five new ministerial implementation groups (MIGs) established to deal with the specific aspects of the coronavirus response. It was thus initially felt that a coordinated response to the public

---

6 Clare Dyer, "Pandemic preparedness: Government hasn't released full report of exercise, say campaigners," *BMJ*, 2020, 371: m4145, DOI: 10.1136/bmj.m4145; David Pegg, "Official report that said UK was not prepared for pandemic is published," *The Guardian*, October 22, 2020.
7 "Exercise Iris Report," last modified June 3, 2020, https://www.gov.scot/publications/exercise-iris-report/.

health emergency required all four governments to take action within their own areas of responsibility whilst coordinating their action. To this purpose, the four governments jointly published a first Coronavirus Action Plan on March 3, 2020, which they jointly amended a few days later, on March 12, as they decided to move from the "contain phase" to the "delay phase," and on March 16, when people were asked to limit unnecessary social contact and for the most vulnerable to shield.

This led to more consultation and joint working between the UK and devolved governments. Initial guidance on social distancing and closures of pubs, restaurants, and schools was published on a UK-wide basis and the decision to impose a lockdown on March 23 was first announced by the UK Prime Minister before the First Ministers of the three devolved administrations made similar announcements. The Coronavirus Act 2020 became law on March 25 and conferred new powers on devolved ministers in areas such as health, education, and justice. The Scottish Parliament swiftly agreed to a Legislative Consent Motion for the Act to apply to Scotland, with the Scottish Government soon making use of these powers to make new regulations to tackle the pandemic. It was followed by a Coronavirus (Scotland) Act to complement and regulate the use of these emergency powers and introduce provisions to ease regulations and ensure continuity in sectors – such as the NHS, Social Security Scotland, and the Scottish Courts – that may struggle with their statutory requirements. The Act increased protections for tenants against evictions, allowed participants in court proceedings to appear by video link, extended the time limits for criminal proceedings, and provided powers to release some prisoners early among other provisions.

Despite the wide-ranging powers of the Scottish Parliament over public health management in Scotland and its divergent structures, there was therefore a high degree of coordination between the governments in the initial phase of the pandemic. Although the Scottish Government did not rule out adopting a divergent approach if justified by scientific evidence, it nevertheless firmly stated its intention to engage in a four-nation approach to the virus.[8] The few minor differences introduced were meant to reflect the specific circumstances of Scotland,

---

8 In a speech Mike Russell, Cabinet Secretary for the Constitution, Europe and External Affairs, gave to the Scottish Parliament on March 19, 2020 about the UK Government Coronavirus Bill, he noted that "the Scottish Government has made clear that – while we acknowledge the benefits of alignment across all four UK nations – it is also important that devolved matters can be fully analysed and considered against the emerging situation here in Scotland, and the specific measures and action that we and others need to put in place to respond to that." https://www.gov.scot/publications/statement-uk-government-coronavirus-bill/, accessed June 8, 2021.

as was the case, for instance, when the Scottish Government introduced a financial support scheme for fisheries – due to the economic weight of the fishing industries in some coastal communities of Scotland – a month before any other part of the UK did so too.

Scientific Advice Structures as Drivers of Emergency Health Policy Convergence

One reason for this initial level of coordination is perhaps that the structures of emergency scientific advice are very much integrated on a UK-wide basis. Like other devolved nations, Scotland has a Chief Medical Officer (CMO) and a Chief Scientific Advisor who meet regularly with their counterparts for the UK and other devolved nations to share information and provide coordinated advice to government departments in all four nations. Some decisions – like adding anosmia to the list of official coronavirus symptoms or extending the self-isolation period of symptomatic patients from 7 to 10 days, for instance – were made jointly by all CMOs. In addition, expert scientific advisory groups such as the New and Emerging Respiratory Virus Threats Advisory Group (NERVTAG) or the Scientific Pandemic Influenza Group on Modelling are also convened at a UK level through the Scientific Advisory Group for Emergencies (SAGE) that initially provided advice to COBR and to the devolved administrations. Scotland, like the other devolved nations, established its own scientific advisory group, the Scottish Government Advisory Group (SGAG), whose chair is also a participant in SAGE and whose key aim is to interpret SAGE outputs in the specific Scottish context, taking account of demographics, health, population density, NHS capacity and, naturally, the spread and prevalence of the virus. Yet, the latter may differ more widely within the different regions of each nation and are not necessarily a driver of divergence between the devolved nations' approach to crisis management. What appears clearly is that the emergency scientific advisory structures in Scotland and the rest of the UK imply a significant level of information transmission, coordination and exchange leading to broadly consistent views and advice. Scientific advice can therefore be considered as a factor limiting divergence.[9]

---

9 Jess Sergeant, "Co-ordination and divergence, Devolution and Coronavirus," *Institute for Government* (2020): 13, accessed June 8, 2021, https://www.instituteforgovernment.org.uk/sites/default/files/publications/coordination-divergence-devolution-coronavirus.pdf.

In fact, divergent responses to the pandemic started appearing in May 2020, when UK Prime Minister Boris Johnson announced that lockdown measures were going to be eased without specifying that these changes would only apply to England and without any prior consultation of the three devolved administrations. Neither were the First Ministers of the devolved nations consulted as the slogan used in efforts to fight the coronavirus pandemic was changed from "Stay Home" to "Stay Alert" on May 10, perhaps damaging the already low level of trust between the devolved administrations and the UK government. The more complex and nuanced messages required by a gradual easing of lockdown measures in the four nations also coincided with a decrease in the frequency of the aforementioned Civil Contingencies Committee held through COBR and which was the principal mechanism for coordination in the early stages of the pandemic. As the spread of the virus was brought under control, the frequency of the meetings was reduced and so was the communication between governments. The UK government's decision to terminate the Ministerial Implementation Groups (MIGs) – to which ministers from the devolved administrations were routinely invited – without prior consultation also reduced the scope for communication and cooperation between the different governments in the country.

Perhaps as a consequence of reduced communication between the different administrations, Boris Johnson's announcement of the easing of lockdown measures and new "Stay Alert" message was rejected by the three devolved nations in their subsequent statements and they each published their own separate plans for easing lockdown restrictions, leading to different sets of rules applying to different parts of the country. While the UK government set out three phases for easing lockdown restrictions, Scotland had four, Northern Ireland five, and Wales a traffic light system. This set the tone for things to come and the months that followed were marked by greater variation between the nations in their management of restrictions. Some differences were a matter of timing, with non-essential shops, gyms, pubs, and restaurants or schools being allowed to reopen or being closed again at different times, while others were more substantive, with variations in the number of people and number of households allowed to meet, as well as differences in restrictions on outdoor and indoor meetings.

Although all administrations cited epidemiological evidence to back this, there is little evidence that differences in the spread and prevalence of the virus were the most significant drivers for policy divergence. An IfG study states that "the scientific imperative behind territorially differentiated approaches was weaker in the UK than in other countries,"[10] citing evidence that a comparison of excess deaths between March and May 2020 found that all regions of the UK had excess death rates above 30%, whereas this was only the case of seven out of 20 regions in Italy and two out of 13 regions in France. It also found greater variation within England itself than between the four nations of the UK. In fact, excess deaths were lower in Scotland than in England and do not explain why restrictions were stricter in Scotland than in England when the opposite might have been expected.

Political Drivers of Divergence: Economics, Trust and the Constitution

These inconsistencies in the different territorial approaches to restrictions in the four nations of the UK are easily explained by the wider socio-economic consequences of the pandemic on each nation. The management of the pandemic entails finding difficult compromises between public health and the socio-economic impact of restrictions introduced to contain the virus and protect the population. These are political decisions which involve the responsibility of the ministers as they make choices with far-reaching consequences for which they will be held accountable by their own legislatures and voters. This implies that they will be made in good faith but that they will be balanced against socio-economic considerations. The UK government's response to the coronavirus can be perceived as having prioritized economic considerations more than its Scottish counterpart as it allowed non-essential retail outlets, as well as pubs and restaurants, to remain fully open for much longer periods of time. It also reopened schools to younger pupils, despite SAGE's warnings that there was no clear evidence that it was safe, in order to allow people to return to work, and it encouraged those working from home to return to their offices earlier in order to stimulate spending in city centers. Yet, one of the main differences between Scotland's devolved government and its UK counterpart is that it is not responsible for the macro-economic consequences of the crisis as these are among the matters reserved to Westminster. The UK government will be more mindful of the debt incurred by ongoing furlough schemes, which it will eventually be held accountable for, and of the impact of lockdown restrictions on the wider UK economy. The fate of the incumbent Conservative government in future elections depends in large part on its economic record. Holyrood on the other hand is

---

10 Jess Sergeant, "Co-ordination and divergence, Devolution and Coronavirus," 13.

primarily funded by an annual block grant calculated according to the Barnett Formula,[11] the amount of which is affected either positively or negatively by any changes to public spending levels in England. This means that although the Scottish government will naturally be wary of the potential consequences in Scotland of a UK economic slowdown, it will be more removed from the direct economic consequences of Covid. The Scotland Act of 2016 devolved a wide range of financial powers, including full control over income tax rates and thresholds, as well as receipts from the first 10p of the standard rate of VAT and the first 2.5p of the reduced rate of VAT in Scotland. Yet, Scotland's devolved administration has no borrowing capacity and its decisions are therefore dependent upon UK decisions on economic support. With health being Scotland's biggest spending obligation, its budget is potentially more affected by the pandemic's impact on public health and it is no wonder then that it should adopt a more cautious approach. In fact, SNP governments have enjoyed much greater financial powers than their predecessors in office but have used them sparingly. This is in part due to the SNP's strategy for independence which seeks to argue in favor of the economic benefits of independence, counter the criticisms of its opponents, and reassure undecided voters through its sound management of the economy. The Scottish government's more cautious management of the pandemic is therefore partly due to the latter's potential budgetary repercussions and is in keeping with the SNP's cautious management of the economy as part of its ultimate independence strategy.

As governments weigh the importance of each factor in their decision-making processes, they remain aware that their capacity to implement reforms and policies are also dependent on the levels of trust among voters in their legislatures, especially where short-term sacrifices are involved and long-term gains are less perceptible.[12] Trust is both necessary to introduce reforms and to ensure compliance with rules and regulations.[13] Yet, maintaining trust is made more dif-

---

11 The Barnett Formula is a mechanism used by the British Treasury to calculate the annual block grants allocated to Scotland, Wales, and Northern Ireland. It is intended to reflect changes in spending levels allocated to public services in England and Wales and to give each one of the four nations the same public spending ratio per person. It takes into account annual changes in UK government departments' spending levels, the relative population of the devolved administration, and the extent to which the UK government departments' services are devolved.
12 Sofie Marien and Marc Hooghe, "Does political trust matter? An empirical investigation into the relation between political trust and support for law compliance," *European Journal of Political Research* 50 (2011): 267–91, DOI: 10.1111/j.1475-6765.2010.01930.x
13 OECD, "Trust in government, policy effectiveness and the governance agenda," *Government at a Glance 2013*, OECD Publishing (2013), accessed June 8, 2021, https://doi.org/10.1787/gov_glance-2013-6-en.

ficult by the diversification of news sources and the faster flow of information across society through more recent technological developments, internet, and social networks.[14] This has created a more complex environment for governments which have to maintain an acute awareness of their public image, the importance of public communication, and the levels of trust in governmental action among the general public.

The impact of a breakdown in the levels of trust voters have in their government was illustrated by the backlash to political figures' breaches of travel restrictions and social distancing.[15] Compliance with the strict rules and regulations imposed during the pandemic came to be seen as reliant upon the trust that the population had in their legislatures and any breaches of these rules by governmental figures raised concerns about governmental transparency, accountability, and equality. When the Prime Minister's Chief Adviser Dominic Cummings was found to have travelled with his family from London to his parents' home in Durham and then to Barnard Castle while experiencing COVID-19 symptoms during the first lockdown in May 2020, the media coverage and public outcry that ensued ultimately led to his undoing despite Boris Johnson's support. The UK Government's defense of Dominic Cummings was widely condemned by scientists as undermining essential public health messaging. A study published in *The Lancet* in August 2020 further provided evidence that what it called the "Cummings effect" corresponded to a decrease in public confidence which had adverse consequences on public adherence to guidelines, which were essential to control infection rates and mortality. It concluded that "public trust in the government's ability to manage the pandemic is crucial as this trust underpins public attitudes and behaviors at a precarious time for public health,"[16] While many MPs called on Dominic Cummings to resign, a YouGov poll published in *The Guardian* that month showed that 71% of people polled thought he had broken lockdown rules and 59% thought he should resign.[17] Yet, the UK government's decision to support Dominic Cummings despite the

---

14 OECD, "Transparency, communication and trust: the role of public communication in responding to the wave of disinformation about the new coronavirus," OECD Publishing (2020), accessed June 8, 2021.

15 Kenneth Newton, "Government communications, political trust and compliant social behaviour: the politics of Covid-19 in Britain," *Political Quarterly* 91–3 (2020): 502–13.

16 Daisy Fancourt, Andrew Steptoe, and Liam Wright, "The Cummings effect: politics, trust and behaviours during the Covid-19 pandemic," *The Lancet* 396 (2020): 464–65, accessed June 8, 2021, DOI: 10.1016/S0140-6736(20)31690-1.

17 Heather Stewart, Rowena Mason, and Kate Proctor, "Tory unrest increases pressure on PM adviser to resign," *Guardian*, May 27, 2020.

outcry that ensued his breach of Covid regulations contrasts with the attitude adopted by the Scottish government in similar cases. The SNP government's more cautious approach suggests that it was wary of the impact that any misstep might have on levels of public confidence.

Scotland's SNP government was not immune from questioning of its accountability and fairness but its reactions to breaches of regulations by its own members indicate how highly it valued public trust in its actions. First, Scotland's Chief Medical Officer, Catherine Calderwood, was called to resign by First Minister Nicola Sturgeon in April 2020 after she was found to have visited her second home despite travelling restrictions. The First Minister explained her decision in the following terms: "What was at the forefront of my mind was how firstly I continue to have the best advice to enable me to deal with this virus, but also how I ensured that the confidence of the public in the advice that we are giving them was maintained."[18] Then in October 2020, she also suspended Margaret Ferrier, SNP MP for Rutherglen and Hamilton West, and called for her to resign after she was found to have travelled between London and Glasgow following a positive test result for COVID-19. Finally, the First Minister issued a public apology after she removed her face mask to talk to some of the attendees at a wake in March 2021.

These episodes – together with the Scottish government's more cautious approach to rules and regulations than its UK counterpart despite there being little evidence of differences in the prevalence and spread of the virus on each side of the border – illustrate the importance given by the Scottish government to the public's perceptions of its actions during the pandemic. They suggest that trust in the government's actions was not only believed to be necessary to ensure public compliance to rules and regulations in Scotland, but also that public trust represents a key aspect of the SNP's governance strategy. Indeed, public confidence in the SNP's ability to govern has been a key element of its independence strategy for the last two decades. Prior to devolution, the SNP unsuccessfully sought to win a majority of Scottish seats at Westminster, which it aimed to use as a mandate for independence. With the introduction of devolution in 1999 and a Scottish Parliament elected on a semi-proportional electoral system, the SNP was able to move away from the fringes of political power – where it had heretofore been confined by Britain's first-past-the-post system – and its strategy for independence came to rest upon government office in Holyrood. Not only did the Scottish Parliament make the prospect of an electoral majority more likely

---

18 Severin Carrell, "Nicola Sturgeon reveals she asked chief medical officer to resign," *The Guardian*, April 6, 2020.

due to its semi-proportional electoral system but it also provided the SNP with a unique Scottish political platform. As the only Scottish party with no UK counterpart, the SNP has benefited from an advantageous position in Scotland's devolved landscape. It has been able to appear as the only party to speak for Scotland's distinctive interests outside of any UK-wide concerns. This has been key to winning over voters in Holyrood elections, which most voters view as elections primarily concerned with Scottish issues, contrary to Westminster general elections where wider UK concerns determine voters' electoral choices.[19] Once in government, the overall government strategy and aim of the SNP administration has been focused on creating positive conditions for independence. Not only did the SNP use the Scottish Parliament as an institutional mechanism through which to hold an independence referendum, but it has also attempted "to use government office to build autonomy and support for independence through effective government performance."[20] Perceptions of the SNP governments' performance have thus been central to the party's independence strategy and the pandemic provided an opportunity for the SNP to compare favorably to its UK counterpart and build trust in its ability to govern an independent Scotland.

Trust is a highly subjective phenomenon which hinges upon the confidence of citizens in the actions of a "government to do what is right and perceived fair."[21] It depends on the congruence between citizens' perceptions of what is fair or not fair and the perceived performance of a government.[22] Yet, because it does not depend on the actual performance of a government according to a set of objective criteria but rather its perceived performance according to a set of subjective criteria that may vary from one person to the other, trust can therefore only be measured by perception surveys asking citizens whether they trust a government, leader, institution or party. Bouckaert argues that trust in government can be analyzed at three levels: a macro-level, broadly relating to political institutions and the functioning of democracy, a meso-level corresponding to trust in policy, and a micro-level that can broadly be defined as perception of

---

19 John Curtice, "The electorate and elections," in Gerry Hassan, *The story of the Scottish Parliament at twenty* (Edinburgh: Edinburgh University Press, 2019).
20 Peter Lynch, *The history of the Scottish National Party*, second edition (Cardiff: Welsh Academic Press, 2013).
21 David Easton, *A systems analysis of political life* (New York: John Wiley Publishing, 1965).
22 Geert Bouckaert and Steven van de Walle, "Comparing measures of citizen trust and user satisfaction as indicators of 'good governance': difficulties in linking trust and satisfaction indicators," *International Review of Administrative Sciences* 69, no. 3 (2003): 329–43, DOI: 10.1177/0020852303693003.

service delivery.[23] Measures of trust in the Scottish government's actions during the first year of the pandemic can thus be analyzed following Bouckaert's taxonomy.

It is firstly interesting to note that, at a macro-level, there are stark differences in the level of trust that the Scottish public has in the Scottish Government as compared to the trust they have in the UK government. A series of nine ComRes polls between December 2020 and May 2021 asking whether respondents felt either favorable or unfavorable towards the Scottish Government in Holyrood found that 47.5% on average felt favorable and 31.5% unfavorable, with 21% answering that they felt neither favorable nor unfavorable.[24] The same polls asked respondents in Scotland whether they felt favorable or unfavorable to the UK Government in Westminster and found that only 26% of respondents felt favorable towards the UK Government and that 53% felt unfavorable, with 21% feeling neither.[25] Interestingly, the time period for this series of polls corresponds to the mass vaccination campaign launched by the UK government and suggests that trust in the UK Government among Scottish respondents was little improved by its success or by that of the furlough scheme which alleviated much of the financial burden borne by Scottish businesses throughout the pandemic. By May 31, 2021, 38.6% of the UK population and 38% of the Scottish population was fully vaccinated, while 59.2% of the UK population and 59.9% of the Scottish population had been given a first dose of the vaccine.[26] This compared very favorably to other European countries: only 16.8% of the French population and 18.2% of the German population was fully vaccinated by the same date.[27] Yet, in December 2020, when the vaccination campaign was first launched, 57% of respondents declared that they had an unfavorable opinion of the UK Government and 53% still responded similarly in May 2021.

Bouckaert's taxonomy argues that at a meso-level, trust relates to policy-making, that is to say the ability of governments to manage economic and social issues and to generate positive expectations of the future. This level thus assess-

---

23 Geert Bouckaert, "Trust and public administration," *Administration* 60 – 1 (2012): 91 – 115.
24 What Scotland Thinks, accessed June 8, 2021, https://whatscotlandthinks.org/questions/to-what-extent-do-you-feel-favourably-or-unfavourably-about-the-scottish-government-in-holyrood/.
25 What Scotland Thinks, accessed June 8, 2021, https://whatscotlandthinks.org/questions/to-what-extent-do-you-feel-favourably-or-unfavourably-about-the-uk-government-in-westminster/.
26 UK Government, "Coronavirus (Covid-19) in the UK," accessed June 8, 2021, https://coronavirus.data.org.uk.
27 Our World in Data, "Coronavirus (Covid-19) vaccinations," Statistics and research, accessed June 8, 2021, https://ourworldindata.org/covid-vaccinations

es the Scottish public's perceptions of the SNP government's distinctive response to the pandemic and its more cautious approach (notably its enforcement of stricter restrictions and longer periods of lockdown). The SNP government's response to the pandemic was consistently rated better than the UK government's response, as illustrated by a series of three IpsosMori polls between May 2020 and February 2021 which showed that, on average, 73% of respondents believed that the Scottish Government had handled the coronavirus outbreak well against 30% who believed the same of the UK Government. While only 15% of respondents believed the Scottish Government had handled the pandemic badly, 54% believed the UK Government had handled it badly, suggesting a stark contrast in the levels of confidence secured by each government.[28]

However, another series of Scottish polls asking a similar question about both governments' leaders over roughly the same period showed that the public's assessment of their handling of the crisis had become more negative with time, suggesting that levels of trust had perhaps been eroded with lockdown fatigue. Two IpsosMori polls in May 2020 and November 2020 and one BMG Research poll in March 2021 asked how well or badly Nicola Sturgeon and Boris Johnson had handled the coronavirus outbreak so far.[29] While 82% thought Nicola Sturgeon had handled it "very well" or "fairly well" in March 2020, 74% thought so in November 2020 and only 57% believed so in March 2021. This erosion is also visible in responses to Boris Johnson's handling of the crisis – albeit less so because overall perception of his handling of the coronavirus outbreak was more negative to begin with – as only 24% of respondents believed he handled the outbreak "very well" or "fairly well" in March 2021, down from 30% in March 2020.

Finally, at the micro-level, Bouckaert believes that trust refers to the impact of government on people's daily lives through service delivery. In the case of a pandemic crisis, perceptions of this service delivery will very much depend on successful communication and information. Indeed, Bouckaert suggests that trust is not something that happens to governments but something that they can influence through their actions and policies. The manners and processes to

28 What Scotland Thinks, accessed June 8, 2021, https://whatscotlandthinks.org/questions/how-well-or-badly-do-you-think-the-scottish-government-has-handled-the-coronavirus-so-far/ and https://whatscotlandthinks.org/questions/how-well-or-badly-do-you-think-the-uk-government-have-handled-the-coronavirus-outbreak-so-far/.
29 What Scotland Thinks, accessed June 8, 2021, https://whatscotlandthinks.org/questions/how-well-or-badly-has-nicola-sturgeon-handled-the-coronavirus-outbreak-so-far/ and https://whatscotlandthinks.org/questions/how-well-or-badly-do-you-think-boris-johnson-has-handled-the-coronavirus-outbreak-so-far/.

attain the final results are perhaps as important as the results themselves. Here, Scottish First Minister Nicola Sturgeon's communication skills appear to have been more effective in commanding higher levels of trust. On the contrary, Boris Johnson's initial flippant attitude, and the vague and confusing directives which his government issued, appear to have had a negative impact on the level of trust in his government.

Given that the level of divergence between both governments has on the whole remained low – albeit with a more cautious approach to the pandemic response in Scotland –, the difference in perception of both government leaders' handling of the pandemic can partly be explained by differences in communication skills and partisanship. Data published by the British Election Study Internet Panel of June 2020 showed that perceptions of government competence varied according to political outlook: Conservative voters had the most favorable views of the British government's response to the pandemic and the most unfavorable views of the Scottish government's response, while SNP voters were much more positive in their views of how the Scottish government had handled the pandemic and negative in their perception of the British government's response.[30] The percentage of respondents with positive views of the British Prime Minister and his government remained low but corresponds approximately to the percentage of Conservative voters in Scotland. Indeed, only 21% of respondents in Scotland believed that Boris Johnson was doing well as Prime Minister according to a YouGov poll of November 10, 2020 as opposed to 79% who thought he was doing badly. Similarly, only 22% of respondents declared they felt favorably towards the Prime Minister in a ComRes poll of May 2021, against 60% who felt unfavorably and 13% who felt neither favorably nor unfavorably.[31] The Scottish Conservatives obtained 22% of the vote in the May 2021 Scottish Parliament election, which suggests that the Prime Minister was most popular with those who identified as Conservative.

In sharp contrast to the British Prime Minister, the SNP government's high communication skills and media-savvy First Minister appear to have been much more successful in building trust in Scotland. Nicola Sturgeon's clarity and precision in her daily briefings, her empathetic persona as she addressed children or shared her own distress at being unable to see her family, may have increased confidence in the SNP government's handling of the pandemic.

---

30 Eilidh Macfarlane, "The Impact of the Coronavirus Pandemic on Support for the SNP and Scottish Independence?," *Social Science Research Network*, April 15, 2021, accessed June 8, 2021, http://dx.doi.org/10.2139/ssrn.3827168.
31 What Scotland Thinks, accessed June 8, 2021, https://whatscotlandthinks.org/questions/to-what-extent-do-you-feel-favourably-or-unfavourably-about-boris-johnson/.

Her candor in admitting her government's failings – notably over the discharge of elderly hospital patients to care homes during the first wave of the pandemic – and her manifesto commitment to commission an enquiry into the handling of the pandemic in Scotland – pressing Boris Johnson to move faster in appointing a UK inquiry himself – also helped to neutralize potentially controversial issues. Her high visibility in the media may have contributed to higher levels of confidence in her actions. There was an outcry in September 2020 when the BBC announced that it would stop broadcasting the First Minister's daily briefings on the pandemic. Nicola Sturgeon won plaudits for her communication skills during her televised briefings, her latest updates on the pandemic numbers in Scotland drew in large audiences (attracting on average 275,000 viewers each day), and the corporation duly backtracked on its decision to end them. In fact, her daily appearances and occasional lapses into other subjects as she answered journalists' questions were criticized by some – like Labour peer Lord Foulkes, for instance – as a breach of impartiality rules, and appear to have contributed to raising her profile. Indeed, polls have shown that Scots' positive perceptions of the First Minister even occurred among Leave voters at the European referendum of 2016 and among No voters at the 2014 independence referendum.[32] This may have translated into increased support for the SNP: polls show that support for the SNP started rising after December 2019 with Boris Johnson's election as Prime Minister and remained high throughout the pandemic until the winter of 2021 when it fell slightly before stabilizing to between 46% and 53% of voting intentions. Yet, positive popularity ratings, higher levels of trust, and increased support for the SNP did not translate ultimately into increased support for independence.

Polls suggest that the surge in support for independence which occurred between the spring of 2019 and January 2021 was in fact linked to the lengthy negotiations between the UK Government and the EU Commission over the UK's departure from the EU as well as the prospect of a hard Brexit. A series of 20 consecutive polls (by Panelbase, YouGov, IpsosMori, Survation, ComRes, and JL Partners) published between May 2020 and January 2021 showed that support for independence was consistently ahead of support for the status quo, oscillating between 51% and a record 59%. By February 2021, once Brexit became reality, these trends subsided and polls started showing a clear midway split in public opinion over the constitutional question. A ComRes poll published

---

32 John Curtice, "A coronavirus swing in favour of independence?," *What Scotland Thinks*, July 5, 2020, accessed June 8, 2021, https://whatscotlandthinks.org/2020/07/a-coronavirus-swing-in-favour-of-independence/.

on February 9 2021, only a few days into Brexit, was the first to show a reversal of trends with 52% of respondents supporting the status quo against 48% supporting independence. All following polls have shown a narrow lead for either support for independence or support for the status quo, indicating that the Scottish electorate is now evenly divided over the constitutional future of Scotland.

The pandemic ultimately appears to have had little impact on support for independence. A Panelbase poll for the *Sunday Times* published on March 26, 2021 asked respondents whether the pandemic made them more likely to support or oppose independence and found that 24% declared it made them more likely to support independence, 17% answered that it made them more likely to oppose independence, and a majority of 60% said it made no difference.[33] In fact, if there was perhaps some initial impact on support for independence at the start of the pandemic, it appeared to subside as restrictions dragged on and lockdown fatigue settled over the issue. A series of three YouGov polls published between August 2020 and May 2021 showed that while 43% of respondents in August 2020 expected Scotland would have responded to coronavirus better as an independent country, this figure fell to 38% in March 2021 and 31% in May 2021. On the contrary, the percentage of people who believed Scotland would have responded worse to coronavirus if it were independent rose from 16% in August 2020 to 25% in March 2021 and 31% in May 2021.[34]

Conclusion

Notwithstanding the increasing weariness of the electorate with the duration of restrictions, the May 2021 Scottish Parliament election entrenched a more partisan approach to the constitutional debate and was marked by homecoming electoral trends as the number of seats obtained by each party remained very similar to that of the 2016 Scottish Parliament elections. The results of the pro-independence parties roughly mirrored levels of support for independence in Scotland: between them the pro-independence parties obtained 49% of the constituency vote and 50.1% of the regional vote while the three main unionist parties obtained 50.4% of the constituency vote and 46.5% of the regional vote. Despite

33 What Scotland Thinks, accessed June 8, 2021, https://whatscotlandthinks.org/questions/does-the-covid-19-situation-make-you-more-you-more-likely-to-support-or-oppose-independence/.
34 What Scotland Thinks, accessed June 8, 2021, https://whatscotlandthinks.org/questions/do-you-think-scotland-would-have-responded-to-coronavirus-better-or-worse-as-an-independent-country/.

the SNP's cautious management of the pandemic and communication efforts, the pandemic did not produce any surge of support for independence and other issues dominated the campaign. Much was said during the May 2021 electoral campaign about the different parties' plans for the country's recovery after the pandemic and all parties' manifestos presented recovery as their main objective and policy framework, yet the debate was drowned out by the constitutional question as Scotland's future had now narrowly come to be seen in terms of its constitutional status. More than anything, the May 2021 Scottish Parliament election results confirmed the polarization of the Scottish electorate over the constitutional issue as the campaign was dominated by the SNP's plans for a second independence referendum rather than the pandemic. This suggests that the SNP's strategy for independence based on good governance and public trust in its ability to govern an independent Scotland has limited success. Since its formation of a minority government in 2007, the SNP has attempted to assert its competence over key economic and social issues in order to boost voter confidence in a future independent Scotland. Polls show that a cautious management of the pandemic in Scotland and effective communication have indeed delivered higher levels of public trust in the Scottish government than in the UK government. However, public confidence in the Scottish government's management of the pandemic appears to have had little impact on support for independence and the current polarization of the electorate in Scotland suggests that the outcome of a second independence referendum remains highly uncertain.

Daniel Wincott

9 The Anglo-British State, Welsh Devolution, and the Covid-19 Pandemic in England and Wales

Territorial Riddles, Mysterious Boundaries, and Enigmatic Identities

Introduction

Since the UK is often described as a "unitary state,"[1] we might have expected it to have a unified territorial response to the COVID-19 pandemic. Things did not, however, turn out that way. Instead, hypercentralist responses from the government in London show both its skewed understanding of the UK territorial state and its impoverished ability to cooperate with devolved governments or local authorities in England. The Westminster/Whitehall state's interactions with other governmental authorities within the UK were often highly abrasive. Its inability to generate a unified response to a major pandemic threat starkly exposes flaws and limits in the historic conventional ways of understanding the UK state. Imagining it as a "unitary" state that offers clear powers and authority to any central government able to command a majority at Westminster offers at best a partial perspective on the UK. It is, in many respects, seriously misleading.

The approach adopted here is unusual. It sets pandemic governance in a territorial politics perspective,[2] raising basic questions about dominant "methodologically nationalist" or "nation-statist" social science. Even within a territorial politics frame, the places from which we observe pandemic politics –Wales and English localities – provide an atypical perspective on the UK state. If Wales

---

1 BEIS (Department of Business, Energy and Industrial Strategy), *UK Internal Market* CP 278 para 16, p. 12, https://assets.publishing.service.gov.uk/government/uploads/system/uploads/attachment_data/file/901225/uk-internal-market-white-paper.pdf, accessed August 2 2021.
2 Charlie Jeffery and Daniel Wincott, "The Challenge of Territorial Politics: Beyond Methodological Nationalism," in *New Directions in Political Science*, ed. Colin Hay (London: Macmillan, 2010).

Daniel Wincott, Professor, Wales Governance Centre, School of Law and Politics, Cardiff University.

https://doi.org/10.1515/9783110745085-010

provides our main viewpoint, taking in the Welsh government's interaction with its counterpart in London, we also consider English local authorities and a small group of relatively recently created "metro-mayors".

Partly flowing from the specific approach to territorial political analysis used here, the study also adopts a distinctive "real-time" approach to its examination of pandemic policy. The depth of the challenges posed by the COVID-19 pandemic makes it difficult to keep track of what occurred and how it happened with respect to any government. Standard official sources of evidence concerning the events analyzed here are sparse. We shall see that the UK-level government defaulted to hypercentralism and hyperinnovation, sometimes giving the events themselves a peculiar quality. Consequently, we rely heavily on contemporaneous coverage – often in local or Welsh media – of events that may have seemed peripheral in London. Though this evidence is easily ignored or forgotten, framed in a territorial perspective it takes on more significance.

Historically, Wales has been more tightly integrated with England than Scotland or Northern Ireland. Within the Westminster system, the English local government occupies a strictly sub-ordinate position. Our approach reveals the *modus operandi* of the UK state in places where it senses little basic threat to its territorial integrity. Whitehall and Westminster also show a mix of inability and unwillingness to recognize either devolved Welsh actors or local English ones. Equally, the analysis shows limits to the UK government's capacity to achieve its objectives across territory.

So far from creating the unity suggested by conventional "unitary state" accounts of the UK, Whitehall/Westminster's default hyper-centralism itself became a source of policy variegation. The Johnson administration's use of concentrated power generated differentiation through specialized, *ad hoc* responses to policy dilemmas. It was obsessed with innovation. Its first instinct was to turn to the private sector, especially to people known as entrepreneurs and innovators. The approach had one striking success: the Vaccine Task Force (VTF).[3] More often, hypercentralism, in the name of fitting policy to the specific circumstances of particular situations, had counterproductive consequences. The UK government's pandemic response was often *ad hoc* or arbitrary, reactive, short-term, and often abrasive. It also tended to respond the situation in England, particularly the south-east, rather than other parts of the state.

---

3 "UK Vaccine Taskforce 2020 Achievements and Future Strategy: End of Year Report," *Department of Business, Energy and Industrial Strategy* 1, December 2020, accessed August 2, 2021, https://assets.publishing.service.gov.uk/government/uploads/system/uploads/attachment_data/file/944308/VTF_Interim_report_-_5th_publication.pdf.

In turn, the Westminster/Whitehall state's default hypercentralism is deeply rooted in an Anglo-British state nationalism.[4] Dominant in the London-based media as well as the UK state, Anglo-British identity is also an important element in the highly complex, variegated pattern of mass public attitudes across the UK. Though understandable, the British state's distinctively English preoccupations are often hidden in its leaders' euphemistic language about "the country" or "the nation" and a strange reluctance to mention England (except in relation to football). In effect, England is hidden within Britain, particularly by those who view Britain from a distinctively English perspective. The resulting Anglo-British fusion[5] imparts strange, and sometimes peculiarly fragile, qualities to the UK state.

Policy differentiation, such as the UK's distinct bodies of primary law on health and education, is generally a normal feature of a devolved state. Yet the UK government and Conservative MPs sometimes seemed deeply annoyed by variations in pandemic policy. Westminster Conservatives seem to have been disobliged, bewildered, and even offended by distinct Welsh COVID-19 policies (even when UK government changes created the difference). That those in power at Westminster should be deeply unsettled by the operation of devolution illustrates an element of fragility in their Anglo-British sensibilities. These sensibilities help to make sense of the UK state's difficulty in accurately "reading" its territories and their governance systems.[6]

Finally, while policy differences have been an important aspect of the COVID-19 pandemic, in general, the policies pursued and resulting outcomes were much more similar than internal UK debates suggest. In fact, the conventional wisdom is that intergovernmental coordination was highly effective in

---

4 Daniel Wincott, C.R.G Murray, and Gregory Davies, "The Anglo-British imaginary and the rebuilding of the UK's territorial constitution after Brexit: unitary state or union state?," *Territory, Politics, Governance*, published online May 17, 2021, DOI: https://doi.org/10.1080/21622671.2021.1921613; Daniel Wincott and Gregory Davies, "The Anglo-British imaginary stands in the way of any sensible debate about the future of the UK," *LSE British Politics and Policy Blog*, September 28, 2021, accessed September 29, 2021, https://blogs.lse.ac.uk/politicsandpolicy/anglo-british-imaginary/; Gregory Davies and Daniel Wincott, "Brexit, the Press and the Territorial Constitution," *Social and Legal Studies* 30 (2021): 157, https://doi.org/10.1177/0964663920921922; Ailsa Henderson and Richard Wyn Jones, *Englishness: The Political Force Transforming Britain* (Oxford: Oxford University Press, 2021).
5 Ailsa Henderson and Richard Wyn Jones, *Englishness: The Political Force Transforming Britain* (Oxford: Oxford University Press, 2021), 167–94.
6 Daniel Wincott, "The possible break-up of the United Kingdom," *UK in a Changing Europe*, December 19, 2020, accessed August 2, 2021, https://ukandeu.ac.uk/long-read/the-possible-break-up-of-the-united-kingdom/.

the initial stages of the pandemic,[7] at least once policymakers had begun to grasp its challenges. In part, overarching UK government policies pushed broad commonalities in approach. Perhaps more important, similarities of policy and outcome also result from historic legacies and similarities of outlook.

The chapter has seven further substantive sections. The first briefly addresses national identities across the UK and considers their relation to the state's territorial structure. The subsequent sections analyze, in turn: the UK government's initial pandemic response; the initial effectiveness of Anglo-Welsh intergovernmental co-ordination; changes as the initial lockdown was eased; central-local relations within England; UK vaccine procurement and delivery; and the impacts of COVID-19 on territorial politics in England and Wales. The chapter aims to demonstrate that the initial modest effectiveness of UK-Welsh government co-operation was always matched by elements of fierce conflict. The Johnson administration had notable successes which benefited the whole UK: the VTF and perhaps also its furlough scheme. Abrasiveness and incomprehension often marked the Johnson administration's relations with the Welsh government and some English localities. Perhaps revealing a fragility in its "Anglo-British" orientation, the UK government seemed disinclined to acknowledge – perhaps even unable to recognize – any policy successes of its Welsh counterpart.

The (post-)Brexit Context, National Identities, and the Territorial Structure of the UK State

The Brexit referendum unveiled a complex and variegated set of national identities across the UK. Historic "ethno-national" identities in Northern Ireland tend to pitch British and Irish identities against one another. Today a large growing group identifies with "neither" of these positions. Across Great Britain, sub-state identities (English, Scottish, Welsh) coexist with a putatively "state-wide" British identity. And yet, over Brexit, British identity is linked to opposite attitudes in different parts of the state. That is, in Scotland and Wales, relative emphasis on Britishness was associated with voting to leave the EU, while in England it was linked to voting to remain. Obversely, those with strong English

---

7 Jess Sargeant, "Co-ordination and divergence: Devolution and coronavirus," *Institute for Government IfG Insight* (2020): 4, accessed August 2, 2021, https://www.instituteforgovernment.org.uk/sites/default/files/publications/coordination-divergence-devolution-coronavirus.pdf.   We shall see that the reality was much more complex than this gloss suggests.

identity were more likely to vote leave, while those with strong (especially exclusively) Scottish or Welsh identity tended to vote to stay in the EU.

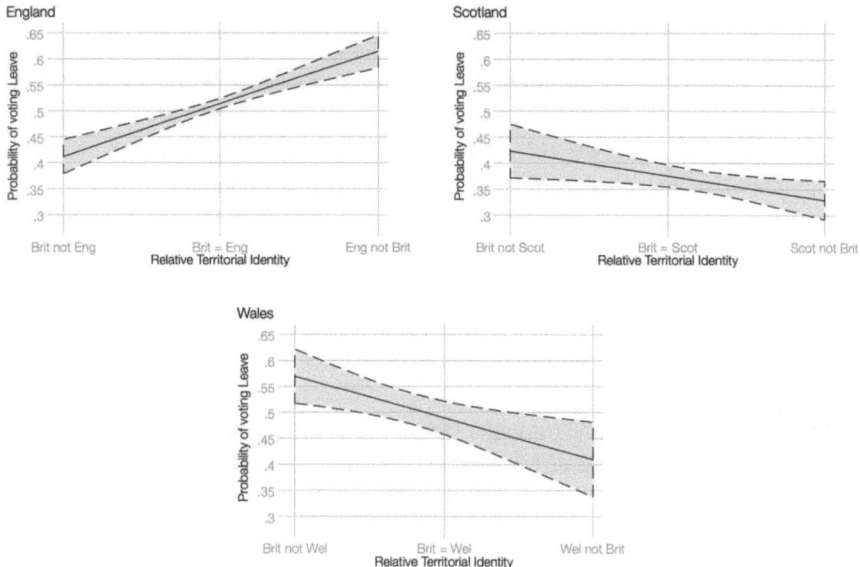

Chart 1: Relative territorial identity and Brexit vote choice. Ailsa Henderson et al., "Analysing vote-choice in a multinational state: national identity and territorial differentiation in the 2016 Brexit vote," *Regional Studies* 55, no. 9 (2021): 1520, accessed August 2, 2021, doi:10.1080/00343404.2020.1813883.

Thus, the political implications of British identity differ across the UK. Delving into the relationship between sub-state identities and Britishness, a further difference emerges. Anglo-Britishness is, typically, a fused identity within which both elements are often thoroughly mixed or muddled. By contrast, being Welsh and British means having attachments to two distinct levels. In terms of national identities, then, each of the UK's sub-state nations or jurisdictions displays distinctly different territorial politics and political identities.

Their distinctive patterns of national identity shape how various groups view the state. The "unitary state" idea has a particularly tenacious hold on how "Anglo-British" politicians and commentators view the UK state.[8] Historically,

---

8 Gregory Davies and Daniel Wincott, "Brexit, the Press and the Territorial Constitution," *Social and Legal Studies* 30 (2021): 157, https://doi.org/10.1177/0964663920921922; Daniel Wincott, C.R.G Murray, and Gregory Davies, "The Anglo-British imaginary and the rebuilding of the UK's terri-

the UK can also be understood as a multi-national "union." It has never been a single legal "unit," having always been constituted of three territorial legal jurisdictions (England & Wales, Northern Ireland, Scotland). For most of its history within its current territorial boundaries, it has included at least one devolved political system (for Northern Ireland from the 1920s to 1972 and since 1999 for Scotland, Wales and (intermittently) for Northern Ireland). Although mostly organized functionally for domestic policymaking in Great Britain, the modern administrative state – known as "Whitehall" – has always encompassed extensive "administrative" devolution of central state functions to Scotland.

Today, the UK is a devolved state with dramatic asymmetries in the powers exercised in each of its four major parts. The UK-wide government also serves as the government for England with respect to all the policy fields devolved to any of the UK's other three governments. Conventionally, the Westminster and Whitehall systems (sometimes known collectively by their postcode in London – SW1) are known as the UK's central government. In effect, however, the state also has three devolved central governments, each with different powers. As well as governing England, a variety of UK-wide powers are "reserved" to SW1, including overarching macro-economic and public finance functions alongside security, defense, and foreign affairs.

There are, it turns out, few ways in which the UK acts as a "unit." Why, then, is the "unitary state" idea so persistent? There is one major respect in which the UK is singular, politically speaking. Ultimately political power is concentrated in a single place: the Palace of Westminster. The principle conventionally known as "parliamentary sovereignty," more formally the "Crown-in-Parliament" (the Monarch, the House of Lords and the House of Commons – a secular Trinity), means that Westminster can make or unmake any law at all. Parliamentary sovereignty is hotly contested both historically and normatively; if accepted parliamentary sovereignty means that the powers – even the existence – of sub-state parliaments and governments are ultimately contingent on – or at the whim of – those in power in SW1. It is, though, vital to note that any formal super-concentration of political authority at Westminster makes the UK a single "unit" in only a particular – even a peculiar – way. Despite repeated anxieties about "post-code lotteries" – the idea that the availability or quality of public services might vary in different neighborhoods, a neuralgic issue in Westminster politics especially in relation to healthcare – there is little evidence that the Anglo-British state as-

torial constitution after Brexit: unitary state or union state?," *Territory, Politics, Governance*, published online May 17, 2021, DOI: https://doi.org/10.1080/21622671.2021.1921613; Ailsa Henderson and Richard Wyn Jones, *Englishness: The Political Force Transforming Britain* (Oxford: Oxford University Press, 2021).

pires to provide the same policy package to all citizens irrespective of where they live.

Generally, the UK state has sought to operate devolution as if it created two independent levels of public policy, one layered over the other. COVID-19 unveiled a reality of blurred lines and jagged edges. Territorial government in the UK is strikingly asymmetrical. It is the fruit of the *ad hoc* development of devolution and decentralization, layered over deep historical legacies of plural national identities and variegation of territorial governance. Brexit ramped up political contention over territorial politics; it amounts to a "behind our backs" reform of the territorial constitution.[9] Key pieces of Brexit legislation passed at Westminster had major implication for devolution. Westminster sovereignty notwithstanding, normally the London parliament only passes legislation that encroaches on devolved policy domains with the consent of the devolved legislatures. Yet the Scottish Parliament withheld consent for both the European Union Withdrawal Act (2018) and the UK Internal Market Act (2020), with the Senedd or Welsh Parliament also withholding consent from the latter piece of legislation. A deeper legacy of ramshackle intergovernmental relations provided a difficult background for the COVID-19 outbreak. Intergovernmental relations also worsened during the pandemic, not least due to ongoing Brexit/post Brexit developments.

This history produced complex patterns of pandemic policymaking across levels of government within the UK. Efforts at intergovernmental coordination came and went – and at times the levels seemed to work at cross-purposes. Table 1 provides a summary of some key COVID-19 policy domains.

Table 1: key COVID-19 policy domains

UK Government	Wales/England
– Furlough	– Health care and social care (note historic
– Universal Credit uplift	patterns)
– Sick pay	– Lockdown and unlocking
– Vaccine procurement	– Local & national boundaries
– [External border control]	– [Variation on external border rules]
– [Test, trace and isolate]	– [Variations in test and trace]
	– Vaccine rollout

---

9 Daniel Wincott, "Brexit is re-making the UK's constitution under our noses," *LSE Brexit Blog 2015–2021*, September 17, 2018, accessed August 2, 2021, https://blogs.lse.ac.uk/brexit/2018/09/17/brexit-is-re-making-the-uks-constitution-under-our-noses/.

The Initial UK Government Response

There is deep controversy attached to the UK's initial pandemic policy response. Whitehall's Civil Contingencies Committee COBR (named for the Cabinet Office Briefing Rooms, sometimes called COBRA) met five times about COVID-19 in January and February 2020.[10] The Prime Minister attended none of these five meetings. The UK government took little practical action before March 2020.

When it did face up to the pandemic, the Johnson administration often opted for new systems, seeking to create resources and products from scratch. From ventilators and vaccines to new large-scale emergency critical care hospitals, from PPE supply chains to the testing and tracing of COVID-19 infections, the UK government's instinct was to invent something new, rather than rely on – and seek to scale up – existing facilities and suppliers. Rather than working with the public sector, local authorities and the universities, it selected private sector innovators (often working outside their existing experience). For example, the pro-Brexit industrialist James Dyson enjoyed a flurry of publicity for his company's response to a UK government appeal for new ventilators. Known as an innovator and famous for novel domestic cleaning devices, Dyson's team designed a wholly new ventilator in 30 days. Despite initially suggesting it would purchase 10,000 machines, by late April 2020, the UK government decided Dyson's ventilators were not needed. Due to "regulatory and legal hurdles" the entrepreneur decided not to make his ventilators available to other countries.[11]

Dyson himself paid the £20 million development costs for his new ventilator that has never been used. But most entrepreneurs proved unwilling to bear costs of this kind themselves. Billions of pounds were spent by the UK Government, a significant proportion on equipment that proved to be unusable.[12] Ineffectiveness and waste shaded into corruption – called out as "cronyism and chumoc-

---

10 Peter Walker, "Boris Johnson missed five coronavirus Cobra meetings, Michael Gove says," *The Guardian*, April 19, 2020, accessed August 2, 2021, https://www.theguardian.com/world/2020/apr/19/michael-gove-fails-to-deny-pm-missed-five-coronavirus-cobra-meetings.
11 "Dyson Covid-19 ventilators are 'no longer required'", *BBC Website*, April 24, 2020, accessed August 2, 2021, https://www.bbc.co.uk/news/business-52409359; Virginia Bottomley, "Dyson's coronavirus response – Sir James Dyson on COVID-19 and developing the CoVent ventilator in 30 days," *Odgers Berndtson*, August 2, 2021, https://www.odgersberndtson.com/en-gb/insights/dysons-coronavirus-response-sir-james-dyson-on-covid-19-and-developing-the-covent-ventilator-in-30-days.
12 Jane Bradley et al., "Waste Negligence and Cronyism: Inside Britain's Pandemic Spending," *New York Times*, December 17, 2020, accessed August 2, 2021, https://www.nytimes.com/interactive/2020/12/17/world/europe/britain-covid-contracts.html.

racy" by the Labour opposition.[13] Major contracts were awarded to companies or individuals close to elected Conservative politicians, using a "high priority lane" – an email inbox accessed by government ministers. The UK government defended its approach as appropriate – even necessary – since the pandemic required high speed procurement.

Existing NHS hospitals expanded critical and intensive care capacity – typically by repurposing existing wards and surgical facilities. In addition, large scale critical care facilities were created at speed. On March 21 and 22 2020 planners visited ExCeL London – an exhibition center in East London; two days later Matthew Hancock, then Secretary of State for Health and Social Care announced the creation of a COVID-19 emergency hospital there. Dubbed the NHS Nightingale Hospital London, it opened on April 3. Intended to be able to receive and to discharge 150 patients a day, the hospital had a capacity for 500 patients and scope to expand to 4000. In April 2020, when the number of first wave COVID-19 patients hospitalized in London peaked, the 19 patients were being treated in the London Nightingale facility. It struggled to recruit sufficient staff, at times leading to potential patients being turned away. Similar facilities were constructed at six other sites in England as well as locations in Wales, Scotland, and Northern Ireland. None was ever used extensively.

Three other aspects of the UK level initial pandemic response merit brief further attention: test and trace, furlough and financial support for businesses under lockdown, and the strategies to develop and procure COVID-19 vaccines. First, the UK did not have a system for testing and tracing virus spread at the start of the pandemic. Again, the UK government turned to the private sector to create and run a new system. Described as "NHS test and trace," the NHS had little to do with the system.[14] Rather than working with existing laboratories, say in the universities, in a dispersed network of smaller scale facilities, three new large-scale test processing centers – known as "Lighthouse Labs" – were created in Milton Keynes, Cheshire, and Glasgow.[15] Lack of capacity led the UK government to suspend community-based testing for COVID-19 on March 12,

13 "Timeline: Covid contracts and accusations of 'chumocracy,'" *BBC*, April 20, 2021, accessed August 2, 2021. https://www.bbc.co.uk/news/uk-56319927.

14 Chris York, "Here's Who is Actually Running NHS Test and Trace," *Huffpost*, September 18, 2020, updated October 15, 2020, accessed August 2, 2021, https://www.huffingtonpost.co.uk/entry/nhs-test-trace-private-sector_uk_5f6099e3c5b68d1b09c77477.

15 Juliette Garside and Rupert Neate, "UK government 'using pandemic to transfer NHS duties to private sector," *The Guardian*, May 4, 2020, accessed August 2, 2021, https://www.theguardian.com/business/2020/may/04/uk-government-using-crisis-to-transfer-nhs-duties-to-private-sector.

2020. By then, COVID-19 was spreading fast in the community, but UK testing capacity remained very limited.[16]

Second, the UK Treasury rapidly generated arrangements for financial support to businesses and individuals who were unable to trade due to COVID-19 restrictions. Collectively known as "furlough," rather than laying employees off, these schemes allowed businesses to keep employees on their books, with the government picking up most of the costs. During the first half of 2020 these schemes were widely praised and appeared to work very effectively.[17]

Third, Chief Scientific Advisor Sir Patrick Vallance instigated a UK government Vaccine Taskforce (VTF) in April 2020. Kate Bingham, a venture capitalist with extensive experience in pharmaceuticals, was appointed swiftly to lead the VTF. It supported vaccine development, quickly secured a range of vaccines-types for the UK, made some provision for international vaccine distribution, and sought to establish a long-term vaccine strategy.[18]

Effective Co-ordination: Only Part of the Story?

The consensus is that the "early phase of the crisis was characterized by close co-ordination between the four governments of the UK."[19] Guided by the UK central government and its system of expert and scientific advisors, political leaders across Great Britain and Northern Ireland initially adopted similar approaches. A UK-wide Joint Action Plan was announced on March 3. Governments did not cancel large-scale events well into March 2020. Major sporting events were cancelled, typically at late notice and by governing bodies rather than Governments. On March 13 the Welsh Rugby Union cancelled the Wales-Scotland rugby international due in Cardiff on March 14. On March 17 the Scotland-Israel football international in Glasgow due on March 26 was postponed until early June.[20] The

---

16 Gareth Iacobucci, "Covid-19: Lack of capacity led to halting of community testing in March, admits deputy chief medical officer," *British Medical Journal*, (2020): 369, m1845, accessed August 2, 2021, https://www.bmj.com/content/369/bmj.m1845.

17 Zoe Williams, "Furlough was a radical success. Now let's talk about universal basic income," *The Guardian*, June 1, 2021, accessed August 2, 2021, https://www.theguardian.com/commentis free/2021/jun/01/furlough-universal-basic-income-covid.

18 "UK Vaccine Taskforce...", 4.

19 Jess Sargeant, "Co-ordination and divergence," 4.

20 Scottish Football Association Joint Response Group, "Coronavirus – Joint Response Group Update 17 March," March 17, 2020, accessed August 2, 2021, https://www.scottishfa.co.uk/news/coronavirus-joint-response-group-update-17-march/.

UK delayed moving to a widespread lockdown, partly because senior scientific advisors argued that an early lockdown would risk "behavioral fatigue." Intuitively plausible though this notion may be, the advisors involved were not behavioral experts. The concept of behavioral fatigue was repudiated by specialist behavioral scientists[21] and the UK population subsequently proved supportive of lengthy, tight lockdown restrictions.

Rather than relying on any existing legal framework for civil contingencies, new legislation – the Coronavirus Act 2020 – was created at speed. Introduced on March 19 and approved by the House of Commons on March 23, it completed all stages in the House of Lords and was enacted by Royal Assent on March 25. The legislation granted significant powers to devolved government ministers; it identified them as pivotal to pandemic management and strengthened their powers. Lockdown was eventually introduced on a coordinated basis across the UK on March 23.

Inter-governmental pandemic management did not run through the standard – rather broken-down and ramshackle – structures for UK-devolved government relations. Early on, during winter and spring 2020, the four central governments coordinated through COBR. Others, such as the mayor of London, also attended some of these meetings.

The pandemic put a premium on scientific advice. Deep uncertainty attached to its characteristics and how the virus might be contained and treated. Each government had its own scientific advisors, though the regular meetings of the four Chief Medical Officers suggest closer collaboration between advisors than governments. Initially, the devolved nations/jurisdictions were not represented as such on the UK government's Scientific Advisory Group on Emergencies (SAGE). Experts representing the devolved governments were given observer status on SAGE and, in May 2020, scientific advisers from each government became official SAGE participants. A new structure, the "Technical Advisory Cell," was created in Wales to fit advice to the devolved context. The Institute for Government illustrated its understanding of "scientific advisory structures in the UK and devolved governments" schematically (Figure 1). Over the pandemic's first year or so, all governments received broadly similar scientific advice.

Given the impact of Brexit on devolved and UK government relations, cooperation during the initial period was notably good. But relationships worsened as the initial lockdown eased between May and August and the various govern-

---

21 Nigel Harvey, "Behavioural Fatigue: Real Phenomenon, Naïve Construct, or Policy Contrivance," *Frontiers in Psychology: Cognition*, November 25, 2020, accessed August 2, 2021, https://doi.org/10.3389/fpsyg.2020.589892.

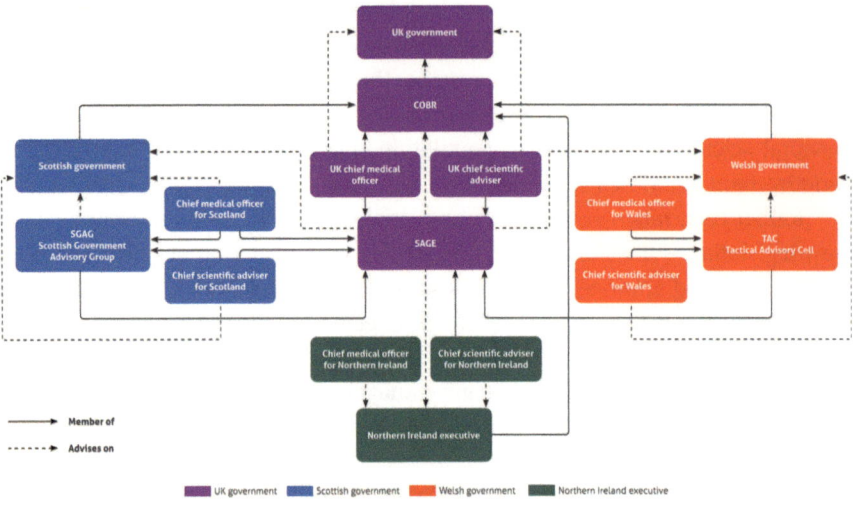

Source: Institute for Government analysis. The Welsh government's CSA for health is a participant in SAGE.

Figure 1: Institute for Government: Structure of Scientific Advice. Jess Sargeant, "Co-ordination and divergence," 16.

ments' policies diverged. Despite some effort to re-establish coordination from August onwards, further significant differences developed alongside a new wave of infection and hospitalization. Intergovernmental relations deteriorated further.

Equally, close attention to the record of UK-Welsh government relations raises questions about the positive mainstream account of coordination, even for the early period. Disputes over the procurement of COVID-19 tests, the development of a COVID-19 testing facility in Cardiff, and tendentious, abrasive public communications about the structure of the health services by then UK government Secretary of State for Health and Social Care, Matthew Hancock, all exemplify these tensions.

There is no evidence of coordination over the procurement of tests for active COVID-19 infection. Public Health Wales (PHW) – the Welsh government's public health agency – negotiated with pharmaceutical company Roche from March 2, 2020 over COVID-19 tests for Wales and the reconfiguration of laboratory machinery to create capacity in Wales to analyze the tests. In early March the Welsh Government set a target of 6,000 tests a day by April 1, rising to 9,000 by the end of that month. For a nation of around three million, that level of testing would have made an ambitious "test trace and isolate" containment strategy possible. Reports of the collapse of a Welsh Government "deal" to purchase

COVID-19 tests emerged on March 28, 2020.[22] The subsequent history is complex, hard to follow, and highly contested.[23] Ultimately, Roche supplied 5,000 tests for the whole UK. Wales received broadly a proportionate share. First, this episode does not show good coordination. Second, the Welsh government and PHW believed the UK government and Public Health England had undermined the Welsh deal. Third, Roche denies ever having a contract – or even an agreement – with the Welsh government. Latterly, that government accepted it had not signed a contract while continuing to insist negotiations with Roche were at an advanced stage, claiming supportive evidence in emails. Equally, there was something naïve, at least, in the Welsh administration's public commitment to a mass testing system when no formal contract for the tests had been finalized.

The Welsh government occluded the terms of this conflict with its UK counterpart. Faced with Freedom of Information requests on it from March 2020 onwards, it refused to make its correspondence public. The reason it offered for doing so on June 5, 2020 is striking. Making the information public "would, or would be likely to prejudice relations with the UK government."[24] As well as seeking to maintain its working relationship with London, the Welsh government may have been covering its own failure to deliver on a promise (although its contemporaneous understanding located most responsibility for the episode with some combination of the UK government and PHE).

Another aspect of test and trace reveals a degree of territorial "muddle": distinct, but overlapping, structures and processes were put in place. The Welsh government had primary responsibility for test and trace in Wales. Even so,

---

22 "Coronavirus testing deal 'collapses' but new plan unveiled," *BBC*, March 28, 2020, accessed August 2, 2021, https://www.bbc.co.uk/news/uk-wales-52078525.

23 https://twitter.com/adavies4/status/1386387587607240706, accessed August 2, 2021. This twitter thread, written by an influential Wales-based home affairs correspondent for Channel 4 television, is richly detailed. It notes PHW head Tracey Cooper reported hearing of a meeting called by the UK government with Roche in mid-March at which the company was instructed to reserve all additional tests "for England" and then "after, by agreement, with the Das" (or devolved administrations). Wales' emerging deal with Roche seemed to be "off." Cooper then had informal negotiations with Alex Sienkiewicz, Director of PHE at Porton Down. PHE sought to borrow equipment from the Welsh Blood Service to increase Covid testing capacity in England. By March 18, Cooper believed, a "deal" had been struck, trading this equipment loan from Wales to England for reinstating Roche's supply of 5,000 weekly tests for Wales. Four days later the Wales-Roche deal was off again. PHW officials believed that "Wales'" 5,000 tests were "intercepted" by PHE Porton Down on March 22. Roche has consistently denied that it "was having similar negotiations with both the UK and Welsh Governments to access the same testing kits."

24 James Williams, "Coronavirus: 'Collapsed' Roche testing deal correspondence withheld," *BBC*, June 9, 2020, accessed August 2, 2021, https://www.bbc.co.uk/news/uk-wales-politics-52977589.

the UK government and PHE reportedly set up a major test venue at Cardiff City's Football Stadium, without informing the Welsh government or PHW.[25] Eventually, it seems, the Welsh government took over the general responsibility for the site. Even then, initially, "Lighthouse Lab" results did not link with Welsh clinical records. The system, developed for England, was not adapted to Wales, limiting its value for Welsh pandemic management.

In mid-April Hancock published an article to celebrate his role creating the new testing center in a leading Wales-focused media outlet. This text is particularly revealing. He claimed credit for the Cardiff drive-through center and called for co-operation and teamwork across "the four-nations."[26] He sought to quash stories about England having priority over Wales for PPE shipments. But the Secretary of State went further, insisting that, in "the end, it's not a Welsh Health Service or an English Health Service but a National Health Service." He did not mention the then recently created "Dragon's Heart" emergency hospital – the third such institution anywhere in the UK. Whether the errors and gaps in Hancock's article were the product of ignorance or a deliberate choice, it is hard to avoid the conclusion that its author's agenda had a partisan element. He may have been gesturing to the potency of the NHS as a UK-wide political symbol. But writing in the Wales-focused media as the first wave COVID-19 deaths were peaking and confusion reigned about the disease, Hancock risked misdirecting his readers about the structure of and responsibility for health services in Wales.

At best the Johnson administration's recognition of and respect for the Welsh government's role was inconsistent. Devolution has never amounted to a coherent system: successive UK administrations have devolved powers to Wales in a piecemeal and often grudging manner. Hancock's comments suggest he struggled to make sense of those powers. At times he, and his colleagues in London, seemed intent on overruling devolution and unpicking its operation. Already in March 2020, its relations with Westminster and Whitehall required a big dose of self-restraint from a Welsh government perspective. It is, of course, hard to define

---

25 Will Hayward, "The flashpoints of the pandemic: the clashes between Wales and Westminster and their life or death consequences," *WalesOnline*, April 10, 2021, accessed August 2, 2021, https://www.walesonline.co.uk/news/wales-news/flashpoints-pandemic-clashes-between-wales-20355424.

26 Matthew Hancock, "We are all on the same team in the battle against coronavirus and we will get through this together," *WalesOnline*, April 19, 2020, accessed August 2, 2021, https://www.walesonline.co.uk/news/politics/matt-hancock-coronavirus-ppe-wales-18113343. Wales-focused media is notoriously weak. Major London-based newspapers publish distinct editions in Scotland, which also has a tradition of high-quality national titles. Neither is true of Wales.

an independent metric for the effective intergovernmental coordination: the assessor's expectations are critical. Even so, if describing effective intergovernmental pandemic coordination as "surprising" is apt, the UK's territorial governance practices must be deeply flawed.

Worsening Relations after the Initial Lockdown

Intergovernmental relations worsened significantly as the initial lockdown eased. In contrast to earlier regular COBR-based contact, communication between the Welsh and UK governments dried up. Though Mark Drakeford, Wales' Labour First Minister, attempted to maintain contact with the Prime Minister, two full months went by without any contact.[27] The UK government lifted restrictions sooner than its devolved counterparts; its key slogan changed from "Stay at Home, Protect the NHS, Save Lives" to "Stay Alert, Control the Virus, Save Lives" in early May. By contrast, the Welsh government retained the earlier – and previously shared – "Stay Home" slogan. In a pre-recorded speech released on May 10, Boris Johnson announced a "conditional plan" to reopen society. Widely derided as confused and confusing, the reopening was also more limited than some had expected. "Freedom" was extended from one to multiple daily episodes of outdoor exercise. New permission was given to drive to parks and beaches for exercise or to sunbathe.[28]

Some English Conservative MPs and the London-based media expressed concerns about cross-border confusion and complexity: their assumption was, it seems, that Welsh authorities should adapt to UK government policy for England. Johnson made little effort to simplify, clarify or explain these policy differences – or even to define the territorial scope of his government's policies. Although typically his "easing" was for England only, Johnson often used the euphemism "this country" or referred to Britain or the UK. The lack of territorial clarity in UK government ministerial statements reflects a complex identity that fuses elements of majority (English) and state (British) nationalism. The imagined community of Anglo-Britain seems to view itself as natural, while seeing other sub-state nationalisms as inherently divisive.

Shortly before Johnson's speech, Daniel Kawczynski – an English Conservative MP in a Welsh border constituency – had complained that the "Welsh As-

---

27 Hayward, "The flashpoints…".
28 "Boris Johnson speech: PM unveils 'conditional plan' to reopen society," *BBC*, May 10, 2020, accessed August 2, 2021, https://www.bbc.co.uk/news/uk-52609952.

sembly and UK Parliament" were "increasingly divergent."[29] Kawczynski said "The Prime Minister has told us we can go to the beach now, but we are then told we can't go to any of our closest beaches because they are in Wales, and the Welsh Government doesn't want us to come."[30] The beaches nearest to his constituency in England are close to equidistant to those in Wales.[31] No doubt these new cross-border policy differences did cause some confusion, but Kawczynski presented any difference as inherently problematic. By stirring up discontent, he added to the confusion and increased tensions over the border. Kawczynski attributed responsibility for confusion solely to the Welsh government, wholly ignoring Johnson's frequent imprecision and inaccuracy in describing the territorial extent of UK government policy. Kawczynski was, it appears, offended and unsettled by the existence of distinct Welsh policies and the attention they drew to the Anglo-Welsh border. The Anglo-centric form of Britishness he displayed is characteristic of many English Conservative MPs.[32]

As COVID-19 infection rates began to rise again in autumn 2020, the disconnection between UK government and devolved policies worsened. The UK Treasury planned to terminate its furlough schemes at the end of October. Without this Treasury support, any lockdown would have immediate harsh consequences for

---

29 Daniel Kawczynski, https://twitter.com/dkshrewsbury/status/1258805950426894336?lang= en, accessed August 2, 2021. Two days earlier the Assembly had changed its name to the Welsh Parliament or Senedd Cymru; it is generally known as "the Senedd" by English speakers. Around the same time Kawczynski had also called for the Assembly's abolition.

30 Quoted in Mark Andrew, "'We can't go to the beach': MP says Welsh Government is undermining coronavirus message," *Shropshire Star*, May 12, 2020, accessed August 2, 2021, https:// www.shropshirestar.com/news/politics/2020/05/12/we-cant-go-to-the-beach-mp-says-welsh-gov ernment-is-undermining-coronavirus-message/.

31 Nation Cymru, "Shrewsbury MP deletes tweet calling for Welsh Parliament to be scrapped after backlash," *Nation.Cymru* October 15, 2020, accessed August 2, 2021, https://nation. cymru/news/shrewsbury-mp-deletes-tweet-calling-for-welsh-parliament-to-be-scrapped-after-backlash/.

32 John Denham, "English Nationalism? Or Anglo-centric British nationalism?," *The Optimistic Patriot blog*, September 22, 2020, accessed October 4, 2021, https://www.theoptimisticpatriot.co. uk/post/629983304244969472/english-nationalism-or-anglo-centric-british; Michael Kenny and Jack Sheldon, "When Planets Collide: The British Conservative Party and the Discordant Goals of Delivering Brexit and Preserving the Domestic Union, 2016–2019," *Political Studies*, first published June 20, 2020, https://doi.org/10.1177/0032321720930986, develops a related argument. They detect a turn from "banal" or "unthinking" unionism to "muscular-" or "hyper-unionism" among English Conservative MPs. My analysis of broadly the same developments focuses more on the default to a Westminster-focused hypercentralism and the blurred lines across Anglo and British identities, which allows the unionism of Conservative MPs to be both banal and muscular all at once.

employment and the viability of businesses. Yet despite warnings about a second wave from SAGE as early as September 21, the Treasury maintained its plan to end the scheme.

Despite the Treasury's commitment to ending furlough, the Welsh government ordered a "firebreak" – a period of renewed restrictions – to begin on October 23. Running into November, past the furlough's planned end-date, the firebreak was designed to be short. The government also preannounced that its postfirebreak restrictions would be light-touch. The potential for a lockdown without Treasury furlough-type support to have a rapid, harsh, and enduring economic impact may have influenced the design of the firebreak. Asked by the Welsh government to adapt its policy to support the firebreak, the Treasury declined to do so.

Shortly thereafter, Treasury policy did change when the UK government introduced new restrictions across England. Hours before furlong was due to end, the Chancellor extended it across the UK.[33] While businesses and workers in Wales did, ultimately, benefit from the change, its mid-firebreak introduction was chaotic. With the Treasury having set the expectation that furlough would end, some employment contracts may have been terminated by businesses anticipating being unable to operate during the firebreak with no support in place. The Johnson administration seems to have been attuned to priorities in England – perhaps even in the south of England. Its policies' impacts elsewhere were, it appears, little more than incidental; other parts of the UK were not its pressing priority.[34]

Other episodes point in a similar direction. The Welsh government gradually introduced local restrictions in September and October 2020, with people told to stay within their local authority boundaries. England, however, had no equivalent restrictions. Drakeford sent Johnson two letters asking him to restrict movement from England into Wales, but received no response.[35] After genomic analysis showed virus outbreaks had been caused by travel from England, the Welsh government eventually banned travel from some parts of that country. The Welsh

33 Rachel Lewis and Amy Wren, "Coronavirus: furlough is back again and lockdown mark II," *Farrier & Co* 2 November 2020, accessed August 2, 2021, https://www.farrer.co.uk/news-and-in sights/blogs/coronavirus-furlough-is-back-again-and-lockdown-mark-ii/.
34 Helen Pidd, "Government accused of being London-centric with Covid support," *The Guardian*, October 22, 2020, accessed August 2, 2021, *https://www.theguardian.com/world/2020/oct/22/ government-accused-of-being-london-centric-with-covid-support*.
35 Joshua Searle, "Coronavirus: FM, Drakeford's full letter to Boris Johnson," *South Wales Argus*, October 13, 2020, accessed August 2, 2021, https://www.southwalesargus.co.uk/news/ 18791211.coronavirus-fm-drakefords-full-letter-boris-johnson/.

authorities made use of England's new 3-Tier system, introduced in mid-October, banning travel from places under its two most restrictive levels.[36] The treatment of borders by the UK government was inconsistent. It was willing to impose its own local border restrictions – English guidance advised people not to cross a tier 3 border – but critical of restrictions imposed by others. A Downing Street official called it "disappointing that the Welsh administration has chosen to act unilaterally."[37]

Localities and Boundaries in England

While taking umbrage at the Welsh government's approach to the Anglo-Welsh border, closer analysis of developments within England reinforces the sense that the UK government objection was not to the use of borders as such. In fact, it had enforced local boundaries within England long before it introduced the new 3-Tier system. That new system was an attempt to replace a variety of bespoke local arrangements previously imposed *ad hoc* by the UK government long before October 2020. The new arrangements also reflected rising cases in London. They seemed to reveal a pattern: the UK government responded to rising infection rates in London and the south-east with England-wide restrictions but used bespoke local restrictions for other places. Outside the south-east *ad hoc* local restrictions had been introduced particularly in places with large minority ethnic and religious communities. They started in Leicester and were then introduced in many places across the north of England.

Leicester's bespoke local restrictions began on July 4, 2020. The city remained under special arrangements until mid-October, when high-level restrictions continued under the new tiered arrangements. Leicester remained locked down for a very long period, given the England-wide restrictions in the autumn/winter of 2020/2021. Cramped, multi-generational living and the role of textile factories in the local economy seem to be implicated in the City's stub-

---

36 Peter Walker et al., "Boris Johnson unveils three-teir Covid restrictions for England," *The Guardian*, October 12, 2021, accessed August 2, 2021, https://www.theguardian.com/world/2020/oct/12/boris-johnson-unveils-three-tier-covid-restrictions-for-england.
37 John Johnson, "No 10 says it is 'disappointed' at Welsh Government plans to close the border to visitors from England," October 15, 2021, accessed August 2, 2021, https://www.politicshome.com/news/article/no-10-welsh-border-plans-coronavirus.

born rates of infection,[38] which England's governmental system failed to address effectively.

Parts of northern England with large Muslim populations had restrictions introduced at very short notice before the celebration of Eid-al-Udha in July 2020.[39] Like Leicester, Greater Manchester was subject to restrictions over a long period. These ranged from *ad hoc* local rules to tight restrictions under the England-wide 3-Tier system and, from November 5, the new England-wide lockdown. Before the extension of furlough, resources were provided to support businesses under tight local restrictions, but not at the 80% of workers' wages provided by the full system. Moreover, the UK government came to *ad hoc* financial arrangements with the various local authorities involved. Andy Burnham, Greater Manchester Mayor, objected to the UK government's approach. The level of financial support was, he argued, too low, given the long-term pressures on local businesses and their employees. Moreover, he objected to the government's approach of "side deals for local areas," arguing that a "fair financial framework' should be set out for Tier-3 areas across England.[40] Burnham engaged forcefully with the UK government, and the resulting high profile gained him the nickname "King of the North."

Hypercentralism meets Devolution: Vaccine Successes Across the UK

Starting in early 2020, a variety of types of remarkably effective COVID-19 vaccinations were developed very rapidly. The UK government adopted a distinctive VTF-centered approach to vaccine development, procurement, and roll-out. It was bespoke, hypercentralized, and drew heavily on private sector expertise, all hallmarks of the Johnson administration.[41] As late as mid-November 2020 critics depicted the VTF as just another example of the "cronyism" they argued characterized much of the Conservative government's COVID-19-related procure-

---

38 David Pittam, "Coronavirus: 'Big problem' at Leicester factories, say workers," *BBC*, July 7, 2020, accessed August 2, 2021, https://www.bbc.co.uk/news/uk-england-leicestershire-53311548; Clarke, "Leicester lockdown …".
39 "Coronavirus: 'The spirit of Eid …".
40 Chris Slater, "Andy Burnham says it's 'not just about the size of the cheque' as 'government offers Greater Manchester millions' for Tier 3 lockdown," *Manchester Evening News*, October 19, 2020, accessed August 2, 2021, https://www.manchestereveningnews.co.uk/news/greater-man chester-news/andy-burnham-says-its-not-19126628.
41 "UK Vaccine Taskforce 2020…".

ment.[42] The VTF was an *ad hoc* creation in response to the "Nation" being surprisingly "ill prepared to deal with pandemics when they arrive," in the words of Sir Richard Sykes (GlaxoWellcome CEO in 1998).[43] In fact, the VTF built on the fragile legacy of a New Labour-era effort – the Jenner Institute – to strengthen UK vaccine development from 1998. Jenner was a government, industry, university collaboration for basic vaccine research, supported for 10 start-up years by funding from GlaxoWellcome. From 2008 the institute "struggled to obtain Government support and eventually ended up at Oxford University."[44]

Against this backdrop, Kate Bingham's VTF leadership was key to its success. The taskforce supported some basic vaccine development and helped scale-up UK vaccine manufacture capacity. While they were being developed and before their effectiveness was known, it procured huge volumes of vaccine across a variety of types. Setting aside arguments about cronyism and ill-preparedness, the VTF was a model high-risk high-reward gamble. Initially pushed by Sir Patrick Vallance, the UK government's Chief Scientific Officer, perhaps uniquely among the UK government's bespoke, *ad hoc* pandemic initiatives, the VTF gamble paid off handsomely, albeit contingent on the underlying science of vaccine development, and proved remarkably quick and effective. The various relevant authorities and institutions worked well across the UK. The Conservative government wrapped a Union Flag around the VTF: Johnson presented vaccine development in particular – especially by "Oxford AstraZeneca" – as a distinctively "British" success.[45] The media mixed wider processes of vaccine testing, approval, developing new UK-based manufacturing capacity, procurement, and roll-out into the same success story. During the first half of 2021, UK vaccine success was explicitly contrasted with slower roll-out in the EU. Senior Conservative MPs, including ministers, attributed the UK's relative success to Brexit. Johnson himself "kept relatively quiet" through a period of vaccine-related UK-EU rows and recrimination within EU-Europe, "content to enjoy a propaganda win over the EU."[46]

---

42 Jolyon Maugham, "Covid-19 contracts smell of cronyism – so I'm taking the government to court," *The Guardian*, November 16, 2020, accessed August 2, 2021, https://www.theguardian.com/commentisfree/2020/nov/16/covid-19-contracts-cronyism-government-court.
43 "UK Vaccine Taskforce 2020...", 4.
44 "UK Vaccine Taskforce 2020...", 4.
45 Boris Johnson, "The Oxford vaccine shows why we and the world need Britain to be global," *The Times*, March 16, 2021, accessed August 2, 2021, https://www.gov.uk/government/speeches/pm-boris-johnson-the-oxford-vaccine-shows-why-we-and-the-world-need-britain-to-be-global.
46 Luke McGee, "Boris Johnson's vaccine strategy gets another boost, while Europe confronts fresh problems," *CNN*, February 25, 2021, accessed August 2, 2021, https://edition.cnn.com/2021/02/25/uk/boris-johnson-vaccine-eu-intl-gbr/index.html. The article quotes David Davis as

The reality of vaccine roll-out was more complicated than the UK government-centered story suggests. Centralized VTF procurement and quick approval allowed for a relatively early start for UK mass vaccination programs. Though they proceeded quickly all across the UK, outwith England, the devolved governments delivered distinct vaccine programs. After a slow start, the Welsh government's approach turned out to be particularly successful. As of June 9, 2021, Wales had the highest proportion of its population with a first dose of vaccine anywhere in the world.[47] Moreover, alongside the UK government, Drakeford's Labour administration gained credit with the public for the COVID-19 vaccination program. Again, Conservatives in London struggled to acknowledge Welsh government successes. They found it hard to share credit for rolling-out vaccinations, still less did they learn lessons from Wales. UK ministers could have argued, legitimately, that vaccine roll-out in Wales depended on UK-wide vaccine procurement. Matthew Hancock went further, revealing his disputatious partisanship or a remarkably thin-skinned anxiety about the perception of greater success in Wales, or both. He claimed the Welsh strategy was contingent on a UK government vaccine "buffer" (and implicitly, therefore, held no lessons for England). "Wrong" said a Welsh government spokesperson: "we hold our own and actually deliver a smaller proportion of vaccine to our centers than other UK nations."[48]

Politics, Public Attitudes, Territoriality, and COVID-19

The structure of sub-state national communities has shaped public attitudes to political leadership throughout the pandemic. To make sense of public responses to their government's COVID-19 policies, the vaccine thread needs to be braided together with our other themes, some specifically pandemic-related,

---

saying "If we were still in the EU now some people would be dead who are not." Early on Hancock had claimed, wrongly, that the UK had been able to approve the Pfizer/BioNTech vaccine earlier than the EU "because of Brexit"; Peter Walker, "No 10 and regulator contradict Hancock's 'because of Brexit' Covid vaccine claim," *The Guardian*, December 2, 2020, accessed August 2, 2021, https://www.theguardian.com/world/2020/dec/02/hancock-brexit-helped-uk-to-speedy-approval-of-covid-vaccine.

47 Ione Wells, "Covid: Matt Hancock says UK approach helped Wales vaccinate quicker," *BBC News*, June 10, 2021, accessed August 2, 2021, https://www.bbc.co.uk/news/uk-wales-politics-57429539.

48 Wells, "Covid: Matt Hancock says…"

others much more deeply rooted – or buried – in the complex, contested, and contradictory terrain of UK territorial politics.

Perhaps reflecting the genuinely hard policy choices he faced as well as his own encounter with COVID-19, many in England gave Boris Johnson the benefit of the doubt.[49] His approval rating across Great Britain benefited from a "rally round the flag" spike in April 2020. It then turned sharply downwards over the summer and autumn of 2020. From around the turn of the year the prospect of effective vaccines flowed into growing evidence of successful roll-out. Johnson's ratings received a "vaccine bounce"; they recovered somewhat from December and by March 2021 had just about returned to a net-positive level.

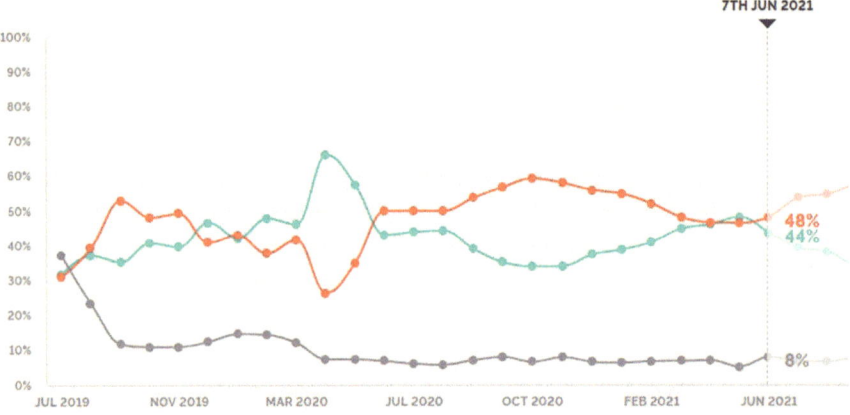

Chart 2: Boris Johnson approval rating. YouGov. Question, "Do you think that Boris Johnson is doing well or badly as Prime Minister?" https://yougov.co.uk/topics/politics/trackers/boris-johnson-approval-rating.

COVID-19 also placed devolved political leaders in the spotlight. Mark Drakeford gained particular new prominence as First Minister of Wales. Historically, Welsh politicians have struggled for recognition, even within Wales. He featured frequently on UK-wide media. After an initial downward blip, Drakeford's popularity grew to match his profile. Like Nicola Sturgeon in Scotland, Drakeford presented a steadier, more cautious persona than Boris Johnson. He was, perhaps, more willing to articulate the dilemmas and difficulties of pandemic management than the UK Prime Minister. Despite the broad similarity of outcomes across Britain, this contrast in tone served him well. Voters in Wales (and Scot-

---

49 Jen Gatskill et al., "Public Trust and Covid-19," *UK in a Changing Europe*, July 24, 2020, accessed August 2, 2021, https://ukandeu.ac.uk/public-trust-and-covid-19/.

land) also credited the UK Government for COVID-19 vaccines, but they were at least as impressed with the devolved government-led vaccine roll-out. They remained much more critical of other aspects of the Johnson administration's pandemic communication and handling of the lockdown. By contrast, Mark Drakeford (again like Sturgeon) received more positive endorsement on these matters.

These differences in public attitudes played out in a set of elections held on May 6. 2021. They encompassed ballots for the devolved parliaments in Scotland and Wales, a range of local elections across England, including for the mayors of several combined authorities or City-Regions and a by-election for the Hartlepool Westminster constituency. Johnson's Conservatives won in Hartlepool, indicating that COVID-19 had not dented their new political competitiveness in the north of England. Equally, the incumbent Labour government performed well in Wales (as did the SNP in Scotland),[50] matching its best-ever haul of 50% of Senedd seats. Perhaps to Johnson's surprise, the devolved governments also gained significant credit for their role in the vaccine roll-out. Despite pandemic outcomes broadly similar to those in England, however, trust in the Welsh government did not pivot on vaccine success. It was also rooted in the perception that they "stood up" for Wales and to the Johnson government during the pandemic.[51]

Conclusion

England has no dedicated devolved government. Instead, the London government has England-only and UK-wide responsibilities. So dominant is England within the UK that these territorial arrangements slip easily from the minds of policymakers and political leaders. The aphorism "devolve and forget" reflects an attitude of mind as well as ramshackle formal institutions. It reflects a complex "fusion" of Englishness and Britishness. There is a deeply-rooted Anglo-centric quality to much nominally British elite discourse. Shakespeare's idea of England as an unconquered, distinctive "sceptred isle" remains a remarkably pervasive today.

---

50 Martin Kettle, "That wasn't quite the resounding Conservative election victory it seemed," *The Guardian*, May 13, 2020, https://www.theguardian.com/commentisfree/2021/may/13/re sounding-conservative-election-victory-local-devolved-polls; Akash Paun, "Elections 2021: what did we learn?," *Institute for Government*, https://www.instituteforgovernment.org.uk/publica tion/elections-2021.
51 This narrative also helps to explain Andy Burnham's comfortable victory in the Greater Manchester Mayoral election.

UK central government struggled to "read" any of the territories it governs.[52] It proved unable or unwilling to specify the territorial extent – limited to England – of many pandemic regulations. English Conservative Ministers seemed reluctant to work with the Welsh government, to acknowledge its policies or respond to its concerns. Conservatives at Westminster repeatedly indulged in abrasive criticism of Welsh COVID-19 policies. They seemed surprised and deeply disconcerted when Welsh and English policies differed. At times English government ministers even appeared to treat Welsh "success" as a threat. Placing the first 18 months of COVID-19 in Anglo-Welsh territorial perspective suggests an instability or fragility about Anglo-British identity. Westminster was wrong-footed by and poorly connected to developments in many parts of England. The patchwork process of devolving power to English City-Regions seemed to stall.

UK constitutional arrangements allow a majority at Westminster to make/unmake any rule for all parts of the state. They allow London to default to hyper-centralism and *ad hoc* territorial interventions. Except for the VTF,[53] hyper-centralized UK-level pandemic responses have proved expensive and, often, unsuccessful. Yet halfway through 2021 Johnson's administration seemed set on course for further centralization of UK policy and politics. Mid-pandemic it devoted considerable time and effort to passing the UK Internal Market Act – legislation that weakened devolution in practice under the guise of extending its scope. Johnson proclaimed his intention to intervene directly in devolved policy matters, bypassing the Welsh (Scottish and Northern Irish) authorities.[54] Refracted through prisms of national identity across the UK, these changes are likely to be viewed differently across England, Wales, Scotland, and Northern Ireland – and lock the UK into an abrasive mode of territorial politics.

---

52 Wincott, "The possible break-up…".
53 "UK Vaccine Taskforce…"
54 Wincott et al., "The Anglo-British Imaginary…"

Conclusion: **The European Union**

Sara Casella Colombeau

10 The COVID-19 Pandemic and its Effects on the Free Movement of People within the E.U.

Assessing the Tensions between the EU and National Political Centers

Introduction

Since the beginning of the COVID-19 pandemic, free movement of people, and more specifically the crossing of international borders, has been high on the agenda, almost everywhere in the world. Restrictions on mobility have been praised by governments all over the world as one of the central means to deal with the pandemic.[1] The European Union was no exception. From the beginning of March 2020, 19 European member states (including four, not belonging to the Schengen area) decided to limit international mobility, including within the Schengen area. These decisions, although uncoordinated, resulted in the unilateral reintroduction of border checks at national borders and consequently at the internal borders of the Schengen area. This reinstatement of border checks did not last long, however. In fact, three phases can be identified: a first phase from March 2020 to June 2020, when restrictions on mobility were the highest, both within the national territories and across international borders; a second phase from June 2020 to January 2021 when most member states lifted the checks at internal borders and sometimes limited internal mobility; and a third phase beginning in January 2021, when member states introduced health requirements (COVID-19 tests and/or quarantine) to cross their national borders.

One could consider that the unprecedent pandemic situation requires an analysis of these reintroductions of border checks as an exception. Yet, this is

---

1 Lorenzo Piccoli, Jelena Dzankic, and Didier Ruedin, "Citizenship, Migration and Mobility in a Pandemic (CMMP): A Global Dataset of COVID-19 Restrictions on Human Movement," ed. Francesco Di Gennaro, *PLOS ONE* 16, no. 3 (2021), accessed September 30, 2021, DOI: 10.1371/journal.pone.0248066.

Sara Casella Colombeau, Associate Professor, Univ. Grenoble Alpes, ILCEA4, 38000 Grenoble, France.

https://doi.org/10.1515/9783110745085-011

not the first time in the recent years that member states have reinstated border checks at internal borders of the Schengen area.[2] Since the beginning of the 2010s there has been a clear acceleration in the reinstatement of border controls at internal borders. Indeed, since the year 2015, and the collective reintroduction of border checks[3] at internal borders to prevent secondary migratory movement, Schengen has been depicted as being "in crisis."[4]

I suggest, then, to reflect on the continuities and discontinuities of this phenomenon. What can be drawn from the history of border checks reinstatement to understand the dynamics at play in today's response to the pandemic? What are the specificities of the reinstatement of border checks during the COVID-19 pandemic? How did the EU institutions and the member states react to the pandemic? Has there been some kind of coordination between member states?

Within this edited volume, this contribution aims at taking a side step to envision the response to the COVID-19 pandemic at the European level and not at the national level. This change of scale might seem at odds with most of the contributions that focus on national responses to the pandemic. But this contribution will seek to reflect on similarities that can be observed in the tensions between political centers.[5] Indeed, the COVID-19 responses given either by member states or the EU regarding individuals' mobility uncover the underlying tensions between political centers at different scales: be it between central government and regional authorities (Comunidades autónomas, nations, etc.), or between the EU political centers (namely EU supranational institutions) and the member states.

This work is then in line with the post-Rokkannian literature which explores the parallel between State formation and transformation on one side and EU integration, in other words European political center formation,[6] on the other. Rokkan analyses the formation of a nation state as the successful attempts by a po-

---

2 Kees Groenendijk, "Reinstatement of Controls at the Internal Borders of Europe: Why and Against Whom?," *European Law Journal* 10, no. 2 (2004).
3 Elspeth Guild et al., "What Is Happening to the Schengen Borders?," *CEPS Paper in Liberty and Security in Europe*, December 2015.
4 Sara Casella Colombeau, "Crisis of Schengen? The Transformation of Border Police Practices at the Schengen Internal Borders in Ventimiglia in 2011 and 2015," *Journal of Ethnic and Migration Studies* 46, no. 11 (2020).
5 Stein Rokkan, *State formation, nation-building, and mass politics in Europe: the theory of Stein Rokkan based on his collected works*, ed. Peter Flora, Stein Kuhnle, and Derek William Urwin (Oxford; New York: Oxford University Press, 1999).
6 Stefano Bartolini, *Restructuring Europe: Center Formation, System Building and Political Structuring between the Nation-State and the European Union* (New York: Oxford University Press, 2005).

litical center to control the functional boundaries and borders of its peripheries. The nation state emerges when the political center succeeds in aligning the military, economic, linguistic, cultural, and political boundaries with its territorial borders. Corresponding to this process of centralization, there is an attempt by peripheries at preserving their distinctiveness and autonomy. State formation is then characterized by this center-periphery tension. Stefano Bartolini analyzes the EU integration as a new political center formation, where the EU political center tries to control its peripheries' boundaries, namely the member states boundaries. This theoretical framework has been used to understand the long-term dynamics of EU internal security.[7] With this theoretical framework in mind, the creation of an area of free movement for individuals can be seen as the successful attempt of the EU political center to remove national borders which are also internal boundaries of the Schengen area. Furthermore, free movement of people within the EU has been associated since the 1990s with compensatory measures, namely the creation of a common external border, whose characteristics are defined by the European political center. In this context, the reintroduction of border checks at internal borders of the Schengen area can be interpreted as resistance by the peripheries (the member states) to the standardization process led by the EU political center.

This chapter will then explore the tension between the EU political center and a national political center, namely France, during the response to the COVID-19 regarding free movement of people. It will investigate how between June 2020 and March 2021, the EU political center tried to remove internal borders of the EU and Schengen area and at the same time how the peripheries—in this context the member states—resisted this removal.

The data used in this chapter were gathered during two main fieldworks at the internal border of the Schengen area between France and Italy in 2008–2009 and then in 2015. The first one consisted in interviews with police officers from the French border police department and the second one in interviews with NGO members, activists working at the border between France and Italy and a police union representative.

Regarding the current COVID-19 "crisis" the analysis was built on official statements and guidelines by the European Commission, secondary literature (notably think-tank reports and analysis), and a review of the recently published articles on the subject.

The first part will present a general overview of the legal definition and implementation of free movement of people within the Schengen area as well

---

7 Denis Duez, "De l'État à l'Union," *Politique européenne* 65, no. 3 (2019).

as the conditions for reinstatement of border checks at internal borders of the Schengen area. The second part will describe how member states responded to the COVID-19 pandemic in a very similar but also very uncoordinated way by reintroducing temporarily border checks at their national borders. Finally, the third part will analyze the EU's response to the mobility issue in time of pandemic crisis.

Schengen Agreement and the Reinstatement of Border Checks

What Does "Free Movement of People" Exactly Mean?

Free movement of people is one of the main achievements of the European integration and had been planned since its inception in the 1950s. However, until the mid-1980s, free movement within the European territory was not defined as the right to cross national borders, but as the right to access national labor markets. It was mainly implemented as the result of the non-discrimination principle between European citizens, perceived most and foremost as workers.

In June 1985, five member states (Germany, Belgium, the Netherlands, Luxembourg, and France) adopted the Schengen Agreement. This agreement gave nationals the right to cross freely while the conditions for free movement of individuals, as we know them today, were set in the Convention Implementing the Schengen Agreement (Schengen Convention) in June 1990. This Convention became effective in 1995 and was implemented in the following years in the different member states. The Convention was later incorporated into EU law with the Treaty of Amsterdam (1997), so that free movement of people was set as a requirement for all new member states integrating the EU.

The Schengen border code, which defines precisely the conditions for crossing the internal borders of the Schengen area and for the exceptional reintroduction of border checks at these same borders, has been revised several times. Free movement of people is defined in Article 22 of the Schengen border code. This article provides that "internal borders may be crossed at any point without a border check on persons, irrespective of their nationality, being carried out." In practical terms, this amounts to a prohibition of checks at border stations which had previously applied to all travelers. Traffic cannot be slowed at internal borders, and all infrastructure blocking traffic has to be removed.

However, as data gathered during a fieldwork in 2008 and 2009 at the French-Italian border show, checks did not disappear entirely after the implementation of the Schengen Convention in the late 1990s. As a captain of the French border police, posted at the French Italian border in Menton, explained: "With the Schengen agreement, we abandoned fixed checks. Many people think there are no more borders, whereas it's just that control went from fixed and systematic to mobile and random."[8]

Contrary to a common presumption, free movement of people does not correspond to the complete removal of checks at internal borders. In fact, border checks never disappeared from Schengen's internal borders.[9] Discriminatory practices based on racial profiling are a recurrent practice of border control,[10] while it is also the case within the Schengen area, especially at borders placed along the migratory routes that cross the European territory.[11] At the specific internal borders that are examined here between France and Italy border checks concentrate on one specific type of travelers: the people who are identified by the police as being migrants or asylum seekers. Border police officers have to respond to a double bind: make free movement a reality by ensuring the fluidity of the Schengen internal border crossing for most of the travelers while controlling immigration at the national borders. As a former work has shown,[12] the result of this double bind is that checks concentrate on people they identify as migrants, and are therefore based on discriminatory practices. The analyses point to the fact that it is crucial to look not only at the legal definition of free movement but also at its implementation.

8 PAF officer from the Pont Saint-Louis office, November 2008.

9 Sara Casella Colombeau, "Policing the Internal Schengen Borders – Managing the Double Bind between Free Movement and Migration Control," *Policing and Society: An International Journal of Research and Policy* 27, no. 5 (2017); Maartje van der Woude and Joanne van der Leun, "Crimmigration Checks in the Internal Border Areas of the EU: Finding the Discretion That Matters," *European Journal of Criminology* 14, no. 1 (2017).

10 Josiah Heyman, "Class and Classification at the U.S.-Mexico Border," *Human Organization* 60, no. 2 (2001).

11 Martina Tazzioli, "Disjointed Knowledges, Obfuscated Visibility. Border Controls at the French-Italian Alpine Border," *Political Geography* 79 (2020), accessed September 30, 2021, DOI: 10.1016/j.polgeo.2020.102155; Sarah Bachellerie, "La traque policière des étranger·es à la frontière franco-italienne (Hautes-Alpes) comme 'maintien de l'ordre social et racial'", *Journal of Alpine Research | Revue de géographie alpine* 108, no.2 (2020), accessed September 30, 2021, DOI: 10.4000/rga.7208.

12 Casella Colombeau, "Policing the Internal Schengen Borders," op. cit: 486.

What are the Conditions for Reinstatement of Border Checks?

The legal condition for temporary reinstatement of border checks are stated in the Schengen border code (articles 25 to 35) adopted in 2016.[13] Member states' administrations that wish to reintroduce a border check can justify it by referring to a "foreseeable threat" (e. g. a high-level political meeting), an "immediate and serious threat," and "persistent serious deficiencies related to Schengen's external borders." The member states' administration must notify the other member states and the Commission about its intention to reintroduce border checks. Some exceptions are defined which give the possibility to member states to reintroduce the border checks before notifying either the Commission or the other member states. These reintroductions have to be temporary, and any case cannot exceed a maximum duration of two years.

However, notifications to the Commission do not constitute a reliable instrument to assess the reality of the reinstatement of border checks. France's use of the notification in 2015 provides a good example of the gap that might exist between formal use of notifications by member states and the reality of the checks. The immigration and asylum EU policy crisis of 2015 reached its peak at the end of the summer when seven member states officially reintroduced border checks at their national borders (Austria, Germany, France, Denmark, Sweden, and Norway). Yet, in France the first measures taken to reinforce the border checks at the France-Italy border had been taken in June 2015. The central authorities decided to reinforce staff numbers and more drastically limit circulation at the internal border of the Schengen area. The reinforcement of staff and controls resulted in the blocking of migrants who had landed on Italian coasts and were trying to travel north towards France and northern Europe.[14] Yet, it was not until October 2015 that the notification was sent to the European Commission. Furthermore, the notification's justification for reintroducing border checks did not mention the ongoing "migrant crisis." It stated the necessity to adjust border checks to the preparation for the COP 21 Climate change conference in November 2015. The reinstatement was later extended until February 26, 2016 amid the state

---

13 For a complete legal analysis of the conditions for reinstatement of border checks in time of Covid-19 outbreak see Daniel Thym and Jonas Bornemann, "Schengen and Free Movement Law During the First Phase of the Covid-19 Pandemic: Of Symbolism, Law and Politics," *European Papers* 5, no. 3 (2020).

14 The effects of these checks were highly visible, and the internal border between Vintimiglia and Menton became the stage for a politization of the migration crisis and its management by French pollical actors (among them the Prime minister Manuel Valls and the interior minister Bernard Cazeneuve), see Casella Colombeau, "Crisis of Schengen?," op.cit.

of emergency declared after the November 2015 terrorist attacks in Paris. From that date, French authorities have never lifted the controls at the internal borders. The "temporary" reintroduction of border checks at internal borders has been on since 2015.[15] This example of reinstatement of internal border checks illustrates the tensions between the Commission's will to enforce the Treaty and the member states' practices of evading these requirements without facing any repercussions. Member states certainly enjoy a lot of autonomy in the enforcement of the Schengen border code.

Another illustration of this gap between the notifications and the reality of the checks is that border checks cannot be fully reintroduced at the land border. Border police simply do not have the means to check every individual willing to cross the national border. The rationale for targeting individuals who are identified as "migrants" by police officers is still very much in place during these reinstatements of border checks periods. Usually the reinstatement of borders simply meant a reinforcement of the border police staff with officials from other police departments. The reinstatement of border checks usually corresponds to a continuation of border practices but with more human resources.

The post-Rokkanian theoretical framework presented in the introduction provides a clear analysis of the legal and practical conditions for reintroducing border checks. The legal framework can be interpreted as the result of the EU political center's will to regulate the peripheries – or member states' attempts at escaping the definition of common external boundaries by reviving their national borders. The EU legal framework officially constrains member states on their sovereign power to control their national borders. This framework has been set to harmonize the conditions for crossing the internal borders of the Schengen area, in "normal" times, as well as in exceptional situations, when member States request the right to reintroduce border checks. But a closer look at the implementation of this legal framework shows that member states still enjoy an important room of maneuver to define the conditions for crossing their national borders. The tensions between the EU political center and the national peripheries can then be observed in the way these legal conditions are implemented.

---

15 Indeed, France' authorities notified the EC on March 31, 2020. This notification was made in continuity with a previous notification dating back from October 2, 2019 and based on national security threat following terrorist attacks.

The COVID-19 Outbreak and Free Movement within the EU

Even considering that border checks have been reinstated in the past it is impossible to ignore that the nature of the free movement has been highly affected by the responses to the COVID-19 pandemic. The following part will examine the relations between the EU institutions and the member states related to reinstatement of border checks at internal borders between March and June 2020.

Reintroduction of Border Checks and Introduction of Restrictions

Between March 11 and March 20 2020, 15 member states reintroduced border checks at their national borders and consequently at the internal borders of the Schengen area. The reintroduction was large-scale, but very heterogeneous. Some states limited this reintroduction to specific border areas, such as Italy. But generally, the scope of the official reintroduction was national. In a very short amount of time, the nature of free movement within the EU changed without any coordination between the member states. Around the same time, the European council adopted an EU-wide travel ban for citizens of non-EU countries. The external borders of the EU were then officially closed to anyone with no European passport. This is the first time a large-scale reintroduction of border checks happened in the EU.

On top of reinforcing border checks, member states also introduced restrictions on entry and exit. These restrictions meant that not only passengers had the validity of their travel or identity documents checked, but new criteria were also introduced to enter national territories. For example, restrictions were introduced on air borders, with the closing of various airports or the suspension of flights from certain countries. On land borders, train services from either some countries or all countries were suspended. And regarding maritime borders, prohibition of entry in ports or waterways, and a ban on cruise ships, were issued.

Restrictions were also introduced concerning some nationalities, including sometimes nationalities from the EU. For example, Austria imposed an intra-EU (and intra-Schengen) entry ban for foreign nationals coming from Italy (from March 7, 2020), Switzerland and Liechtenstein (from March 16, 2020), as well as Germany, Hungary, and Slovenia (from March 19, 2020). Exit bans were also introduced, namely by Belgium, Czech Republic, and Lithuania. These practices are highly unusual.

The legal requirement to notify the Commission or the time limitation for re-introducing the border checks were treated by member state governments "as matters of political good will."[16] The legal requirements of the Schengen border code seem to have played little role in the member states' strategy. This is not new, as former reinforcement of border checks in 2015 showed. And the Commission, the guardian of the Treaty, did not react in a restrictive way towards the un-bidding member states. Here again the tensions between the European center, represented here by the Commission, and the national political centers illuminate the situation. The Commission is not in the position of imposing the requirements that are provided in the legally-binding Treaty. The post-Rokkanian theoretical framework can provide insight to understand that EU integration is a process that comprises unresolved (or temporarily resolved) tensions between the center and peripheries.

In the first phase[17] of the pandemic, between March and June 2020, very few countries had developed a broad-range capacity to test passengers at the border for Covid. Border checks were reintroduced as a public health measure. But instruments were lacking to implement a border check that would be based on health requirements, or testing. Border checks relied then on very broad and non-health-related categories. They were implemented on the basis of already known criteria: travel documents, nationality, administrative or migration status in the territory. As Sergio Carerra and Ngo Chun Luk state, "overall priority [was] given to a 'public policy and internal security' (law enforcement) approach over public health considerations of individuals."[18]

These temporary reinstatements of border checks were decided in a context when the possibility of a total closure of national borders was considered as plausible. We will see in the following section that this border closure fantasy was only possible in the very exceptional situation of the first phase of the COVID-19 outbreak.

---

16 Daniel Thym and Jonas Bornemann, "Schengen and Free Movement Law During the First Phase of the Covid-19 Pandemic: Of Symbolism, Law and Politics," op.cit.: 1154.

17 The three phases under study in this chapter have been presented in the introduction. These phases refer to the set of measures adopted by national governments and EU authorities, and coincide only loosely to the different "waves" of the epidemic. Indeed, the temporality of the different waves varies from one member state to the other.

18 Sergio Carrera and Ngo Chun Luk, "Love thy neighbour? Coronavirus politics and their impact on EU freedoms and rule of law in the Schengen Area," *CEPS paper in Liberty and Security in Europe* 4 (2020): 2.

International and Internal Mobility

Indeed, one of the specificities of the interruption of free movement during the first phase of the pandemic is that these measures were adopted in a context where most of the mobilities were constrained. Lockdown as well as a ban on interregional mobility were introduced in most of the member states with various implementation features. Cross-border mobility was then one of the many measures that were adopted by member states. The main constraint for border police officers to enforce a closed border is the intensity of cross-border traffic. Thirty years after the implementation of the Schengen convention, cross-border traffic is usually so dense at the internal borders of the Schengen area that it is practically impossible to check every individual. But in a context of strong restrictions on mobility at every scale (from local to international), systematic checks at internal border became suddenly feasible. Limitation of free movement within the EU does not have the same impact in a context when these limitations are also implemented within the national territory of the members states.

At the France-Italy border, where border checks were reinforced several times in recent years (mainly in 2011 and 2015), long-time observers acknowledged for the first time during this first phase of the pandemic that systematic checks at the land border were enforced.[19] With the reduction of traffic, police forces could close down one of the two roads that cross the national border between Menton and Vintimiglia, while on the other road every vehicle was checked, reviving a practice that entirely disappeared at the end of the 1990s.

The restraints on international mobility can only be fully implemented if limitations also exist at other levels within the national territory. After the first period, even if border checks, restrictions or health requirements were reintroduced, the lifting of restrictions on free movement never had the same impact, notably because the volume of exchange remained too big to actually control every traveler. The limitation on free movement introduced in the first phase of the pandemic cannot therefore be considered as being the new landmark for the reintroduction of border checks. On the contrary, it shed some light on the reality of these reinstatements in other circumstances. Reinstatement of border checks are never systematic, they consist in reinforcing the number of checks, but following the same logics, depending on the local border context.

---

19 Daniela Trucco, "The Southern French–Italian Border Before, During, and After COVID-19 Lockdowns," *Borders in Globalization Review* 2, no. 1 (2020).

Attempt at Coordinating the Member states' Strategy

Faced with their unilateral and inconsistent decisions, the European Commission encouraged the member states to enhance their coordination. On March 16, 2020, the Commission published *COVID-19 Guidelines for border management measures to protect health and ensure the availability of goods and essential services*.[20] The major concern was to keep the internal market working, by organizing a differentiated regime of mobility. On March 30 the Commission issued another set of guidelines related to the checks at internal borders. Most of this second communication by the EC was dedicated to the conditions for travel for posted and frontier workers. The list of workers who could benefit from a right of mobility in this context was surprisingly long: from health professionals to "food manufacturing and processing and related trades and maintenance workers." These guidelines clearly indicated the type of mobility that was considered as essential by European institutions. Interestingly, the Commission then seemed to come back to a pre-1980s definition of free movement within the EU, when only European workers (and their family) were granted the right to move and work in any member states.

Another set of measures adopted at EU-level was the EU-wide travel ban, when the European Council adopted a "Temporary Restriction on Non-Essential Travel to the EU" on March 16, with the idea that it would encourage the member states to lift the restrictions at intra-Schengen borders.[21] The idea here was to reinforce control at external borders of the EU so that member states felt safe to lift the controls at their own borders.

In the first phase of the COVID-19 outbreak, European institutions therefore acknowledged the legitimacy of member states reintroducing border checks at internal borders but tried to regulate and define common ground for a redefinition of free movement within the EU. By doing so, they participated in a redefinition of free movement this time limited to workers. Interestingly, the European center also defined a new version of free movement that was limited to legal categories forged at the EU level: posted workers defined by the 1996 directive[22] and frontier worker defined by a Council Resolution of June 20, 1994.[23]

---

20 (C(2020) 1753 final), COVID-19 Guidelines for border management measures to protect health and ensure the availability of goods and essential services, March 16, 2020.
21 Sergio Carrera and Ngo Chun Luk, "Love thy neighbour? Coronavirus politics and their impact on EU freedoms and rule of law in the Schengen Area," op. cit.
22 Directive on the enforcement of Directive 96/71/EC concerning the posting of workers in the framework of the provision of services and amending Regulation (EU) No 1024/2012 on admin-

Reopen Europa – Uncertainty in the Definition and Enactment of free Movement

The restrictions and reinstatement of border checks were lifted around the same period in most of the member states during the month of June 2020.

Health Requirement as New Criteria to Enter National Territories

This swift "recovery" for free movement within the Schengen area was the result of intergovernmental negotiations.[24] Most travel bans based on nationality were lifted, with the exception of travelers from the UK in December 2020 due to the outbreak of the "Alpha variant." Between July 2020 and January 2021 border checks at internal borders came back to the pre-COVID-19 outbreak level. With the "second wave" of the virus' diffusion, new mobility restrictions were brought in around the months of October and November 2020. Lockdowns were introduced in Ireland, France, Belgium, and Austria, but they were not associated with intra-Schengen border checks reinstatements.

From the beginning of 2021, restrictions evolved into health requirements to cross the borders. These requirements were defined on an individual basis by member states. They consisted in PCR-Test, isolation, and quarantine. Every time internal measures were reintroduced during the second and the third "wave" of COVID-19 outbreak, member states also adopted measures concerning entry into their territory including from other member states. Measures sometimes differed from one border type to another: generally, PCR-tests were introduced during the second wave at ports and airports, but only around the beginning of the "third" wave at land borders. This disparate landscape of health requirements to cross internal borders of EU territory gave the police force in charge of implementing them a large discretion. An assessment of the reality

---

istrative cooperation through the Internal Market Information System ("the IMI Regulation") – The Enforcement Directive 2014/67/EU.

23 Council resolution of June 20, 1994 on limitation on admission of third-country nationals to the territory of the Member States for employment [Official Journal C 274 of 19.09.1996], https://eur-lex.europa.eu/legal-content/LT/TXT/?uri=CELEX:31996Y0919(02).

24 Daniel Thym and Jonas Bornemann, "Schengen and Free Movement Law During the First Phase of the Covid-19 Pandemic: Of Symbolism, Law and Politics," op.cit.

of border checks at French internal borders provides a good illustration of the phenomenon.

In France, the strengthening of internal border controls during this period was in large part disconnected from health concerns. On October 2, 2020 France notified the Commission that it would extend border controls from November 1 2020 to April 30, 2021. Most of the justification letter referred to terrorist threats and "secondary movements of migrants."[25] In the context of the trial of the 2015 Charlie Hebdo attacks and a new attack aimed at the former offices of the satiric newspaper, French authorities justified the extension of the temporary reintroduction of border controls with reference to terrorist threats more than public health concerns. Concomitantly, police border staff were reinforced at the French-Spanish border.

Health requirements were only introduced in January 2021.[26] From this date, a negative COVID-19 test was required to enter the French territory. Police union were quick to react: systematic checks of this requirement at internal borders would require a strong increase in staff.[27] Due to this practical constrain, the modalities of implementation of this measure varied highly locally. At some internal border all train passengers were checked and had to present a negative COVID-19 test (that was the case in Perpignan for international trains); but at other internal borders (as in Menton, at the French-Italian border for example), very few passengers were checked on health requirements grounds.[28] Most border police checks observed by local NGOs targeted individuals identified as "migrants," as it was before the pandemic.

During the second phase of the pandemic continuity regarding border checks was the main feature. The only diverging aspect emerged in January 2021 with health requirements. Their implementation varied greatly and depend-

---

25 Prolongation of the temporary reintroduction of border controls at the French internal borders in accordance with Articles 25 and 27 of Regulation (EU) 2016/399 on a Union Code on the rules governing the movement of persons across borders (Schengen Borders Code), 7138/1/20 REV 1, October 6, 2020.

26 Décret n° 2021–99 du 30 janvier 2021 modifiant les décrets n° 2020–1262 du 16 octobre 2020 et n° 2020–1310 du 29 octobre 2020 prescrivant les mesures générales nécessaires pour faire face à l'épidémie de covid-19 dans le cadre de l'état d'urgence sanitaire.

27 "Covid-19: vers un contrôle généralisé à la frontière italienne? Impossible, selon les syndicats de police," France 3 Provence-Alpes-Côte-d'Azur, January 31, 2021, accessed September 30, 2021, https://france3-regions.francetvinfo.fr/provence-alpes-cote-d-azur/alpes-maritimes/menton/covid-19-la-police-va-t-elle-pouvoir-controler-tout-le-monde-a-la-frontiere-italienne-1933627.html.

28 Interview with a local NGO activist.

ed on local border area contexts and border police discretion. Indeed, at ports and airports, health requirements were checked much more systematically.

At the borders where the main pre-pandemic concern was migratory control (e. g. the France-Italy border), this concern remained the main stake from the beginning of the second phase. Local contexts greatly influenced the implementation of border checks.[29] Health requirements were also introduced during this phase at borders but only where it was practically feasible to enforce them: at port and airports entries. On land borders where it was impossible to systematically check the passengers, these requirements were not fully implemented. Implementation capacities therefore appear as a key feature of border checks in "normal" time and as in a time of "crisis."

The COVID-19 Certificate: Coordination More than Harmonization of Conditions for Cross-border Travels

EU institutions continuously argued for enhanced cooperation regarding free movement. Discussion among member states started in January 2021 when the Greek Prime minister suggested creating a common document testifying that people were vaccinated. This "green" certificate would allow travelers to cross internal borders without any testing or quarantine. Southern member states, whose economies rely on tourism, declared their support for this measure (Malta, Italy, Spain, and Portugal). The Commission's proposition[30] issued on March 17, 2021 was to create a standard for common recognition of health conditions to travel: travelers would be able to either present a proof of vaccination, a negative COVID-19 test or a proof of recovery from the disease. Once again, member states took unilateral decisions regarding this certificate and some countries, such as Iceland, introduced vaccination certificates or bilateral agreements to facilitate the travel of vaccinated citizens (Greece, Cyprus, and Israel for example).

The proposal of the Commission was to create this certificate without making its use mandatory. Member states also remained free to impose a quarantine to green certificate holders but they had to justify it to the Commission, and they

---

29 Sara Casella Colombeau, Mathilde Darley, and Elsa Tyszler, "Filtrer, diviser," in *La police des migrants. Filtrer, disperser, harceler*, ed. Babels et al. (Paris: Le Passager Clandestin, 2019).
30 Proposal for a Regulation of the European Parliament and of the Council on a framework for the issuance, verification, and acceptance of interoperable certificates on vaccination, testing, and recovery to facilitate free movement during the COVID-19 pandemic (Digital Green Certificate). COM/2021/130 final.

could introduce health requirements for all the people who did not hold this green certificate. The EU digital covid certificate was finally adopted by the European parliament on June 8, 2021 and became available in all EU countries from July 1, 2021. This certificate was delivered to people who had either "recovered from COVID-19," "been vaccinated against COVID-19" or "received a negative test for COVID-19." This certificate was free and non-obligatory. It could be digitally stored on a mobile device or in a paper format. The certificate only provided an EU-wide recognition of either testing, vaccine or recovery, but member states could still have varying criteria of entry. For example, some countries accepted people who had been vaccinated with the four vaccines recognized by the EU (Pfizer/BioNTech, Moderna, AstraZeneca, and Johnson & Johnson) but some states (Hungary and Greece for example) also accepted Spoutnik V and Sinopharm vaccines. Member states also had the choice to accept a rapid antigen test or not, and to decide upon the period of time to consider these tests as valid (48 or 72 hours for example).[31] The Council only formulated recommendations for the use of these rapid antigen tests, but no obligation of recognition for member states. In Norway, non-vaccinated people can enter the country if they justify it, but have to isolate for seven days before passing a first PCR test. With this certificate the EU institutions tended towards the harmonization of criteria to cross the internal borders of the Schengen area. But member states still enjoyed a rather important room of maneuver to define the condition of entry to their territories.

Airlines companies did not wait for governments' decision to create their own passports. International Air Transport Association issued a "travel pass": a platform which compiled all the health requirements of the different countries in the world to enter their territory. Users had to download an application, create a verified identity profile, and upload all the travel information of their next flight. These applications centralized both the passport information and the health information (result of test for example). Air France also created its own travel pass in March 2021. Private actors have long been involved in the definition or the implementation of border checks. Airline companies had been involved since the mid-1980s[32] in controlling the identity and travel documents of their customers. With the introduction of carrier sanctions legislations, airline

---

31 "Frontières: où peut-on se déplacer en Europe depuis la France?", Toute l'Europe, September 23, 2021, accessed September 30, 2021, https://www.touteleurope.eu/societe/frontieres-ou-peut-on-se-deplacer-en-europe-depuis-la-france/.
32 Virginie Guiraudon, "Logiques et pratiques de l'Etat délégateur: les compagnies de transport dans le contrôle migratoire à distance,"' *Cultures & Conflits* 45 (2002), accessed September 30, 2021, DOI: 10.4000/conflits.773.

companies are deemed responsible if they allow an undocumented migrant to enter a country's territory, and have to pay for his or her deportation in addition to a fine. To prevent such costs, airlines companies introduced identity checks at the point of departure, which are usually realized after the official control point, just before entering the plane.

While the COVID-19 certificate could only be used in the EU, the IATA "travel pass" was a world-wide instrument. Considering that the coordination between member states only resulted in the exchange of verified information and not in a harmonization of entry criteria, private actors had every opportunity to also provide a coordination instrument, especially as the latter would apply much more broadly at international level.

Conclusion

Transnational mobility was highly affected by the COVID-19 crisis and several points on the EU and national political centers' responses to this crisis can be emphasized.

First, for many years (from the 1990s to the 2010s), the reinstatement of border checks appeared as being part of the routine of the implementation of free movement of people. They were mainly unnoticed. From the mid-2010s however, the reinstatement of border checks at internal borders of the Schengen area have come to be increasingly politicized. The implementation of border checks remained the same, but the way the member states executive chose to communicate about it changed. The reintroduction of border checks was then interpreted as convenient criticism towards European rules over migration and, more broadly, European integration. Criticisms over Schengen corresponded to the will of some governments to regain their sovereignty over "Brussels," the EU political center. Tension between European and national political centers was also observed during the COVID-19 pandemic. This tension was never so visible as during the first phase. The fantasy of a total border closure during the first phase of the pandemic was exceptional, but only because they were accompanied with restrictions to mobility within the territory. Translocal, transregional and then transnational traffic was so limited, that systematic checks at internal borders of the Schengen area were made possible. As a result, restrictions to mobility cannot only be analyzed at the international level or even the European level; one also has to consider the other restrictions to mobility that were taken at the national level.

Secondly, this tension between center and periphery can be observed in the uncoordinated nature of the member states' reactions. The alteration of

free movement as a response to the COVID-19 outbreak was characterized by a lack of coordination between member states, but associated with a strong inter-dependence. Member states' responses consisted of unilateral decisions to reintroduce border checks and to lift them at the end of the first lockdown period, then to reintroduce them in a very heterogeneous way, deciding upon health requirements or restrictions for individuals to cross the internal borders. There was obviously a lack of cooperation at the EU level regarding free movement in this context but it has to be assessed in the general framework of the EU's reaction to the pandemic and the fact that, generally speaking, the member states reacted individually to the crisis.

EU institutions enjoyed very few powers to manage the internal borders of the EU territory and the instrument that was implemented, the COVID-19 certificate, was a coordination tool more than a harmonization one as the Commission was torn between the necessity to enforce a legal requirement stated in the Treaty and the fear that a strict enforcement of the rules regarding the reinstatement of borders would lead the member states to change the Schengen border code in order to enhance their autonomy.

List of contributors

Pierre-Alexandre Beylier is Associate Professor in North American Studies at Grenoble-Alpes University. In 2013, he completed a PhD at Paris 3-Sorbonne Nouvelle University entitled "The Canada/US Border Since 9/11: Continuity and Change" for which he received the Award of the French Association of Canadian Studies. His book – *Canada/Etats-Unis: les Enjeux d'une Frontière* – was published in May 2016. His work now focuses on border communities and the issues of mobility, representations and identity. His latest publications include "Cross-Border Mobility in *Ambos Nogales* since Trump's Election" in *The Journal of Borderlands Studies* and "Cross-Border Live in an American Exclave: Point Roberts and the Canada/US Border" in *BIG Review*.

Charles Breton is Executive Director of the Centre of Excellence on the Canadian Federation at the Institute for Research on Public Policy in Montréal. He holds a PhD in political science from the University of British Columbia. His latest publications include "Does International Terrorism affect Public Attitudes toward Refugees? Evidence from a Large-scale Natural Experiment" in the *Journal of Politics* and "Realignment and voter issue preferences in Quebec's 2018 provincial election: a conjoint experiment" in *French Politics*.

Giliberto Capano is Professor of Political Science and Public Policy at the University of Bologna. He has been the co-founder of the International Public Policy Association. He is currently a member of the Executive Committee of the European Consortium of Political Research. He has (co-)authored nine monographical studies and (co-)edited sixteen books. He specializes in comparative public policy, policy design, comparative governance and higher education policy. His last books are *Convergence and Diversity in the Governance of Higher Education: Comparative Perspectives* (co-editor with D. Jarvis), Cambridge University Press, 2020; and *Guide to Modern Public Policy* (co-editor with Michael Holwett), Edward Elgar, 2020.

Sara Casella Colombeau is Associate Professor in politics at the department of Foreign languages at the Grenoble-Alpes University. She has previously held several post-doctoral positions, at the University of Edinburgh, Aix-Marseille-University, the University of Montreal and the French Collaborative Institute for migration. Her work focuses on border policies, both at the French and European level, and on the State's attempt to detect, monitor and control unauthorized migration on French territory. She is currently editing a collective volume, an Atlas on free movement, to be published in 2022 by Armand Colin editions.

Sarah H. Gordon is Assistant Professor in the Department of Health Law, Policy, and Management at Boston University School of Public Health. She is a health services researcher who studies health insurance coverage, access to care, and health equity in the U.S., with a specific focus on the Medicaid program. Dr. Gordon is a senior advisor in the Office of the Assistant Secretary for Planning and Evaluation at the U.S. Department of Health and Human Services. However, this chapter was conceived and drafted while Dr. Gordon was employed at Boston University, and the findings and views in this article do not reflect the official views or policy of the Department of Health and Human Services.

https://doi.org/10.1515/9783110745085-012

Nicole Huberfeld is Edward R. Utley Professor of Health Law at Boston University School of Public Health and Professor of Law at Boston University School of Law. Her scholarship explores the intersection of health law and constitutional law, often addressing health reform (especially Medicaid), federalism, federal spending power, and the needs of vulnerable populations. She is the author of two health law casebooks and many book chapters and articles, including coauthoring "What Is Federalism in Healthcare For?" (*Stanford Law Review*, 2018), a 5-year study of the federalism dynamics of the implementation of the Affordable Care Act, and "Federalizing Medicaid" (2011), cited in the first Supreme Court decision on the ACA.

David K. Jones was Associate Professor at the Boston University School of Public Health. He is the author of *Exchange Politics: Opposing Obamacare in Battleground States* (2017). His work has appeared in the *New York Times*, the *Washington Post*, and the *Wall Street Journal*, among other newspapers. He was awarded the Academy-Health Outstanding Dissertation Award and the John D. Thompson Prize for Young Investigators by the Association of University Programs in Health Administration.

Michelle Falkenbach, PhD is a postdoctoral associate in the Department of Public and Ecosystem Health at Cornell University. Her latest publications include a co- edited volume entitled the *Populist Radical Right and Health: National Policies and Global Trends* and a co-authored book *Ageing and Health: The Politics of Better Policies*. Her research has been published in the *International Journal of Health Policy and Management,* the *European Journal of Public Health, Health Policy and Technology, Government and Opposition*, as well as other outlets.

Anna Malandrino is a postdoctoral scholar and adjunct professor of public policy analysis at the University of Bologna, and a postdoc scientific collaborator at the University of Bern. She specializes in public policy, public procurement, policy compliance and education policy. She has recently published, among others, in the *Journal of Comparative Policy Analysis* and *European Policy Analysis.*

Michel Martínez Pérez is Associate Professor in Spanish/Catalan Studies, at the University Toulouse Capitole. The former Director of the Department of Languages and Civilizations (DLC) between 2017 and 2021, he has been the head of the Hispanic World Law Degree at the European School of Law since 2013. He is a permanent member of FRAMESPA (UMR 5136-CNRS) and an associate member of CRIMIC (Sorbonne-University). He specializes in contemporary Spain and has written a thesis on the Chunta Aragonesista political party (1986 – 2004). He is the author of articles on peninsular nationalisms, Catalan-speaking Aragon, plurilingual and plurinational Spain and, more generally, on Catalan studies.

Véronique Molinari is Professor of British Studies at Grenoble Alpes University and co-Director of the research center ILCEA4 (Institut des langues et cultures d'Europe, Amérique, Afrique, Asie et Australie). Her research focuses on the various forms of women's political participation and British politics. Her latest publications include *Using and Abusing Science* with C. Besson (CSP, 2016), "The Northern Irish Assembly and the Abortion Issue, 1967 – 2017", *Études irlandaises*, 45 – 2 | 2020, 77 – 99, and *Mobilising Voters in the United States and the United Kingdom: political strategies from parties and grassroots organisations (1867 – 2020)*, with G. Benedetti, (De Gruyter, 2021).

Dr. Valerià Paül is Associate Professor at the Department of Geography of the University of Santiago de Compostela (Galicia, Spain). Previously, he was Assistant Professor at the University of Western Australia (2014–15). He holds a PhD in Geography from the University of Barcelona and has received University of Barcelona Special Awards both for Bachelor Studies (2002) and for Doctoral Studies (2007). His research interests include regional planning and management with a focus on open spaces, protected and mountain areas and development; historical and cultural geography of landscape; agriculture, food and rural studies; political geography; and tourism (specifically, cultural, natural and rural tourism). He has participated in numerous projects earned by public competitive applications, usually working on inter-disciplinary rural and regional studies; these projects have been funded by the European Union and Australian, Spanish, Galician and Catalan governments.

Paisley Sim is the Director of Research and Operations of the Canada Grid initiative of the Transition Accelerator based in Montreal, Canada. She was previously a Research Associate at the Institute for Research on Public Policy where she focused on federalism and intergovernmental relations at the Centre of Excellence on the Canadian Federation. Prior experience includes working for Alberta Premier Rachel Notley, as a special advisor to Alberta's Minister of Justice and Solicitor General, and in the non-profit arts world. She holds a conservatory diploma, a bachelor of fine arts from Concordia University, and a master in public policy from McGill University's Max Bell School of Public Policy.

Fiona Simpkins is Associate Professor in Contemporary British History, Politics and Society at the University Lumière of Lyon, France. Her main areas of research are devolution, nationalism, unionism and the constitutional debate in Scotland. She has published her research in a variety of books and journals, including the *Revue Française de Civilisation Britannique* and *Observatoire de la Société Britannique*.

Dr. Juan-M. Trillo-Santamaría is a Lecturer at the Department of Geography of the University of Santiago de Compostela (Galicia, Spain). His research has benefited from research stays in international centers in France, the Netherlands and the UK. He holds a PhD in Humanities from the University Carlos III of Madrid (European mention) and has received University of Carlos III Special Awards both for Bachelor Studies and for Doctoral Studies. His approach to Border Studies has emphasized the geographical tradition with a comprehensive spatial analysis of social, political, economic and cultural processes related to the production and reproduction of borders. His academic interests include cross-border cooperation and multilevel governance, historical and cultural geography, tourism and geopolitics. He is currently a Co-Editor for Europe of the *Journal of Borderland Studies*.

Roberto Vila-Lage is a PhD candidate at the Department of Geography, University of Santiago de Compostela (Galicia, Spain). He holds a BA degree in Economics from the University of A Coruña, a BA degree in Geography and Spatial Planning and a MA in Spatial Planning, Management and Development from the University of Santiago de Compostela. Roberto's doctoral project focuses on the study of cooperation across external (Galicia-North of Portugal) and internal (Galicia-Asturias / Galicia-Castile and Leon) Spanish borders and is funded by a research grant from the Spanish Ministry of Science, Innovation and Universities obtained through a publicly-competitive process.

Birte Wassenberg is Professor in Contemporary History at Sciences Po at the University of Strasbourg and member of the Research Unit Dynamiques européennes (UMR). She holds a Jean Monnet Chair, is deputy director of the Franco-German Jean-Monnet Center of Excellence and the director of the Master in Border Studies, International Relations. From 1993 to 2006 she was responsible for cross-border cooperation at the *Région Alsace*. Her research fields are: border regions, Euro-scepticism and the history of European organizations, especially the Council of Europe. She is also a former student from the College of Europe, promotion Charles IV, (1992–1993).

Daniel Wincott is Blackwell Professor of Law and Society in Cardiff University's School of Law and Politics. He Directs the ESRC's Governance after Brexit programme. Recent publications, written with various colleagues include "Voluntary Action Territory and Timing: The Council of Social Service for Wales, Periodisation and the New Historiography of the 'British Welfare State'" in *Journal of Social Policy*, "The Anglo-British imaginary and the rebuilding of the UK's territorial constitution after Brexit: unitary state or union state?" in *Territory, Politics, Governance* and "Analysing vote-choice in a multinational state: national identity and territorial differentiation in the 2016 Brexit vote", in *Regional Studies*.

Bei Fragen zur Produktsicherheit wenden Sie sich bitte an:
If you have any questions regarding product safety,
please contact:

Walter de Gruyter GmbH
Genthiner Straße 13
10785 Berlin
productsafety@degruyterbrill.com